Infections of Leisure

David Schlossberg

Editor

Infections of Leisure

Springer-Verlag

New York Berlin Heidelberg London Paris
Tokyo Hong Kong Barcelona Budapest

David Schlossberg, M.D., F.A.C.P.
Professor of Medicine
Medical College of Pennsylvania
and
Director, Department of Medicine
Episcopal Hospital
Philadelphia, PA 19125-1098, USA

With eight illustrations.

Library of Congress Cataloging-in-Publication Data
Infections of leisure / David Schlossberg, editor.
    p.   cm.
    Includes bibliographical references and index.
    ISBN 0-387-94069-3.—ISBN 3-540-94069-3
    1. Communicable diseases—Popular works.   2. Leisure—Health
aspects.   3. Zoonoses.   I. Schlossberg, David.
    [DNLM: 1. Infection—etiology.   2. Disease Vectors.   3. Zoonoses.
4. Leisure Activities.   WC 195 I438 1993]
RC113.I54 1993
616.9′0471—dc20
DNLM/DLC
for Library of Congress   93-3831

Printed on acid-free paper.

Production managed by Chernow Editorial Services, Inc. and managed by Henry Krell; manufac-
    turing supervised by Jacqui Ashri.
Typeset by Best-set Typesetter Ltd., Hong Kong.
Printed and bound by Edwards Brothers, Inc., Ann Arbor, MI.
Printed in the United States of America.

9 8 7 6 5 4 3 2 1

ISBN 0-387-94069-3 Springer-Verlag New York Berlin Heidelberg
ISBN 3-540-94069-3 Springer-Verlag Berlin Heidelberg New York

This book is dedicated to Elzbieta

". . . but this is wine
That's all too strange and strong;
I'm full of foolish song,
and out my song must pour."

Guys and Dolls, Frank Loesser

Preface

Many of us spend our leisure time hiking, sailing, snorkeling, and camping. We like to sample new foods, pamper our pets, and travel to magical places. All these pursuits enrich our lives but carry attendant risks. This book details the infections that complicate exposure to vacation climates, pets, recreational activities, and exotic cuisine.

There are many infectious disorders that fit this category, and they frequently overlap. Thus, touring a tropical paradise affords one the opportunity to eat poisoned food, swim in contaminated waters, and sustain serious injury from marine life. The Great Outdoors adds arthropod-borne infection and polluted water to the dangers of zoonoses. Clearly, risks are multiple, and a comprehensive guide is necessary. This book attempts to organize the wealth of information about these interesting and varied infections in a convenient and accessible format.

Contents

Contributors

BRUNO B. CHOMEL, D.V.M., PH.D., Department of Epidemiology and Preventative Medicine, School of Veterinary Medicine, University of California, Davis, CA 95616, USA

MARK A. CLEMENCE, M.D., Division of Geographic Medicine, University of Virginia Health Sciences Center, Charlottesville, VA 22908, USA

BURKE A. CUNHA, M.D., Department of Medicine, Division of Infectious Disease, Winthrop and Women's Hospital, Mineola, NY 11501, USA

DAVID L. DWORZACK, M.D., Departments of Medicine and Medical Microbiology, Creighton University School of Medicine, Omaha, NE 68131-2197, USA

DANIEL B. FISHBEIN, M.D., Center for Disease Control, Division of Viral and Rickettsial Disease, Atlanta, GA 30333, USA

JAMES G. FOX, D.V.M., Division of Comparative Medicine, Massachusetts Institute of Technology, Cambridge, MA 02139, USA

ELLIE J.C. GOLDSTEIN, M.D., 2021 Santa Monica Boulevard, Santa Monica, CA 90404, USA

CRAIG E. GREENE, D.V.M., M.S., College of Veterinary Medicine, University of Georgia, Athens, GA 30602, USA

J.K. GRIFFITHS, M.D., St. Elizabeth's Hospital, Boston, MA 02135, USA

RICHARD L. GUERRANT, M.D., Division of Geographic Medicine, University of Virginia Health Sciences Center, Charlottesville, VA 22908, USA

RICHARD F. JACOBS, M.D., Department of Pediatrics, Arkansas Children's Hospital, Little Rock, AR 72202-3591, USA

ROBERT S. JONES, D.O., M.S.C., Section of Infectious Diseases, School of Medicine and Hospital, Temple University, Philadelphia, PA 19104, USA

GERALD T. KEUSCH, M.D., Department of Medicine, New England Medical Center Hospital, Boston, MA 02111, USA

JOHN W. KREBS M.S., Center for Disease Control, Division of Viral and Rickettsial Disease, Atlanta, GA 30333, USA

MATTHEW E. LEVISON, M.D., Departments of Medicine and Infectious Disease, The Medical College of Pennsylvania, Philadelphia, PA 19129, USA

BENNETT LORBER, M.D., Section of Infectious Diseases, School of Medicine and Hospital, Temple University, Philadelphia, PA 19104, USA

JAY P. SANFORD, M.D., Antimicrobial Therapy Inc., Dallas, TX 75206, USA

GORDON E. SCHUTZE, M.D., Department of Pediatrics, Arkansas Children's Hospital, Little Rock, AR 72202-3591, USA

MARTIN S. WOLFE, M.D., Traveller's Medical Service, Washington, DC 20037, USA

1
In the Garden

Burke A. Cunha

Introduction

There are many potential infectious diseases that one may acquire while in the garden. People have gardened for years without ever becoming infected, whereas others have become infected with rather limited time spent in the garden. Being in the garden presents a series of complex possibilities from the standpoint of infectious disease, and the likelihood of one acquiring an infectious disease while gardening depends on many factors. Gardens are usually adjacent to or near the home and may be the closest many people get to being in the great outdoors, especially in urban or suburban environments. The time spent in the garden is not nearly as important as the age and condition of the gardener, his friends, or family (1–5).

Gardening may be a salutary experience for the healthy, but can be more dangerous to a patient with impaired immunity. For example, if a compromised host should contract coccidiomycosis, histoplasmosis, or the organism responsible for cat scratch fever, he or she would be at increased risk for dissemination. Elderly patients are fortunately relatively safe in terms of acquiring diseases in the garden. While elderly individuals can still acquire a variety of these infections from the soil, animals, or animal-related insect bites, as a group they are not at increased risk for acquiring disorders solely on account of their age. Of course, if earth excavations or construction are taking place nearby, if the area had *Legionella*, and if the wind was right, then an elderly person would be more likely to acquire and have a more severe case of Legionnaires' disease than their younger gardening counterparts.

Since many gardens are an extension of the home, children of various ages frequent the garden or the land close to the house alone or with gardening adults. Many infectious diseases acquired in the garden are age-specific, e.g., small children are more likely than adults to get *Strongyloides* or hookworm infections. The plant filled garden is not only visited by humans, but may be a stopping point or refuge for birds and animals. Because of its close proximity to the house, household pets frequently wander freely throughout the backyard and the garden. Even if one do not have pets, it is not uncommon that pets from the neighbourhood will spend varying lengths of time and perform various bodily functions while passing through the garden.

Therefore, if dogs, cats, or rodents are in the area, it is wise to consider that the garden and yard present the potential for contact with these animals or their excreta. Birds may fly over, nest above, or be found sick or dead in the garden. A great potential for histo-plasmosis or blastomycosis is present from bird droppings in wood stacked for winter, or in nests near the soil. To add another dimension of complexity to the problem, one need only consider the confounding variable of household pets meandering through the external environment and then coming into contact with their owners in a variety of ways. *Toxocara* organisms may be picked up by a dog or cat by ingestion and later transmitted via petting to children. A stray neighborhood cat giving birth in or near the garden immediately sets the stage for transmission of Q fever. The possibilities are almost endless. Lastly, there are the soil and plants themselves which, after all, are the foundations of a garden. What the soil contains is largely a function of the animal life in the area as well as the particular location of the garden.

For example, if the garden is located near moist, humid environments, such as riverbanks in the South, then blastomycosis becomes a diagnostic consideration. In contrast, if the garden is in the Southwest, then coccidiomycosis or even plague, if the appropriately infected rodent is in the area, also become diagnostic possibilities. Contact with rose bush thorns or sphagnum moss should immediately suggest the possibility of sporotrichosis. In the southeastern United States where soil in moist areas may be contaminated with hookworm or *Strongyloides* larvae, these worms add to the number of potential diseases that can be acquired when unprotected skin comes into contact with the soil. The *Ioxides* ticks that transmit Lyme disease in endemic areas may be found in lawn grass adjacent to the garden, so Lyme disease may literally be acquired in your own backyard or garden.

Therefore the soil, either through the kinds of organisms that normally reside in specific locations, e.g., the spores of coccidiomycosis or the larvae of hookworm, is an infectious disease hazard that needs to be reckoned with. One must also consider the contribution made by various animals to the soil, either by their presence or by contamination with their body fluids. One can easily appreciate the great array of infectious diseases that confronts the person simply slipping out of the house and walking across the yard to do a bit of gardening!

The Diagnostic Approach

In trying to analyze diagnostic possibilities in someone who has become ill and has spent time in the garden, it is necessary to consider the diagnosis from three different perspectives. First, one should consider the potential nature of the contact, either passive or active, that has befallen the individual. If there has been extensive soil contact, then sporotrichosis is the most likely diagnostic possibility. If piles of stacked or old moldy wood have been moved in association with wood gardening, then blasto- and histoplasmosis become additional possibilities. Nearby excavations with aerosolization of soil and water may suggest the possibility of Legionnaires' disease. If the patient resides where Lyme disease is endemic, then this diagnosis should be considered with the appropriate clinical presentation. Similarly, as mentioned in the introduction, specific locations suggest specific soil organisms, e.g., hookworm, coccidiomycosis, histoplasmosis, etc. Additionally, potential animal contact needs to be considered from a variety of standpoints. The person's own pets and their interaction with insect vectors and other animals in the area should be carefully ascertained and considered. In the absence of one's own pets, one needs to consider the pets in the neighborhood as well as any wild animals interacting with the gardener or the gardener's pets. One should inquire specifically about dead birds or animals the gardener may have found and buried in the garden. Specific inquiry should be made about potential contact with rodents or rabbits in the wild or runaway pets in the area. Only rarely will a disease be actively transmitted from an animal to a human, and the situations are usually straightforward if the proper questions are asked. For example, a dog bite suggests the possibility of *Pasteurella multocida*, DF-2 infection, or even rabies in the appropriate setting. Little kittens licking or scratching small children as well as adults raise the spectre of cat scratch fever, etc. As has been mentioned previously, some infectious diseases may be acquired actively or passively, e.g., sporotrichosis may be acquired by simply handling sphagnum moss, or may be actively acquired as the result of a puncture wound from the thorn of a rose. The epidemiological associations with infectious diseases acquired from plants, soil, or animal vectors are presented in Table 1.1.

The second step in the diagnostic process is to use end organ involvement by the infectious disease process to limit diagnostic possibilities and suggest specific disease entities. For example, if the patient presents with lymphadenopathy and a history of garden contact, then diagnostic possibilities are narrowed to toxoplasmosis, cat scratch fever, sporotrichosis, and occasionally, Lyme disease. Kitten or cat contact increases the likelihood of these lesions being due to cat scratch fever and toxoplasmosis, whereas nodular lymphangitis immediately suggests sporotrichosis. Obviously, there are many causes of adenopathy that have nothing to

TABLE 1.1. Epidemiological considerations in the garden.

	Infectious diseases	
Focus/vector	Passively acquired	Actively acquired
Soil/Plants	Sporotrichosis	Sporotrichosis
	Blastomycosis	Legionnaires' disease
	Histoplasmosis	
	Strongyloidosis	
	Hookworm	
Animals		
Cats	Toxoplasmosis	Cat scratch fever (CSF)
	Q fever	*Pasteurella multocida*
	Tularemia	Rabies
	CLM (Ancylostoma)	
	VLM (*T cati*)	
	Strongyloides	
	Campylobacter	
	Giardiasis	
	Yersinia	
	Salmonella	
	Dermatophytes	
Dogs	Group A streptococci	*P multocida*
	VLM (*T canis*)	DF-2
	CLM (Ancylostoma)	Rabies
	Leptospirosis	
	Brucellosis	
	Cryptosporidium	
	Dirofilaria immitis	
	Salmonella	
	Giardiasis	
	Oomphylobacter	
	RMSF (via tick bite)	
	Listeria	
	Dermatophytes	
Birds	Blastomycosis	
	Histoplasmosis	
	Cryptococcosis	
	Q fever	
Rabbits	Tularemia	Tularemia
	Brucellosis	
Rats	Leptospirosis	Rat bite fever
Rodents	Plague (via flea bite)	
	Relapsing fever (via tick bite)	
	Lyme disease (white-footed mouse)	
	Leptospirosis	
	Salmonella	
	LCM (hampsters)	

do with gardening or being in the garden, and the clinician must always be careful to consider the usual causes of lymph node involvement. However, if the adenopathy may be associated with gardening, then diagnostic possibilities are greatly reduced. If there are other associated findings, this also helps to limit diagnostic possibilities. It is a good diagnostic principle in infectious disease as well as in internal medicine to combine two diagnostic findings, even if they are nonspecific, to increase diagnostic specificity. For example, if the patient with axillary adenopathy had in addition a mild nonexudative pharyngitis and a few atypical lymphocytes, then the likelihood of acquired toxoplasmosis is enhanced. Similarly, the likelihood of Lyme disease being present in a patient with lymph node enlargement is enhanced if the patient has a facial nerve palsy. The more variables that one can combine, the easier it is to arrive at a definitive diagnosis. For example, if a patient presented with an ill-defined infiltrate on chest x-ray, with abdominal pain and a cough, accompanied by mental confusion and some diarrhea, then the chances of that individual having Legionnaires' disease are very high. These would not be the findings that would be found in a patient with other atypical pneumonias, i.e., Q fever, psittacosis, or mycoplasma. The diagnosis of worms producing cough or pneumonitis during their pulmonary migration phase may be a much more challenging diagnostic problem. Once again, by looking for associated features, one can increase diagnostic specificity and limit the differential diagnosis. For example, if a nonspecific pulmonary infiltrate was associated with eosinophilia, then strongyloides becomes a very likely explanation for the patient's problem. Mental confusion, especially in a young child, with persistent eosinophilia, may suggest visceral larval migrans (VLM) as a cause for the patient's complaints, especially if there has been a history of cat or dog contact. The differential diagnosis of infectious diseases by organ involvement is presented in tabular form in Table 1.2. The clinician should remember that other diseases may produce similar end organ dysfunction and clinical manifestations, but the table is particularly helpful if gardening is an important epidemiological factor to consider in assessing the patient's problem.

Laboratory tests represent the third and last approach to making the diagnosis. With all of the diseases potentially acquired by working in the garden, the clinician needs to establish a working diagnosis as described above, and arrive at a definitive diagnosis by ordering the appropriate, specific tests. Aside from the specific laboratory tests needed to make a diagnosis, the clinician needs to have some clues that suggest the proper tests to be ordered in the individual patient. Therefore, nonspecific tests are most helpful when applied in the appropriate clinical context and combined with epidemiological and/or characteristic end organ manifestations. For example, anemia in a small child from a rural area of the southeastern United States should immediately prompt a search for

TABLE 1.2. Infectious disease diagnostic considerations by organ involvement.

Skin	Lungs	Lymph nodes
CLM	Legionnaires' disease	Toxoplasmosis
Lyme disease	Q fever	Cat scratch fever
RMSF	Psitticosis	Sporotrichosis (nodular)
Dermatophytes	Difofilaria	Lyme disease
Histoplasmosis (*E nodosum*)	Helminths	
Tularemia		
P. multocida		
Group A streptococi		
Strongyloides		

Eye				Central Nervous System
Fundi	Cranial Nerves		Conjunctival Suffusion	Lyme Disease
VLM	Lyme disease		RMSF	VLM
Toxoplasmosis			Leptospirosis	Toxoplasmosis
			Relapsing fever	Cat scratch fever
				Legionnaires' disease

Pharynx	Gastrointestinal Tract	Liver
Toxoplasmosis	Strongyloides	Legionnaires' disease
Cat scratch fever	Cryptosporidia	RMSF
Lyme disease	Campylobacter	Q fever
	Yersinia	Psittacosis
	Giardia	Lyme disease
		Leptospirosis
		Histoplasmosis
		Cat scratch fever

Spleen
Q fever
Lyme disease
Psittacosis
Histoplasmosis

hookworm or strongyloides. The liver is involved in many infectious disease processes and therefore the finding of abnormal liver function tests is an important clue to a whole range of infectious diseases. With respect to the gardening population, an increased bilirubin in a patient with pneumonitis may suggest Legionnaires' disease, and in a patient with conjunctival suffusion should suggest leptospirosis. Mild increases in the alkaline phosphatase or the serum transaminases may occur with such dissimilar diseases as toxoplasmosis and Rocky Mountain spotted fever. If the patient has an atypical pneumonia, i.e., an ill-defined infiltrate and mild to moderately abnormal liver function tests, then diagnostic possibilities are quickly narrowed to Legionnaires' disease, psittacosis, and Q fever. Once again, it is important not to interpret diagnostic tests in a vacuum, but rather to combine them with some other factor in the history of physical diagnosis that quickly limits the diagnostic possibilities and provides the rationale for the working diagnosis. The finding of sterile pyuria, for example, usually suggests genitourinary tuberculosis as well as a wide variety of renal interstitial and tubular disorders. However in a gardener, sterile pyuria may point to brucellosis or leptospirosis rather than the usual diagnostic considerations. Once again, sterile pyuria should not be taken as the sole diagnostic finding, but rather it should be combined with other features to make clinical sense of diagnostic possibilities. Therefore, sterile pyuria with increased transaminases enhances the diagnostic probability of the patient having leptospirosis, whereas low pain and pain on palpation of the gastrocnemius muscles in a patient with unexplained fever and sterile pyuria points more to a diagnosis of brucellosis. Infectious disease diagnostic considerations by laboratory or roentgen findings are presented in tabular form in Table 1.3 (1–5).

TABLE 1.3. Infectious disease considerations by lab/roentgen findings.

↑ WBC	Chest x-ray
Group A streptococci	Infiltrates
↓ Platelets	Q fever
RMSF	Legionnaires' disease
Atypical lymphocytes	Histoplasmosis
Toxoplasmosis	Blastomycosis
Eosinophilia	Ascariasis
Strongyloides	Tularemia
VLM	Coin Lesion
Group A streptococci	Dirofilaria
Ascariasis	Abnormal Brain CT Scan
Hookworm	VLM
Anemia	Abnormal Urinalysis
Hookworm	Legionnaires' disease
Strongyloides	Leptospirosis
Histoplasmosis	Brucellosis
↑ LFTs (Alkaline phosphatases/transaminases)	Abnormal CSF
Legionnaires' disease	Toxoplasmosis
RMSF	Lyme disease
Q fever	LCM
Leptospirosis	Cat scratch fever
Toxoplasmosis	VLM
↑ Bilirubin	Leptospirosis
Legionnaires' disease	RMSF
Leptospirosis	Feces (smear, stain, culture)
	Giardia
	Campylobacter
	Yersinia
	Ascariasis
	Hookworm
	Strongyloides
	Salmonella
	Cryptosporidia

Specific Infectious Diseases

Sporotrichosis

The classic fungus associated with the soil is *Sporothrix schenckii*. A suppurative lymphangitis in the skin and subcutaneous tissues is characteristic of this disorder. *S schenckii* is a dimorphic fungus, which on culture produces conidia arranged in a "daisy" cluster on the top of a conidiophore. *S schenkii* is characterized in culture by the characteristic appearance of these daisy-like clusters. In tissue the organism assumes the yeast form, which is oval or cigar shaped. The organism may be introduced via thorns or splinters through minor abrasions in the skin. Usually the infecting trauma is minor and has been associated with such diverse activities as the picking of berries and/or the weaving of baskets (6). Alcoholics seem particularly prone to developing sporotrichosis, so this diagnostic point should be kept in mind when assessing patients who work in gardens and consume alcohol. Sporotrichosis begins as a small papular nodule which gradually enlarges and becomes a pustule that ulcerates. Spread is from distal to proximal along the lymphatics, and the lesions are characteristically not painful. Extradermal sporotrichosis is unusual, but hematogenous dissemination to the lungs, bones, and joints does occur (1). The diagnosis is usually clinical with specific confirmation by tube or latex agglutination tests. While other diseases may resemble sporotrichosis, e.g., tularemia, the indolent course of the illness along the lymphatic distribution with "bridges" of normal skin between unpainful lesions is highly suggestive of sporotrichosis (6–8).

Histoplasmosis

Histoplasmosis has a wide distribution but is most heavily concentrated in North America along the Ohio and Mississippi River valleys. A humid environment is key to the survival of this fungus in the environment, and decayed tree material contaminated by bat or bird droppings provides an ideal milieu for the survival of the organism. The spores may be aerosolized by manipulation of histoplasmosis containing wood, and the airborne spores may affect individuals far from the site of the initial focus of infection. Excavation, cleaning, or demolition of bird dropping-contaminated organic material usually results in an acute pneumonitis in a nonimmune individual. Obviously the use of bird droppings as fertilizer in the garden enhances the likelihood of acquiring acute pulmonary histoplasmosis in nonimmune individuals (9–13). Most patients have a self-limiting flu-like illness, but patients with chronic diseases, e.g., diabetes mel-

TABLE 1.4. Clinical spectrum of histoplasmosis.

Hematological	Pulmonary	Ear, Nose, and Throat
Thrombocytopenia	"Thick-walled" cavities	Nose ulcers
Anemia	Apical infiltrates	Lip ulcers
Leukopenia	Coin lesions	Gum ulcers
Pancytopenia	Histoplasmosis	Mouth ulcers
Splenomegaly	Hilar adenopathy	Tongue ulcers
Generalized adenopathy	"Buckshot" calcifications	Laryngeal ulcers
Eosinophilia	Miliary calcifications	
	"Marching cavities"	
	Mediastinal fibrosis	
	Obstruction of pulmonary/ artery vein*	
	Obstruction of superior vena cava*	
Dermatological	Cardiac	Neurological
Erythema nodosum	Endocarditis	Chronic meningitis
Erythema multiforme	Pericarditis	Focal cerebritis
Skin ulcers	acute	Spinal cord compression*
	subacute	
	fibrinous	
Gastrointestinal		Other
Esophageal obstruction*		Adrenal insufficiency
Granulomatous hepatitis		
Diarrhea		
Intestinal ulceration		

* Secondary to lymph node compression/mediastinal fibrosis
Adapted from reference 15, with permission.

litus or HIV, may be predisposed to dissemination. Disseminated histoplasmosis may be acute, subacute, or chronic depending on the size of the inoculum and the status of the patient's host defenses. Acute pulmonary histoplasmosis resembles a flu-like illness in symptomatic individuals. Erythema nodosum in a patient with a mild flu-like illness in the proper epidemiological context raises the possibility of histoplasmosis. Disseminated histoplasmosis resembles tuberculosis. However in the AIDS patient, reactivation of pre-existing histoplasmosis or progressive disease presents with a septicemic picture with hepatic and renal involvement that may progress to a shock-like state. HIV patients should be particularly careful to avoid gardening situations where histoplasmosis is likely to be lurking (1). Definitive diagnosis is by culture, tissue biopsy, or serological tests for *H capsulatum* (Table 1.4) (9–15).

Other fungi are very uncommon or only distantly related to gardening per se. Blastomycosis and cryptococcosis are unusual and are associated with typical clinical findings which should lead one to the diagnosis (Table 1.5) (1,5).

TABLE 1.5. Differential diagnosis of histoplasmosis.

	Histoplasmosis	Tuberculosis	Blastomycosis
Fever			
Double quotidian fever	−	±	−
Laboratory Tests			
Pancytopenia	+*	+	−
Hypergammaglobulinemia	−	−	−
Leukemoid reaction	−	+	−
Chest x-ray			
Miliary calcification	+	±	−
Hilar adenopathy	+	−	−
Pleural effusion	−	+	−
Abdominal x-ray			
Liver/splenic calcification	+	−	−
Organ involvement			
Meningitis	+*	+	−
Oropharyngeal ulcers	+*	±	−
Pulmonary infiltrates	+	+	±
Endocarditis	+	−	−
Addison's disease	+*	+	−
Granulomatous hepatitis	+	+	±
Splenomegaly	+*	±	±
Generalized adenopathy	+	±	−
Intestinal ulcers	+*	±	−
Bone/joint lesions	−	+	+
Glomerulonephritis	−	−	−
Epididymo-orchitis	−	+	+
Granulomatous prostatitis	+	−	+
Skin ulcers	+*	±	+
Erythema nodosum	+	+	±

* Only in disseminated histoplasmosis
Adapted from reference 15, with permission.

Legionnaires' Disease

Legionnaires' disease can only be acquired in the garden if the organism is in soil that is being excavated nearby and there is airborne spread of the organism to the garden area. Legionnaires' disease is varied in its distribution; Legionnaires' disease is common in some areas, while the disease is unheard of in other locations. *Legionella* is most common in the late spring and early fall and may begin with a flu-like illness. The course may be subacute or fulminant, and usually the illness presents as a pneumonia. However, a nonpulmonary form, i.e., Pontiac fever, is a manifestation of *Legionella* infection without associated pneumonitis. More typically, however, the disease presents as a community-acquired pneumonia. Legionnaires' disease should be considered in the diagnosis of all community-acquired pneumonias, and specific diagnostic features should be looked for to arrive at a working diagnosis (16). The clue to all of the atypical pneumonias lies in their extrapulmonary manifestations, since they are all systemic infections. With *Legionella*, the patient's extrapulmonary manifestations commonly include changes in mental status, nonspecific abdominal pain, or diarrhea. In contrast to *Mycoplasma* pneumonia, Legionnaires' disease is not associated with otitis or pharyngitis. If the patient has a temperature in excess of 102° F on presentation to the physician, and the patient does not have an arrhythmia, does not have a pacemaker, or is on beta-blockers, then a pulse-temperature deficit provides the single most important clue to the diagnosis. Relative bradycardia is present in virtually all cases of *Legionella* presenting with a temperature of >102° F, and if the pulse is charted with a temperature, a pulse-temperature deficit is readily seen by simple inspection (17). However if one desires to calculate if there is relative bradycardia present, then one takes the temperature in degrees fahrenheit, takes the last number and subtracts one, takes that number and multiplies by ten, and adds that sum to 100. For example, if the temperature is 105° F, the 5 is reduced to 4, multiplied by 10 = 40, and added back to 100, which is 140. Therefore, a pulse with a temperature of <140 in a patient with 105° F temperature, indicates a pulse-temperature deficit even if the patient is "tachying along" at 120 beats/minute. The chest x-ray is not characteristic, but it usually "behaves" in a typical way. Legionnaires' disease on chest x-ray is characterized by a rapidly progressive asymmetrical infiltrate(s). While not all *Legionella* behaves in this fashion, it is nonetheless the most typical roentgen manifestation (17). In terms of laboratory tests, a decreased serum phosphate, when present, is a most helpful finding. A decreased serum sodium appears to be more commonly associated with Legionnaires' disease than with other pneumonias, but is not specific for *Legionella* infections. A decrease in sodium on the basis of SIADH may occur with any pulmonary process, whether it be infectious, inflammatory, or neoplastic. In contrast, a depressed serum phosphate is uniquely associated with Legionnaires' disease (17). An elevated bilirubin in association with an atypical pneumonia is more helpful and limits diagnostic possibilities to pneumococcal pneumonia and *Legionella*. The serum transaminases are almost always modestly elevated in patients with *Legionella* pneumonia, and this is also true for other *Legionella* species. This is another important laboratory clue to the presence of an atypical pneumonia, since only *Legionella*, Q fever, and psittacosis are frequently associated with abnormal liver function tests in contrast to *Mycoplasma* pneumonia. Therefore, a working diagnosis can be readily obtained by combining the aforementioned features, while a definitive diagnosis depends upon demonstrating the organism with DFA of sputum or pleural fluid, or by IFA serological methods. The organism may also be cultured directly from sputum or appropriate samples of lung or pleural fluid. The differential diagnostic features of *Legionella* are presented in tabular form in Table 1.6 (16–19).

TABLE 1.6. Diagnostic features of atypical pneumonias.

Manifestations	Mycoplasma pneumonia	Legionnaires' disease	Psittacosis	Q fever	Tularemia
Symptoms					
Mental confusion	−	⊕	⊖	−	−
Headache	±	⊕	+	+	⊕
Meningismus	−	−	+	+	−
Myalgias	⊕	⊖	+	+	⊕
Ear pain	±	−	⊕	⊕	−
Pleuritic pain	±	+	±	±	−
Abdominal pain	−	+	−	−	−
Diarrhea	±	+	±	±	−
Hoarseness	−	−	−	−	−
Signs					
Rash	± (erythema multiforme)	−	± (Horder's spots)	±	±
Raynaud's phenomenon	±	−	−	−	−
Nonexudative pharyngitis	+	−	−	−	−

Hemoptysis	–	+	+	–	–
Lobar consolidation	–	±	±	±	±
Cardiac involvement	±	±	±	±	–
Splenomegaly	–	–	+	–	–
Relative bradycardia	–	+	+	+	–
Chest Film Findings					
Infiltrate	Patchy	Patchy/consolidation	Patchy/consolidation	Pleural-based	Ovoid bodies
Bilateral hilar adenopathy	–	–	–	–	+
Pleural effusion	± (small)	±	±	–	+ (bloody)
Laboratory Findings					
White blood cell count	←	←	Normal	Normal	Normal
Hypophosphatemia	–	+	–	–	–
Increase in SGOT/SGPT	–	+	+	+	–
Cold agglutinins	+	–	–	–	–
Microscopic hematuria	–	⊕	–	–	–

Adapted from reference 17, with permission.

Q Fever

Q fever is another cause of pneumonitis in the gardener who comes into contact with animals or aerosolized animal products. Q fever has a wide distribution, and the organism *Coxiella burnetii* has been found in a variety of animals. Gardeners should know that *Coxiella* has been isolated in wild birds, squirrels, mice, rabbits and cats (1). Ticks and other arthropods that feed on small domestic animals harbor the organism. The small animals are usually asymptomatic, but at parturition their placenta is usually heavily infected. Dissemination of the organism is via the airborne route, and the organism may persist in the soil for up to 6 months. The inhalation of infected aerosols is the most common route by which humans develop Q fever pneumonia. *C burnetii* is a pleomorphic, gram-negative, coccobacillus that is highly resistant to dessication. Only a single organism is required to cause human infection (20). Most individuals exposed to *C burnetii* develop a self-limiting flu-like illness. However, Q fever is in the differential diagnosis of atypical pneumonia. The typical clues to Q fever pneumonia are a nonproductive cough with mild hemoptysis. Except for viral influenza pneumonia, no other atypical pneumonia is associated with hemoptysis (1). Diarrhea may occur, as with *Legionella* or *Mycoplasma* pneumonia, as do other nonspecific symptoms such as fever, chills, arthralgias, and myalgias. However, Q fever is characterized by severe headache which is common only with psittacosis among the atypical pneumonias. Physical examination is unrevealing, but the chest x-ray usually reveals characteristic pleural-based ovoid infiltrates. The diagnosis is by serology, and the complement fixation test is most frequently used. Occasionally, the disease may become chronic, and the prime manifestation of chronic Q fever is Q fever endocarditis (20–23).

Lyme Disease

Ioxides ticks are widely distributed geographically and require high surface humidity associated with coastal or river areas. The white-footed mouse as well as other small mammals are the primary reservoir of *Borrelia burgdorferi*, the organism responsible for Lyme disease. The larvae of the *Ioxides* tick, reaching high numbers in late summer and early fall, feed preferentially on small animals. Raccoons and rodents are preferentially attacked by the nymphal stage of the *Ioxides* tick. It is the nymphal form of the tick that is responsible for Lyme disease in humans (1,5). Lyme disease acquired from tall grasses or even a lawn infested with the *Ioxides* ticks results in the characteristic skin lesion of erythema chronicum migrans (ECM) in up to 75% of patients. The larval and nymphal forms of the tick are small and need to be in contact with the host for at least 24 hours in order to transmit the spirochetes to the host.

Because the ticks are so small, only 50% of patient can recall being bitten by the tick. Two to 3 weeks after the tick bite, ECM develops in most patients and is the clinical marker for the disease. Although stage 2 Lyme disease, characterized by cardiac or neurological involvement may occur, it would be difficult to associate these clinical presentations with the antecedent tick exposure. Lastly, stage 3, which is characterized by chronic Lyme's arthritis, develops long after the infection and when the exposure in the yard, garden, or woods may be forgotten. ECM is so characteristic that there are few diseases that can be confused with these lesions, if present. The lesions are erythematous, may be associated with some itching, and are warm but not painful. The lesions clear spontaneously within several weeks. Associated with ECM may be nonspecific symptoms of a flu-like illness, with fever, malaise, and pharyngitis, or patients may have a mild meningoencephalitis. Since *B burgdorferi* is a neurotrophic spirochete, neurological manifestations early in stage 1 Lyme disease are not uncommon. The hallmark of neuroborreliosis is seventh nerve involvement, which may be unilateral or bilateral. No other cranial nerves have been associated with Lyme disease. Facial nerve palsy is the most specific and consistent abnormality. Many patients with facial paralysis have an aseptic meningitis profile if CSF is analyzed when the patient has cranial nerve involvement. Chronic neuroborreliosis may occur as a late manifestation. However, the association of peripheral nerve involvement, e.g., polyneuritis, is characterized by dysethesias, paresthegias, and hyperesthesias of the extremities in association with pain in a radicular distribution (24–27). The association of a peripheral and a Bell's palsy would be highly suggestive of Lyme disease in a gardener or anyone else. The diagnosis of Lyme disease may be made clinically if the characteristic ECM lesion is present. In the absence of ECM, IgM titers against the organism, or one or more spirochetal antigens suggest the diagnosis. An elevated IgG titer should be interpreted with caution, since the majority of these patients represent prior exposure to the antigen and inactive clinical disease. The clinical features of Lyme disease are shown in Table 1.7 (24–28).

TABLE 1.7. The clinical picture of lyme disease.

	Dermatological	Neurological	Rheumatology	Cardiac
Stage 1	Erythema chronicum migrans (ECM)	Possible headache, myalgias	Arthralgias	None
Stage 2	Multiple and/or recurrent ECM	Meningoencephalitis, peripheral neuritis	Arthralgias	Carditis
Stage 3	Acrodermatitis chronica atrophicans (ACA)	Chronic encephalitis, meningitis	Chronic arthritis	Cardiomyopathy

Adapted from reference 28, with permission.

Toxoplasmosis

Toxoplasmosis may be acquired by contact with a cat. Mature oocysts are excreted only by cats and may be ingested after direct contact with material contaminated by feline excreta. Cats having toxoplasmosis may excrete millions of oocysts in the first 1 to 3 weeks of the illness. The oocystes become infectious after sporolation, however oocysts may remain infectious for several months in warm moist soils. Immuno-competent adult hosts usually develop acute acquired toxoplasmosis. In the normal host, toxoplasmosis usually presents as a mono-like illness characterized by asymmetrical adenopathy, fever, malaise, arthralgias, and pharyngitis. Toxoplasmosis must be differentiated from EBV in-fectious mononucleosis as well as CMV mononucleosis. This is usually done on the basis of specific serological tests. The IgM IFA test may be positive 1 to 2 weeks after infection, reaching peak titers 1 to 2 months after the initial infection. Such patients should have negative CMV IgM and EBV serologies. In the immunocompetent adult, acute toxoplasmosis is usually self-limited, whereas in immunocompromised hosts the disease may be widely disseminated. Similarly, pregnant females should avoid gardening if they have negative IgG antitoxoplasmosis titers by serologi-cal testing. Since toxoplasmosis is usually asymptomatic in pregnant individuals, and fetal abnormalities are common, it is critical that preg-nant woment avoid obvious contact with cats for the pregnancy as well as the not so obvious contact with potentially infected garden soil (29–33).

Cat Scratch Fever

Cat scratch fever, also known as cat scratch disease, is a zoonosis as-sociated with cats. The organism appears to be a pleomorphic fastidious gram-negative bacillus. Cat scratch fever is less common in household cats than in cats that roam freely outside of the house. The cat scratch organism enters the host through a small break in the skin. Kittens are more likely to harbor the organism than adult cats, and licking is more common than scratching as a mechanism for causing cat scratch fever (34). The initial lesion on the skin may be unremarkable, and patients often cannot associate the mechanism by which the organism was in-oculated and the subsequent illness. Patients develop adenopathy 1 to 2 weeks after the lick, scratch, or bite. Malaise and fever accompany the regional adenopathy characterised by microabscesses pathologically. Pharyngitis, splenomegaly, and encephalopathy occur in some patients. Hepatic involvement with cat scratch fever is distinctly unusual, whereas fever and fatigue are common features (1,5). AIDS patients develop peculiar pedunculated nodules, and the disease may resemble Kaposi's sarcoma in these individuals. Disseminated disease has also been reported in the HIV population. Cat scratch fever may present with meningoence-phalitis as well a peripheral polyneuritis. The diagnosis of cat scratch fever is made by obtaining a positive skin test result on the patient with the appropriate animal contact history. Definitive diagnosis is made by demonstrating the characteristic histology on the lymph node biopsy specimen, or demonstrating the organism by silver stains in tissue speci-mens (34–38).

Rocky Mountain Spotted Fever

Rocky Mountain spotted fever (RMSF) is caused by *Rickettsia rickettsii* and is transmitted to humans via tick bites from dogs and wild rodents. Its peak incidence is in the late spring and early summer, and consists of fever, headache, myalgias, and a characteristic rash. The rash typically begins on the wrists and ankles 3 to 5 days after the tick bite. The rash moves centrally as the patient's illness progresses, and the petechial lesions increase in number. Important clues to RMSF include a selective swelling on the dorsum of the hands and feet, periorbital edema with or without conjunctival suffusion, and the characteristic rash. A variety of nonspecific laboratory tests, when analyzed in concert, may suggest the diagnosis. Typically, one looks for thrombocytopenia and mildly abnormal liver function tests. The rash is characteristic in its appear-ance and distribution. The differential diagnosis includes toxic shock syndrome, meningococcemia/meningococcal meningitis, leptospirosis, dengue fever, and atypical measles Table 1.8 (1,2). The diagnosis of RMSF may be complicated by abdominal pain, diarrhea, meningismus, or hepato-splenomegaly, which may cause diagnostic confusion. The diagnosis of RMSF depends on the presence of the rash initially, and is confirmed by appropriate serology, e.g., the indirect hemagglutination, indirect immunofluorescence, latex agglutination, or complement fixa-tion. The ticks that transmit RMSF, i.e., *Dermacentor*, are larger and more easily recognizable than the ticks that transmit Lyme disease. In the summer, if one spends time in a tick-infested area, frequent checks of the body for ticks is essential. Repellents and protective clothing may help, but one should carefully check one's body and remove them aseptically (39–43).

Ascarids

Ascaris lumbricoides is the most common helminthic infestation. *A lumbricoides* resides in the jejunum and is the largest nematode causing infection in humans. Moist soil is necessary for the eggs to remain in-fectious after a two-week period of embryonation in the soil. While ascariasis is a worldwide problem, children living in rural areas of the southeastern United States are most commonly affected. The eggs are

TABLE 1.8. Differential diagnosis of rocky mountain spotted fever.

Signs and symptoms	RMSF	Meningococcal meningitis	Dengue	Leptospirosis	Atypical measles
Mental confusion	±	±	−	±	−
Headache	+++	+++	++	+++	−
Photophobia	+	+	+	−	−
Myalgia/arthralgia	+++	++	+++	+++	+
Nausea/vomiting	+	+	−	−	−
Abdominal pain	±	−	−	±	−
Rash	petechial-ankles wrists, palms, soles	"palpable" petechiae-asymmetrical	petechial-truncal	maculopapular-truncal	urticarial, maculopapular-truncal
Jaundice	±	−	−	±	−
Splenomegaly	+ (50%)	−	−	±	−
Periorbital edema	++	−	−	−	−
Conjunctival suffusion	+	−	−	+	−
Abnormal LFTs	±	−	−	++	−
Eosinophilia	±	−	−	−	+++
Chest film	−	−	−	−	+

Adapted from reference 43, with permission.

highly resistant in the soil and may last for up to 6 years in the environment. After ingestion, the eggs hatch in the small intestine. The larvae invade the mucosa and migrate via venous channels to pulmonary circulation. After entering the alveoli and ascending the tracheal bronchia tree, they return to the gastrointestinal tract to reach adulthood in the small intestine. Most infestations are asymptomatic clinically, however in the first 1 to 2 weeks following ingestion of the infected eggs, a hypersensitivity lung reaction resulting in cough and pneumonitis frequently occurs during the migratory phase through the lungs. Pneumonitis may last days or weeks and is usually associated with eosinophilia, possibly resulting in Loeffler's syndrome. Ascariasis may obstruct hollow structures contiguous with the small bowel, e.g., the appendix, biliary ducts, pancreatic ducts, etc., and produce infections in those areas. Diagnosis is by examination of stool samples for the characteristic mamillated eggs, which are typically present in large numbers. The adult worms may also be seen on contrast studies of the small bowel as filling defects, or in the postevacuation films as linear structures containing barium. Ascariasis should be considered in young children who have migratory pulmonary infiltrates in association with a peripheral eosinophilia (3–6).

Hookworm

Hookworm is caused by two intestinal nematodes, *Ancylostoma duodenale* or *Necator americanus*. In contaminated soil, eggs hatch within 24 hours and become rhabdidiform larvae. After 5 to 10 days incubation in warm, moist soil, the rhabdidiform larvae develop into filariform larvae which are capable of surviving 2 to 4 weeks in the soil. It is the filariform larvae that penetrate exposed skin. The filariform larvae then migrate to the lungs and from there enter the small intestine where they mature into adults. In the soil of the rural southeastern United States, the heavy rainfall and high humidity are ideal for the life cycle of these nematodes. Patients usually present with symptoms attributable to anemia, which is a function of their worm burden and consequent blood loss. Hyperproteinemia and peripheral edema may also complicate a worm infection. Nonspecific abdominal complaints are common, but the pulmonary phase of the infection is usually asymptomatic in contrast to ascariasis. Diagnosis is by finding the characteristic oval eggs in a direct stool smear. Light infections require stool concentration techniques, fresh stools should be examined immediately since worm eggs may hatch into rhabdidiform larvae resembling the rhabdidiform larvae of strongyloides (1,6).

Strongyloides

S stercoralis has a distribution similar to that of ascariasis. *Strongyloides* is unique among the nematodes, being capable of autoinfection because of its peculiar triphasic life cycle. *Strongyloides* penetrates the skin in a manner analogous to hookworm, and goes through a pulmonary phase similar to that of ascariasis or hookworm. While still in the intestine, the rhabdidiform larvae may develop into infectious filariform larvae which in turn penetrate the colonic mucosa, reinfecting the host. This autoinfective cycle leads to hyperinfestation by this nematode. Chronic *Strongyloides* infection in an immunocompetent host may be asymptomatic or the patient may complain of nonspecific abdominal complaints with or without diarrhea. Characteristic of *Strongyloides* are multiple urticarial lesions, or a pruritic linear serpiginous rash which is common on the trunk or buttocks. The pulmonary migration phase of the parasite is asymptomatic in normal hosts but may be the predominant clinical manifestation in immunocompromised hosts. In compromised hosts, the association of migratory pulmonary infiltrates with peripheral eosinophilia may provide a clue to the diagnosis. The diagnosis may be made by demonstrating filariform larvae in sputum in immunocompromised patients. IgE levels are often elevated in association with peripheral eosinophilia. Definitive diagnosis is by demonstrating the rhabdidiform larvae in duodenal fluid or concentrated stool specimens (4–6).

Toxocara

Toxocara canis in dogs, and *T cati* in cats are responsible for toxocariasis in humans. Toxocariasis occurs when the eggs containing the infective larvae are ingested and hatched in the small intestine. The larvae reach the liver via the port of circulation, then reach the lungs and re-enter the general circulation. Since the larvae are in the general circulation, wide dissemination is the rule with this helminth, e.g., liver, brain, heart, lungs, etc. The larvae survive for months or years in the host, but disappear from the lungs and liver relatively quickly, while concentrating in the white matter of the brain. *Toxocara* larvae in the brain are protected from the host's defense mechanisms. The organism covers itself with collagenous capsules, and the larvae remain viable even within well-encapsulated granulomas. Clinically, *Toxocara* infection manifests itself as visceral larval migrans (VLM) or ophthalmic larval migrans (OLM). The syndromes usually occur in very young children who present with pulmonary or neurological symptoms. VLM should be suspected in children with unexplained behavioral disorders or unexplained onset of focal or generalized seizures, especially if associated with peripheral eosinophilia. Children with VLM may also have liver enlargement and diffuse polyclonal hypergammaglobulinemia. If the parasites migrate and localize to the eye, involvement is typically unilateral and is commonly manifested by a painless loss of vision. OLM occurs in adults but is more common in children. It is thought that light infestations of *Toxocara* result in OLM, whereas heavy infestations result in VLM. The best diagnostic test for VLM is by ELISA. VLM should be considered in any child with a history of contact with a dog or cat, or who has peripheral eosinophilia and neurological abnormalities in the absence of pulmonary abnormalities (44–48).

Conclusions

Gardening is a wonderful pastime and a very peaceful way to enjoy oneself. However, the garden may be a treacherous place for very young compromised hosts when one takes into account the infectious potential residing in the soil, as well as the insect vectors on plants and animals. The location of the garden, and the characteristics of the soil, i.e., moist and warm, play a part in determining its infectious potential. The most important factor in making the garden an infectious and dangerous place is the number and interaction of animals, whether they be pets or wildlife, that temporarily use the garden as part of their daily activities. The clinician should always ask about garden exposure to help narrow the diagnostic possibilities for the patient. The diagnostic approach should utilize epidemiological principles in concert with clinical clues, which together should suggest a reasonable list of diagnostic possibilities. Organ involvement and specific laboratory tests will further narrow the differential diagnosis and will determine the specific tests necessary to make a definitive diagnosis.

References

1. Gorbach SL, Bartlett JG, Blacklow NR (eds): *Infectious Diseases.* Philadelphia, W. B. Saunders, 1992.
2. Braude AI (ed): *Infectious Diseases and Medical Microbiology*, 2 ed. Philadelphia, W. B. Saunders, 1986.
3. Heoprich PD, Jordan MC. *Infectious Eiseases*, 4 ed. Philadelphia, J. B. Lippincott, 1989.
4. Manson-Bahr PEC, Bell DR (eds): *Manson's Tropical Diseases*, 19 ed. Philadelphia, Bailliere Tindall, 1987.
5. Mandell GL, Gordon-Douglas R Jr, Bennett JE (eds): *Principles and Practice of Infectious Diseases*, 3 ed. New York, Churchill Livingstone, 1985.
6. CDC: Multistate outbreak of sporotrichosis in seedling handlers, 1988. *MMWR* 1988; 37:652.
7. D'Alessio DJ, Leavens LJ, Strumpf GB, et al. An outbreak of sporotrichosis in Vermont associated with sphagnum moss as the source of infection. *N Engl J Med* 1965; 272:1054–1058.
8. Powell KE, Taylor A, Phillips BJ, et al. Cutaneous sporotrichosis in forestry workers. *JAMA* 1978; 240:232.
9. Furcolow ML. Environmental aspects of histoplasmosis. *Arch Environ Health* 1965; 10:4.

10. Goodwin RA, Des Prez RM. Histoplasmosis. *Am Rev Respir Dis* 1984; 157:1.
11. Brodsky AL, Gregg MD, Loewenstein MS, et al. Outbreak of histoplasmosis associated with the 1970 Earth Day activities. *Am J Med* 1973; 54:333.
12. Leznoff A, Frank H, Telner P, et al. Histoplasmosis in Montreal during the fall of 1963, with observations on erythema multiforme. *Can Med Assoc J* 1964; 31:1154.
13. Schlech WF, Wheat LJ, Hol JL, et al. Recurrent urban histoplasmosis, Indianapolis, Indiana. *Am J Epidemiol* 1983; 118:301.
14. Medeiros AA, Marty SD, Tosh FE, Chin TDY. Erythema nodosum and erythema multiforme as clinical manifestations of histoplasmosis in a community outbreak. *N Engl J Med* 1966; 274:415.
15. Cunha BA. Histoplasmosis. *Infect Dis Prac* 1986; 9:1–8.
16. Yu VL, Kroboth FJ, Shonnard J, et al. Legionnaires' desease: New clinical perspective from a prospective pneumonia study. *Am J Med* 1982; 73:357.
17. Johnson DH, Cunha BA. *Legionella* chlymcia and *Mycoplasma* pneumonia— Postgraduate *Med* 1993; (in press).
18. Johnson RD, Raff M, van Arsdall J. Neurologic manifestations of Legionnaires' disease. *Medicine* 1984; 63:303.
19. Cunha BA. Atypical pneumonias. *Postgrad Med* 1991; 90:89–101.
20. Clark WH, Lennette EH, Railsback OC, et al. Q fever in California. VII. Clinical features in one hundred eighty cases. *Arch Intern Med* 1951; 88:155.
21. Leedom JM. Q fever: An update. *Curr Clin Top Infect Dis* 1980; 1:304.
22. Murray HW, Tuazon C. Atypical pneumonias. *Med Clin North Am* 1980; 64:507.
23. Sawyer LA, Fishbein DB, McDade JE. Q fever: Current concepts. *Rev Infect Dis* 1987; 9:935.
24. Steere AC, Hutchinson GJ, Craft JE, et al. The early clinical manifestations of Lyme disease. *Ann Intern Med* 1983; 99:76.
25. Steere AC, Schoen RT, Taylor E. The clinical evolution of Lyme arthritis. *Ann Intern Med* 1987; 107:725.
26. Halperin JJ, Pass HL, Anand AK, Dattwyler RJ. Nervous system abnormalities in Lyme disease. *Ann NY Acad Sci* 1988; 539:24.
27. Halperin JJ. Luft BJ, Anand AK, et al. Lyme neuroborreliosis: Central nervous system manifestations. *Neurology* 1989; 39:753.
28. Cunha BA. It's Lyme disease season. *Emerg Med* 1991; May, 1991.
29. Remington JS, Desmonts G. Toxoplasmosis. In: Remington JS, Klein JO (eds): *Infectious Diseases of the Fetus and Newborn Infant*, 3 ed. Philadelphia, W. B. Saunders, 1990.
30. Townsend JJ, et al. Acquired toxoplasmosis. *Arch Neurol* 1975; 32:335.
31. McCabe R, Remington JS. Toxoplasmosis: The time has come. *N Engl J Med* 1988; 318:313.
32. McCabe RE, Brooks RG, Dorfman RF, Remington JS. Clinical spectrum in 107 cases of toxoplasmic lymphadenopathy. *Rev Infect Dis* 1987; 9:754.
33. Dorfman RF, Remington JS. Value of lymph node biopsy in the diagnosis of acute acquired toxoplasmosis. *N Engl J Med* 1973; 289:878.
34. Warwick WJ. Cat-scratch syndrome: Many diseases or one disease? *Prog Med Virol* 1967; 9:256.

35. Moriaty RA, Margileth AM. Cat-scratch disease. *Infect Dis Clin North Am* 1987; 1:575.
36. Margileth AM. Cat-scratch disease: Nonbacterial regional lymphadenitis. The study of 145 patients and review of the literature. *Pediatrics* 1968; 42:803.
37. Hall AV, Roberts CM, Maurice PD, et al. Cat scratch disease in patients with AIDS: Atypical skin manifestations. *Lancet* 1988; 3:453.
38. Daniels WB, MacManay FG. Cat-scratch disease: report of one hundred sixty cases. *JAMA* 1954; 154:1247.
39. Harrell GT. Rocky Mountain spotted fever. *Medicine* 1949; 28:333.
40. Hatwick MAW, O'Brien RJ, Hanson BF. Rocky Mountain spotted fever; epidemiology of an increasing problem. *Ann Intern Med* 1976; 84:732–739.
41. Helmick CG, Bernard KW, D'Angelo LJ. Rocky Mountain spotted fever: Clinical, laboratory, and epidemiological features of 262 cases. *J Infect Dis* 1984; 150:480–486.
42. Salgo MP, Telzak EE, Currie B, et al. A focus of Rocky Mountain spotted fever within New York City. *N Engl J Med* 1988; 318:1345–1348.
43. Cunha BA. Rocky Mountain spotted fever. *Emerg Med* 1988; November:- 129–138.
44. Beaver PC. The nature of visceral larval migrans. *J Parasitol* 1969; 55:3.
45. Schantz PM. Toxocaral larva migrans now. *Am J Trop Med Hyg* 1989; 41:21.
46. Zinkham WH. Visceral larva migrans. A review and reassessment indicating two forms of clinical expression: Visceral and ocular. *Am J Dis Child* 1987; 132:627.
47. Huntley CC, Costas MC, Lyerly A. Visceral larval migrans syndrome; Clinical characteristics and immunologic studies in 51 patients. *Pediatrics* 1965; 36:523.
48. Taylor MRH, Keane CT, O'Connor P, et al. The expanded spectrum of toxocaral disease. *Lancet* 1988; 1:692.

2
On the Farm

JAY P. SANFORD

Introduction

One only has to go to an airport or drive on the interstate highway system to appreciate that for many Americans, travel and leisure are an integral aspect of our lives. This chapter will focus on the farm as a vacation or leisure locus.

In consideration of infections which can be acquired in the farm environment, for many diseases it may be important to define where the farm is located, in what season of the year will potential exposure occur, and what activities will individuals be engaged in while on the farm. The potential risks for acquiring many infections are much less if the leisure time on the farm is spent in a rocking chair on the porch listening to the grass grow than those associated with hands-on involvement in farm activities which bring one in contact with fields, animals and equipment. In this chapter, the assumption is made that activities will be more active than passive. There may be some overlap with infections of leisure which are more associated with camping or fishing; however, those infections which are associated primarily with farming or ranching will be emphasized (Table 2.1).

Viral Infections

Arboviral Infections

As defined by the World Health Organization, "Arborviruses are viruses which are maintained in nature principally, or to an important extent, through biological transmission between susceptible vertebrate hosts by hematophagous arthropods; they multiply and produce viremia in the vertebrates, multiply in the tissues of arthropods, and are passed on to new vertebrates by the bites of arthropods after a period of extrinsic

TABLE 2.1.

A. Viral Infections
   1. Arboviral infections
      a. Colorado Tick Fever
      b. La Crosse virus encephalitis
      c. Eastern equine encephalitis
      d. Western equine encephalitis
      e. St. Louis encephalitis
   2. Rabies
   3. Orf/Milker's Nodule
B. Rickettsial Infections
   1. Q fever
C. Bacterial Infections
   1. Leptospirosis
   2. Tularemia
   3. Brucellosis
   4. Campylobacteriosis
   5. Listeriosis
D. Pig Bites
E. Fungal and Parasitic Organisms

incubation." From this definition it can be appreciated that the term "arbovirus" is used in the epidemiologic sense. Transmission by vectors is not correlated with viral nucleic acid content and morphology. As a result, for taxonomic purposes the term arbovirus has been eliminated; however, it remains clinically and epidemiologically useful. There are currently more than 530 antigenically distinct "arboviruses"; 60 have been isolated in the United States and Canada, of which 16 are associated with human disease. The majority of agents contain single-stranded RNA although the virus of Colorado tick fever contains double-stranded RNA.

"Arbovirus" infection of vertebrates is usually asymptomatic. The viremia stimulates an immune response which terminates the viremia. In arboviral infections encountered in the United States and Canada, infection in humans represents an incidental occurrence which is not essential to the basic maintenance cycle of the virus.

Most human "arbovirus" infections are also asymptomatic. When disease is produced, the spectrum of illness is varied both in predominant features and in severity (Table 2.2).

Colorado Tick Fever

Epidemiology. Colorado tick fever (CTF) is transmitted to humans by the bite of the adult hard-shelled wood tick, *Dermacentor andersoni*. CTF virus has been isolated from 10 to 25% of *D andersoni* collected in

TABLE 2.2. Major clinical syndromes, associated arboviruses, vectors, seasonality, geographic distribution.

Clinical syndrome	Arbovirus	Vector	Seasonality	Geographic Distribution
Fever, malaise, myalgia	Colorado tick fever	Tick (*Dermacentor andersoni*)	March–September (mostly May–June)	Rocky Mountain region of United States and Canada, 4000–10,000 feet
Fever, aseptic meningitis, encephalitis	LaCrosse virus (California complex)	Mosquito (*Aedes triservatus*)	June–October	North central states, New York, eastern seaboard, Mississippi River valley
	Eastern equine encephalitis	Mosquito (*Culiseta melanura, Aedes sollicitans, Aedes albopictus*)	Late summer–early fall	Eastern seaboard, eastern New York, Ontario, western Michigan (? South Dakota)
	Western equine encephalitis	Mosquito (*Culex tarsalis*)	Early–mid summer	Throughout the U.S.
	St. Louis encephalitis	Mosquito (*Culex pipiens-quinquefasciatus* complex, *Culex tarsalis*)	Mid summer–early fall	Ohio-Mississippi River valley, eastern Texas, Florida, Kansas, Colorado, California

endemic areas. The virus is maintained in nature by transovarial transmission. Human exposure occurs from late March through September, mostly in May and June in mountain forest areas between 4,000 and 10,000 feet altitude. While not important in the epidemiology of CTF, the virus persists within erythrocytes of convalescent patients for as long as four months (12). Transfusion-associated CTF has been reported (27).

Clinical Manifestations. The incubation period is usually 3 to 6 days. In 90% of patients, a history of tick bite within 10 days of illness can be obtained. Persons affected are those whose activities, such as horseback riding, bring them in contact with *D. andersoni*. The disease may occur at any age, although in one series 40% were 20 to 29 years of age (12). The illness is characterized by the sudden onset of severe aching of the muscles in the back and legs, chilliness usually without true rigors, rapid rise in temperature to 102 to 104°F, headache with pain on movement of the eyes, and photophobia. The physical findings are not specific, but include tachycardia (proportionate to the fever), flushed facies and variable conjunctival injection. Occasionally the spleen is palpable. Five to 12% of patients may have a maculopapular or petechial rash, usually predominantly on the arms and legs. The fever often (one-half of patients) lyses abruptly after about two days. After an afebrile period of about two days, the fever recurs, may be higher than in the first phase and may last another three days. Convalescence of more than three weeks is reported in 70% of patients over the age of 30, while convalescence is more rapid in individuals under age 20.

Three to seven per cent of patients may have aseptic meningitis or encephalitis (23). Hemorrhagic fever with epistaxis, gastrointestinal bleeding and purpura have been reported in children.

Laboratory Features. The most important laboratory finding is moderate to marked leucopenia. At the onset of illness the total leucocyte count may be normal but by the fifth to the sixth day it is usually 2,000–3,000 per μl (although in one-third of patients it may remain about 4,500 per μl). The leucopenia is characteristically associated with proportionate decrease in lymphocytes and granulocytes. Erythrocyte values remain normal. Mild increases in aspartate aminotransferase (SGOT) and creatine phosphokinase are reported.

Diagnosis. The diagnosis is based upon epidemiologic and clinical findings. Almost one-half of patients diagnosed as Rocky Mountain spotted fever in Utah were subsequently shown to have CTF. The diagnosis can be confirmed by virus isolation or fluorescent antibody staining of erythrocytes.

Treatment. The treatment is symptomatic. None of the currently available antiviral agents is effective.

Prognosis. Only three deaths have been reported, all with hemorrhagic signs.

Arbovirus Meningoencephalitis

Four arboviruses are recognized as important causes of meningoen-cephalitis, the California serogroup (LaCrosse virus), Eastern equine encephalitis (EEE), Western equine encephalitis (WEE) and St. Louis encephalitis (SLE). The spectrum of infection includes inapparent infection, fever with headache, aseptic meningitis and encephalitis. Between 1,500 and 2,000 cases of encephalitis are reported in the United States each year (27). In the absence of epidemics 5 to 10% (75 to 200 cases) are confirmed as "arboviral". In non-epidemic years, LaCrosse virus is responsible for two-thirds to three-fourths of the cases.

LaCrosse Virus Encephalitis

Epidemiology. LaCrosse virus (LCV) infection occurs in the north central states, New York, the eastern seaboard and the Mississippi River valley (Fig. 2.1) (27). The virus is maintained by transovarial transmission in

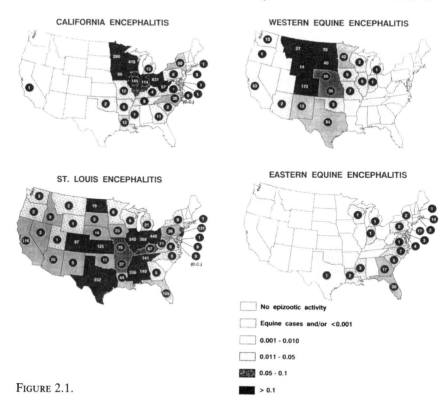

FIGURE 2.1.

woodland mosquitoes, *Aedes triseriatus*, which breed in tree holes in hardwood forests and have adapted to discarded tires. The virus over-winters in the eggs of *A. triseriatus*. Chipmunks and gray squirrels serve as amplifier hosts. LCV encephalitis occurs between June and October, most often involving boys (60%) 5 to 10 years of age (60%) who live in rural areas (2).

Clinical Manifestations. There are two clinical patterns of LaCrosse virus disease (2). One is a mild form with a two- to three-day prodrome of fever, headache, malaise, and gastrointestinal symptoms. About the third day the temperature increases to 104° F, and the patient becomes lethargic and develops meningeal signs. These findings abate gradually over a seven- to eight-day period without overt sequelae. The second pattern, a severe form which occurs in at least one-half of the patients, begins abruptly with fever, headache and vomiting, followed shortly by lethargy and disorientation. During the first two to four days the course is rapidly progressive with the occurrence of seizures (50 to 60%), focal neurologic signs (20%), pathologic reflexes (10%) and coma (10%). Focal neuro-logic signs may include asymmetric flaccid paralysis. Uncommon findings have included arthralgia and rash. Beginning about the fourth day and proceeding over the next three to seven days, there is progressive im-provement, with almost all patients becoming afebrile, seizure-free, and ready for discharge from the hospital within two weeks after onset.

Laboratory Features. In contrast to most viral infections, peripheral leucocyte counts range from 7,000 to 30,000 per µl (median 16,000 per µl) with neutrophilia. Cerebrospinal fluid examination reveals 10 to 500 cells per µl, usually with a predominance of mononuclear cells, protein con-centrations of less than 100 mg/dL, and normal sugar concentrations. Electroencephalograms (EEGs) are abnormal in at least 80% of patients, revealing slow delta-wave activity. In one-half of the patients the abnor-mality is asymmetric, suggesting focal destructive lesions. Brain scans using [^{99}Tc]pertechnetate and computed tomography (CT) also may be abnormal, and temporal lobe localization has been observed.

Diagnosis. Serum and CSF should be tested for LCV IgM antibodies. Serum capture IgM enzyme-linked immunoabsorbent assay (ELISA) tests detected 83% of cases on admission in LaCrosse encephalitis. Early specific diagnosis eliminates the need for brain biopsy to exclude herpes encephalitis which is suggested by the temporal lobe localization.

Treatment. Initial seizure activity is frequently prolonged and difficult to control. The most effective anticonvulsant medication has been parenteral diazepam. Patients with the severe form of disease should be discharged on anticonvulsants such as phenobarbital for six to 12 months.

Prognosis. The case fatality ratio is low (2% or less); however, one-third of patients may have abnormal neurologic findings at the time of discharge. During the early convalescent period, emotional lability and irritability are common. In one series, recurrent seizures occurred in one-quarter of the patients who had seizures during the acute phase. In this same series EEGs were abnormal in one-third of patients evaluated one to eight years after their acute illness. In another series, 15% had sequelae, predominantly personality or behavioral problems.

Other Arbovirus Encephalitides (Eastern Equine, Western Equine, St. Louis)

Epidemiology. The geographic distribution of the other arboviral en-cephalitides is shown in Fig. 2.1. Different mosquitoes serve as vectors (Table 2.1) (27).

The transmission of EEE involves *Culiseta melanura* mosquitoes and swamp-dwelling birds, e.g., red-winged blackbirds, sparrows, pheasants. Transmission by pecking has been shown in domestic pheasant flocks. *C melanura* rarely feed on horses or humans, and other mosquitoes, especially *Aedes sollicitans,* a salt-marsh mosquito which is an avid human feeder, have been postulated as the epidemic vectors. In June 1991, EEE virus was isolated from *Aedes albopictus* in Florida. *Ae albopictus* has the potential for becoming an important epidemic vector. The epidemiology of overwintering and maintenance between outbreaks remains unknown. Equine animals and human beings are "dead ends" in the transmission cycle. In the northeastern United States, epidemics occur in the late summer and early fall. Epizootics in horses precede the occurrence of human cases by one to two weeks. The disease affects mainly infants, children, and adults over 55 years of age. There is no sex preponderance. Inapparent infection occurs in all age groups, suggesting that the decreased likelihood of developing overt infection in the 15- to 54-year age group is not the result of decreased exposure. The ratio of inapparent infection to overt encephalitis approximates 25:1. Epidemics of St. Louis encephalitis fall into two epidemiologic patterns. One is found in the west, where mixed outbreaks of Western equine encephalitis and St. Louis encephalitis have occurred primarily in irrigated rural areas. The vector has been *Culex tarsalis.* The second pattern occurred in the original St. Louis outbreak and the numerous subsequent epidemics. These outbreaks have been more urban in location and are characterized by the occurrence of encephalitis in older persons. Among sporadic cases in the west, men predominate 2:1 due to greater occupational exposure. In the United States, WEE virus is found in virtually all geographic areas. The disease occurs mainly in early and midsummer. Wild birds, which develop viremia of sufficiently high titer to be able to infect mosquitoes that feed on them, are the basic reservoir. *Culex tarsalis* is the principal vector in the western United States. In areas east of the Appalachian Mountains the virus has been repeatedly isolated from *Culiseta melanura*; however, the importance of this species has been questioned, since it is not primarily a human-biting mosquito. The ratio of inapparent infection to disease, as evidenced by serologic survey studies, varies from 1:1 in infants and 58:1 in children to 1150:1 in adults. Approximately one-fourth of patients are less than 1 year of age. The highest attack rates occur in persons 55 years or older.

Clinical Manifestations. The clinical features of "arbovirus" encephalitis are indistinguishable between etiologic agents but differ among age groups. In infants under 1 year of age, the only consistently noted symptom is sudden onset of fever, which is often accompanied by convulsions. Convulsions may be either generalized or focal. Typically the fever ranges between 102 and 104°F. Other physical findings may include bulging of the fontanelle, rigidity of the extremities and abnormalities in reflexes.

In children between 5 and 14 years of age, headache, fever and drowsiness of two to three days' duration before medical attention is sought are common. The symptoms may then subside or become more intense and may be associated with nausea, vomiting, muscular pain, photophobia and, less frequently, convulsions (less than 10% except in LaCrosse virus encephalitis). The child is found to be acutely ill, febrile and lethargic. Nuchal rigidity and intention tremors are often present, and on occasion muscular weakness can be demonstrated.

In adults, the initial symptoms commonly include the abrupt onset of fever, nausea with vomiting and severe headache (24). The headache is most often frontal but may be occipital or diffuse. Mental aberrations, represented by confusion and disorientation, usually appear within the subsequent 24 hours. Other symptoms may include diffuse myalgia and photophobia. The abnormalities found on physical examination relate predominantly to the neurologic examination, although conjunctival suffusion is frequently seen and skin rashes may occur. Disturbances in mentation are among the most outstanding clinical features. These range from coma through severe disorientation to subtle abnormalities detected only by cerebral function tests such as the subtraction of serial sevens. A small proportion of patients show only lethargy, lying quietly, apparently asleep unless stimulated. Tremor is common and is observed more frequently in individuals over 40 years of age. The tremors vary in location and may be continuous or intention in type. Cranial nerve abnormalities resulting in oculomotor muscle paresis and nystagmus, facial weakness and difficulty in deglutition may occur and are usually present within the initial several days. Objective sensory changes are unusual. Hemiparesis or monoparesis may occur. Reflex abnormalities are also common; these include exaggerated palmomental reflexes, and suck and snout reflexes. Superficial abdominal and cremasteric reflexes are usually absent. Changes in the tendon reflexes are variable and inconstant. The plantar response may be extensor and fluctuates almost hourly. Dysdiadochokinesia often exists.

The duration of the fever and neurologic symptoms and signs varies from several days to a month but usually ranges from four to 14 days. Clinical improvement generally follows the subsidence of the fever within several days unless irreversible anatomic changes have occurred.

Laboratory Findings. Erythrocytes are usually normal. Total leucocyte counts often reveal both a slight to moderate leucocytosis (occasionally greater than 20,000 leucocytes per µl) and neutrophilia. Examination of the cerebrospinal fluid usually reveals several hundred cells per µl, but on occasion cloudy cerebrospinal fluid with cells in excess of 1,000 per µl may be seen. Within the first several days of illness, polymorphonuclear neutrophils may predominate. The initial cerebrospinal fluid protein is usually only slightly elevated but on occasion may exceed 100 mg/dL. The level of spinal fluid sugar is normal; a significant decrease should raise serious consideration of an alternative diagnosis. As the illness progresses, mononuclear cells in the cerebrospinal fluid tend to increase so that they predominate and the protein concentration may increase. Other laboratory studies have been reported only sporadically, but abnormalities may include hyponatremia, often due to the inappropriate secretion of antidiuretic hormone, and elevation in serum creatine phosphokinase.

Diagnosis. Specific diagnosis requires the isolation of the virus or detection of antibodies with a rising titer between the acute phase of disease and convalescence. Antibodies can be detected by hemagglutination inhibition, complement fixation, or virus neutralization techniques. Because approximately 40% of patients with SLE have antibodies detectable by hemagglutination inhibition at the onset of illness, acute serum for serologic studies should be submitted promptly to a competent laboratory. ELISA tests for the detection of specific IgM antibodies in CSF or serum provide a means of early specific diagnosis.

Treatment. As with LaCrosse virus encephalitis, treatment consists of supportive care. Current antiviral agents are not effective.

Prognosis. The mortality rate in Eastern equine encephalitis with clinical disease exceeds 50% (17). In the most severe cases, death occurs between the third and fifth days. Children under 10 years of age have a greater likelihood of surviving the acute illness, but they also have a greater likelihood of developing severe disabling residuals: mental retardation, convulsions, emotional lability, blindness, deafness, speech disorders and hemiplegia.

In recent outbreaks of St. Louis encephalitis the mortality rate has varied from 2 to 12%. Subjective complaints, including nervousness, headaches and easy fatigability and excitability, appear to be the most common residuals. Late organic defects such as speech defects, difficulty in walking and disturbances in vision were demonstrated in approximately 5% of patients three years following infection.

In Western equine encephalitis the fatality rate approximates 3% (7). The incidence and severity of sequelae are related to age. Sequelae among very young infants are frequent (appearing in 61% of a group of patients less than 3 months old) and severe; they consist of upper motor neuron impairment, involving the pyramidal tracts, extrapyramidal structures, and cerebellum, and result in behavioral problems and convulsions. Both the incidence and severity of sequelae diminish rapidly after 1 year of age. Adults may complain of nervousness, irritability, easy fatigability and tremulousness for six months or longer after the acute illness. Probably not more than 5% of adults have sequelae which are sufficiently severe to be of practical significance. Postencephalitic seizures are rare.

Rabies

Although human rabies is rare in the United States, animal bites, both wild and domestic, are common, hence decisions regarding post-exposure antirabies prophylaxis are also common.

Epidemiology. In the United States, wild animal rabies is the major problem, with approximately 5,000 cases being reported annually (Fig. 2) (18). At least five major rabies epizootics are occurring in the United States: three in skunks, one in the north central states, one in the south central states and one in northern California; and two in raccoons, one in the northeastern, the other in the southeastern states (Fig. 3) (10). Rabid

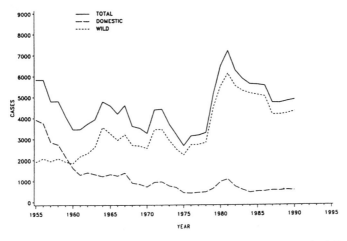

FIGURE 2.2 Rabies in wild and domestic animals, by year, in the United States and Puerto Rico.

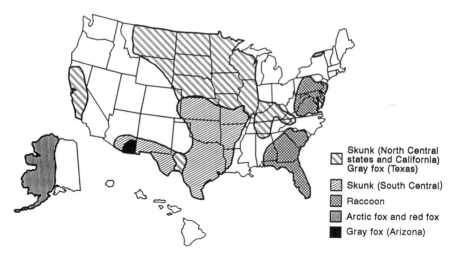

Skunk (North Central states and California)
Gray fox (Texas)

Skunk (South Central)

Raccoon

Arctic fox and red fox

Gray fox (Arizona)

FIGURE 2.3 Rabies epizootics in the United States.

bats accounted for 15% of reports. In 1989, wild animals were shown always to be the source of cat and dog infections. Rabid cats accounted for a greater proportion of bites requiring post-exposure prophylaxis. Rabid cats are more likely to exhibit aggressive behavior than dogs. Rabid cats and dogs died a mean of three days after the bite. Human rabies cases are almost always attributable to bite exposure (penetration of teeth through the skin) and only rarely to non-bite exposure (in the U.S. only 2% of cases between 1946 and 1987). Not all people bitten, even by proven rabid animals, develop rabies. Development of rabies depends upon the severity of exposure and site of the bite. Dog, cat or wolf bites on the hands or legs have a 3 to 20% likelihood of developing rabies.

Clinical Manifestations. The incubation period in rabies is more variable than that for any other acute infection. In most series, 25% are 30 days or less, 50% 31 to 90 days, and 10% greater than 90 days. Recently incubation periods as long as six to seven years have been documented (23). The first symptoms are usually mild and non-specific: constitutional, respiratory, gastrointestinal or central nervous system (headache, irritability). A specific symptom which may occur early is pain or paresthesias at the bite site (present in 16 to 80%). Following two to 10 days of non-specific symptoms, the patient develops acute neurologic disease. This may be characterized by agitation, hallucinations, thrashing about, running or other bizarre behavior (80%). From 17 to 80% of patients will show hydrophobic symptoms. In about 20% of patients, the clinical course may be marked by paralysis. Paralytic rabies is more common after exposure to bats. The acute neurologic syndrome usually ends with coma and respiratory arrest after two to seven days.

Laboratory Features. Routine laboratory tests are of little value in the diagnosis of rabies. The cerebrospinal fluid shows a pleocytosis in up to 90% of patients, the cell count usually being about 75 per µl and seldom more than 300 cells per µl. Early the protein content is normal, but it increases moderately during the course.

Diagnosis. The most rapid way to diagnose human rabies is to examine skin and saliva. The preferred technique for skin is a full thickness biopsy from the posterior aspect of the neck just above the hairline. Using fluorescent antibody staining, rabies antigen is sought in nerve fibers in the plexus surrounding hair follicles. The sensitivity is greater than with corneal impressions. Saliva is examined by intracerebral inoculation into mice.

Treatment. The mainstay of treatment is intensive care. Trials with interferon and ribavirin intravenously and intrathecally have been tried without success.

Post-Exposure Prophylaxis (4). All wounds should be cleaned immediately and thoroughly with soap and water. This has been shown to protect 90% of experimental animals.

Post-exposure prophylaxis guide, United States, 1991.

Animal Type	Evaluation and Disposition of Animal	Recommendations for Prophylaxis
Dogs, cats	Healthy and available for 10-day observation	Don't start unless animal develops sx, then immediately begin HRIG + HDCV or RVA
	Rabid or suspected rabid	Immediate vaccination
	Unknown (escaped)	Consult public health officials
Skunks, raccoons, bats, foxes, most carnivores	Regard as rabid	Immediate vaccination
Livestock, rodents, rabbits, hares	Almost never require antirabies rx	Includes squirrels, hamsters, guinea pigs, gerbils, chipmunks, rats, mice

Post-exposure prophylaxis schedule (unvaccinated persons).

Immunizing Product	Regimen
HRIG*	20 IU/kg, if feasible infiltrate ½ of dose around the wound(s), the rest IM in gluteal area. Not in same syringe as vaccine.
Vaccine: HDCV or RVA*	1.0 ml IM in deltoid area (only acceptable site in adults and older children; younger children, outer aspect of thigh) (never in gluteal area). Days 0, 3, 17, 24, 28

*HRIG = Human rabies immune globulin (Hyperab, Imogam Rabies; HDCV = human diploid cell vaccine, rabies (inactivated) (Imovax Rabies); RVA = rabies vaccine absorbed (inactivated, liquid) (should not be used intradermally)

Prognosis. Only three recoveries have been documented.

Parapoxvirus Infections (Orf/Milker's Nodule)

Two parapoxviruses of domestic animals occasionally cause infection in humans: orf virus (scabby mouth), normally a disease of sheep and goats, and milker's nodule virus (pseudocowpox), normally a disease of cattle (9).

Epidemiology. Orf is a common disease of sheep and goats, while milker's nodule virus occurs in dairy herds in all parts of the world. Both are occupational diseases acquired by contact with infected sheep or cows. Infection occurs through abrasions of the skin.

Clinical Manifestations. The lesions of orf are rather large nodules which may be multiple and the surrounding base is erythematous. The lesions are painful. There is often regional adenopathy and low-grade fever. The lesions of milker's nodule are hemispherical cherry-red to purple nodules which appear five to seven days after exposure. They may be up to 2 cm in diameter and may umbilicate but do not ulcerate. They are relatively painless but may itch. There may be moderate regional adenopathy. The lesions disappear in four to six weeks.

Diagnosis. The diagnosis is made on epidemiological and clinical grounds. Characteristic virions can be demonstrated on electron microscopy.

Rickettsial Infections

Q Fever

Q fever [named query, or unknown, fever by Derrick, who was investigating an outbreak of febrile illness in meat packers in Brisbane, Queensland, Australia in 1935 (6). The Q is not for Queensland, as many assume] is caused by a rickettsial-like organism, *Coxiella burnetii*.

Epidemiology. Q fever is a zoonosis which occurs worldwide. The most common animal reservoirs are cattle, sheep and goats, although many species of animals, birds and arthropods have been found infected. Infected animals are usually asymptomatic. *C burnetii*, which are resistant to drying, are shed in the urine, feces and milk. The organism is also present in large quantities in the birth products of animals, up to 10^9 organisms per gram of placenta in infected sheep; in Nova Scotia exposure to parturient cats has resulted in several outbreaks. The primary mode of transmission to humans is by inhalation of infected aerosols, a single organism being infectious for humans. Viable organisms have been isolated from soil for up to 150 days. While unpasteurized milk may contain *C burnetii*, transmission by ingestion of such has not been proven.

Similarly, many species of ticks including *Dermacentor andersoni* have been found to be infected and may be important in transmission among animals. They are not a source of human infection. Although there is one report of human-to-human transmission in a household, such is most uncommon and isolation is not recommended.

Clinical Manifestations. The usual incubation is three weeks, with the usual range being nine to 39 days. While usually considered as a pulmonary illness, the most common form is probably an undifferentiated self-limited illness of a few days to two weeks (5). Other clinical syndromes include primarily pneumonia, hepatitis and endocarditis (14). The incidence of pulmonary involvement varies between 0 and 90%. The onset may be abrupt or gradual. The most common symptoms are fever, often with rigors, headache, myalgia and arthralgia. Cough is relatively uncommon, being present in one-fourth of patients with radiographic infiltrates. When present, the cough is usually non-productive. Pleuritic chest pain occurs in one-fourth of patients. Gastrointestinal symptoms, nausea, vomiting and diarrhea, may occur but are less common. In contrast to other rickettsial diseases, skin rashes are rare. Other than fever, findings on physical examination are limited. Inspiratory rales may be heard. Hepatomegaly occurs in 10 to 65%. Splenomegaly occurs in about 5% of patients. The illness has a typical course of two to four weeks, although fever may continue for as long as nine weeks. Q fever hepatitis may be manifest only by laboratory abnormalities or may resemble viral hepatitis. Jaundice is uncommon. Q fever endocarditis is rare, especially in the United States. Clinical features are those of culture-negative endocarditis (22).

Laboratory Findings. Routine hematologic tests are non-diagnostic. The erythrocytic sedimentation rate may be normal. Radiographic findings are variable; segmental pleural based infiltrates often with small pleural effusions are common. Multiple rounded opacities are reported after exposure to infected cat placentas. On liver biopsy, lesions range from focal necrosis to non-caseating granulomata.

Diagnosis. The diagnosis is usually based on serological tests since isolation presents a significant laboratory hazard. Complement fixation tests employing paired serum specimens are most widely used although the enzyme-linked immunoabsorbent assays (ELISA) to detect IgM antibodies are more sensitive. IgM antibodies may persist for at least a year, hence may not be indicative of acute infection (22).

Treatment. There have been no controlled therapy trials of antimicrobial agents. No agents are -cidal, although several are -static for *C burnetii*. The usual recommended treatment for other than endocarditis is doxycycline 100 mg po twice daily or tetracycline 500 mg four times daily (adults) or erythromycin for two weeks (14).

Prognosis. Most infections resolve spontaneously. Except for Q fever endocarditis, the prognosis is excellent.

Bacterial Infections

Leptospirosis

Leptospirosis is a term applied to disease caused by all leptospiras regardless of specific serotype (21). The genus *Leptospira* contains only one species, *interrogans*, which is subdivided into two complexes: the interrogans complex, which contains all the pathogenic strains, and the biflexa comples, which includes saprophytic strains. The interrogans complex now contains about 240 serotypes, at least 23 of which occur in the United States.

Epidemiology. Leptospirosis is thought to be the most widespread zoonosis in the world. It has been reported from all regions of the United States, including arid areas such as Arizona. Infection occurs in a wide range of domestic and wild animal hosts. Infection in animals may vary from inapparent infection to severe fatal disease. A carrier state, in which leptospiras persist in the kidneys and are shed into the urine for months, develops in many animals and is key in the epidemiology.

Survival of leptospiras is governed by factors including pH of the urine of the host, pH of soil or water into which they are shed, and ambient temperature. Leptospiras in most "urine spots" in soil retain infectivity for six to 48 hours. Acid urine permits only limited survival; however, if the urine is neutral or alkaline and is shed into a similar moist environment which has low salinity, is not badly polluted with microorganisms or detergents, and has a temperature above 72° F, leptospiras may survive for several weeks. Human infections can occur either by direct contact with urine or tissue of an infected animal or indirectly through contaminated water, soil or vegetation. The usual portals of entry in humans are abraded skin, particularly about the feet, and exposed conjunctival, nasal and oral mucous membranes. Swallowing contaminated water during immersion has been associated with high attack rates. The previously held concept that organisms could penetrate intact skin has been questioned. While leptospiras have been isolated from ticks, these arthropods appear to be unimportant in transmission.

With the ubiquitous infection of animals, leptospirosis in human beings can occur in all age groups, at all seasons, and in both sexes. However, it is primarily a disease of teenage children and young adults (about one-half of patients are between the ages of 10 and 39), occurs predominantly in males (80%) and develops most frequently in hot weather (in the United States one-half of infections occur from July to October). In the United States, United Kingdom, Europe and Israel, water- and cattle-associated leptospirosis is most common. Swimming or partial immersion in contaminated water such as rural swimming holes has been implicated in one-fifth of patients and has accounted for most of the recent common-source outbreaks.

Clinical Manifestations. The incubation period following immersion has shown extremes of two to 26 days, the usual range being seven to 13 days and the average 10 days.

Leptospirosis is a typically biphasic illness. During the leptospiremic or first phase, leptospiras are present in the blood and cerebrospinal fluid. The onset is typically abrupt, and initial symptoms include headache, which is usually frontal. Severe muscle aching occurs in most patients, the muscles of the thighs and lumbar areas being most prominently involved, and often is accompanied by severe pain on palpation. Patients often complain of leg pain with walking. The myalgia may be accompanied by extreme cutaneous hyperesthesia (causalgia). Chills followed by a rapidly rising temperature are prominent. Following the abrupt onset, the leptospiremic phase typically lasts four to nine days. Features during this interval include recurrent chills, high spiking temperatures (usually 102° F or greater), headache and continued severe myalgia. Involvement of one organ system may predominate, often leading to initial misdiagnosis. Such symptom complexes most commonly include hepatitis, nephritis, atypical pneumonia, influenza or "viral" gastroenteritis. Anorexia, nausea and vomiting are encountered in one-half or more of the patients. Occasional patients have diarrhea. Pulmonary manifestations, usually either cough or chest pain, have varied in frequency of occurrence from less than 25% to 86%. Hemoptysis occurs but is uncommon in the United States and Europe, while it is a common feature, being noted in 40% of patients in Korea and China (15).

Examination during this phase reveals an acutely ill, febrile patient, with a relative bradycardia and normal blood pressure. The most characteristic physical sign is conjunctival suffusion, which usually first appears on the third or fourth day. It may be associated with photophobia, but serous or purulent secretion is unusual. Less common findings may include pharyngeal injection, cutaneous hemorrhages, and skin rashes which, even when they occur, are not prominent. The rashes may be macular, maculopapular or urticarial and usually occur on the trunk. Uncommon findings are splenomegaly, hepatomegaly, lymphadenopathy or jaundice. The first phase terminates after four to nine days, usually with defervescence and improvement in symptoms. This coincides with the disappearance of leptospiras from the blood and cerebrospinal fluid.

The second phase has been characterized as the "immune" phase and correlates with the appearance of circulating IgM antibodies. The clinical manifestations of this phase show greater variability than those during the first phase. After a relatively asymptomatic period of one to three days, the fever and earlier symptoms recur and meningismus may develop. The fever rarely exceeds 102° F and is usually of one to three days' duration. It is not uncommon for fever to be absent or quite transient. Even when symptoms or signs of meningeal irritation are absent, routine examination of cerebrospinal fluid after the seventh day has revealed pleocytosis in 50 to 90% of patients. Less common late features include iridocyclitis, optic neuritis and other nervous system manifestations, including encephalitis, myelitis and peripheral neuropathy.

Laboratory Features. Leucocyte counts vary from leucopenic levels to mild elevations in anicteric patients. Regardless of the total leucocyte count, neutrophilia of greater than 70% is frequent during the first stage. Acute hemolytic anemia, presumably due to hemolysins produced by leptospiras, may occur, especially in jaundiced patients. Thrombocytopenia (less than 30,000 platelets per *m*l) may occur.

Urinalysis during the leptospiremic phase reveals mild proteinuria, casts and an increase in cellular elements. In anicteric infections, these abnormalities rapidly disappear after the first week. Proteinuria and abnormalities in the urine sediment usually are not associated with elevations in blood urea nitrogen. Since the anicteric form of the disease often has gone undiagnosed, estimates of the frequency of azotemia and jaundice are probably high. Azotemia has been reported in approximately one-fourth of patients. In three-fourths of these patients, the blood urea nitrogen is less than 100 mg/dL. Azotemia is usually associated with jaundice. The serum bilirubin levels may reach 65 mg/dL; however, in two-thirds of patients the levels are less than 20 mg/dL. During the first phase, one-half of the patients have increased serum creatine phosphokinase (CK) levels, with mean values of five times normal. Such increases are not seen in viral hepatitis, and a slight increase in transaminase with a definite increase in CK suggests leptospirosis rather than viral hepatitis.

Diagnosis. Diagnosis is based upon culture or serologic tests. Whole blood should be inoculated immediately into tubes containing semisolid medium, such as Fletcher's or EMJH medium. If culture medium is not available, leptospiras reportedly will remain viable up to 11 days in blood to which anticoagulants, preferably sodium oxalate, have been added. Direct examination of blood or urine by dark-field methods has been employed; however, this method so frequently results in failure or misdiagnosis that it should not be employed. Serologic methods are applicable during the second phase; antibodies appear from the sixth to the twelfth days of illness. Two serologic methods are commonly used: a macroscopic or slide agglutination test, which is easy to perform but lacks specificity and sensitivity, and hence is suitable for screening only, and the microscopic agglutination test, which is more complicated but also more specific. An IgM-specific dot-ELISA (enzyme-linked immunosorbent assay) has been effective in diagnosing leptospirosis in an endemic area. Serologic criteria for diagnosis include a fourfold or greater rise in titer during the course of illness. Cross-agglutination reactions between various serotypes commonly occur so that the infection serotype often cannot be determined with certainty without isolation of leptospiras.

Treatment. A variety of antimicrobial drugs, including penicillin, streptomycin, the tetracycline congeners, chloramphenicol, erythromycin and ciprofloxacin are effective in vitro and in experimental leptospiral infections. A controlled trial of intravenous penicillin (1.5 million units every six hours for seven days) clearly demonstrated shortening of duration of fever and creatinine elevation, shortening of hospitalization, and prevention of leptospiruria, even when treatment was started after the fifth day of illness. In contrast, a randomized trial of high-dose penicillin was not beneficial in jaundiced patients. Doxycycline (100 mg orally taken twice daily for seven days), when started within four days of onset of symptoms, significantly shortened the duration of fever and most other symptoms and decreased the frequency of leptospiruria in patients with mild illness. Doxycycline (200 mg orally taken once per week) is also highly effective in preventing disease in an area of high prevalence. Azotemia and jaundice require meticulous attention to fluid and electrolyte therapy. Since the renal damage is reversible, patients with azotemia should be considered for peritoneal hemodialysis. Exchange transfusion may be beneficial in the management of patients with extreme hyperbilirubinemia.

Prognosis. The mortality rate in reported cases in the United States has varied annually between 2.5 and 16.4%, averaging 7.1%. Age is the most significant host factor related to increased mortality. In a representative series, the mortality rate rose from 10% in men less than 50 years of age to 56% in those over 51 years of age. Deaths are usually secondary to gastrointestinal hemorrhage or to renal failure.

Tularemia

Tularemia is a typical zoonosis, caused by *Francisella tularensis*, a small gram-negative pleomorphic aerobic coccobacillus.

Epidemiology. Tularemia occurs in the northern hemisphere, worldwide except in the United Kingdom. In the United States it has been reported from all states except Hawaii (Fig. 2.4) (8). *F. tularensis* has been isolated from more than 100 species of wild animals (especially rabbits, hares, squirrels, moles, muskrats and beavers), at least nine species of domestic animals (especially sheep, cattle, dogs and cats) and more than 50 species of arthropods (especially ticks, deerflies and mosquitoes). The most common sources of infection in the United States are ticks or deerflies

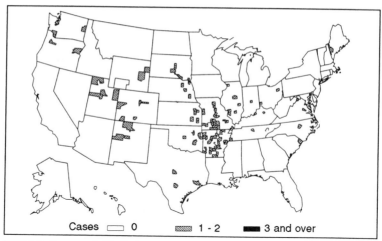

Cases 0   1 - 2   3 and over

Note: Two cases reported in Alaska.

FIGURE 2.4 Reported cases, by county, of tularemia in the United States, in 1990.

and contact with infected animals or their carcasses. In the U.S., the seasonal occurrence is bimodal with peaks in July and December. The summer peak reflects tick-borne disease whereas the winter peak is associated with animal contact, especially rabbits. Less often, people acquire infection from the bite of an animal whose mouth has become contaminated through ingestion of a diseased animal; this accounts for most cases of cat-bite tularemia. Numerous outbreaks associated with exposure to water contaminated by beavers or muskrats have been reported. In Sweden and Finland outbreaks have been associated with handling stored hay or cutting fresh hay (20). This has not been reported in the U.S. In the United States most cases associated with rabbits have been through contact with cottontail rabbits (*Sylvilagus* species). The organism is transmitted between rabbits by the rabbit tick, which rarely bites man. Domestic rabbits have not been implicated in natural disease. While rabbits were responsible for 85 to 90% of cases in the past, more recently tick exposure has been responsible for three-fourths of cases. The most important species are the wood tick (*Dermacentor andersoni*), the dog tick (*Dermacentor variabilis*) and the Lone Star tick (*Amblyomma americanum*).

Clinical Manifestations. Tularemia has been classified into six clinical constellations: ulceroglandular, glandular, oculoglandular, typhoidal, oropharyngeal (anginose) and pneumonic (19). The classification is a matter of convenience an does not indicate any fundamental difference in source of infection or even course of illness or prognosis. In fact, the preconception that tularemia is an ulceroglandular disease may result in failure to recognize it in its other presentations, which represent a quarter to a half of all cases.

Regardless of portal of entry, the mode of onset and general features of tularemia remain the same. The usual incubation period is three to five days (range one to 21). Onset of symptoms is abrupt. Symptoms consist of fever (85%) usually higher than 101°F, chills (52%), headache (45%), cough (38%), generalized myalgia (31%) and vomiting (17%). The high temperature and symptoms usually subside after 24 to 96 hours. After a remission of one to three days, the fever and symptoms recur. Illness then typically continues for two to three weeks longer. During this interval weakness, sweating and weight loss are common.

Forty-five to 85% of patients have the ulceroglandular form of tularemia. Twenty-four to 48 hours after the onset of fever, the area of the lymph nodes draining the site of inoculation becomes painful. The nodes are enlarged, firm and tender, the overlying skin usually inflamed. The inflamed nodes are usually axillary or inguinal, although with tick or mosquito bites on the head, cervical lymphadenopathy occurs. Concurrently or within a day, a local lesion or lesions (about 10% are multiple) are noted. They begin as painful, small, red papules, which progress to a pustule, then to an ulcer with sharp undermined borders and a flat base. Local lesions may occasionally consist of cracked dry skin resembling chapped skin but associated with regional nodes. Over the course of one or two weeks, the ulcers become covered with a dark-colored crust; eventually they heal with a residual scar. Occasionally "sporotrichoid" nodules along lymphatics may develop. If the site of ulceration is an unusual one, such as the shaft of the penis, it is usually misdiagnosed as chancroid or primary syphilis.

Common concurrent findings include pharyngitis (one-third of patients) and respiratory problems (one-half of patients). Sore throat occurs in the absence of a clear reason, e.g., having eaten potentially infected rabbit. The patient may complain of pharyngitis with no physical signs on examination, but half have erythema, and some an exudate. Findings on chest radiographs are abnormal in half of patients, including those who have no symptoms or physical findings. Radiographic findings consist of parenchymal infiltrates, usually in one lower lobe (two-thirds of cases). About a third of patients also have pleural effusions. Hilar adenopathy occurs with variable frequency (3 to 30%). Uncommon associated findings include pericarditis, erythema nodosum and erythema multiforme.

The nodes may persist for long periods, the mean being three months. Half become fluctuant and may develop fistulae. Incision and drainage has on occasion been associated with bacteremia and sepsis. Without treatment, enlarged nodes have persisted as long as three years.

The glandular form (8 to 25% of patients) is virtually identical to the ulceroglandular disease in symptoms and signs, except that an ulcerative lesion is not found.

Oculoglandular tularemia is uncommon—fewer than 5% of reported cases. The portal of entry is the conjunctival sac.

Typhoidal tularemia represents fewer than 5% of reported cases. Clinically it presents as sepsis without localizing features or as a less acute fever of unknown origin. It is not associated with lymphadenopathy. Patients frequently have underlying medical disorders. The diagnosis is often made fortuitously by blood culture. Features in such patients include sterile pyuria (one-third of patients), hyponatremia and elevated serum levels of creatine kinase (with or without rhabdomyolysis). Pulmonary infiltrates occur in half to three-fourths of these patients. Typhoidal tularemia is easily mistaken for severe legionellosis. Thorough questioning for a history of exposure to rabbits or tick bites is essential.

Pneumonic tularemia is a blanket term that encompasses both primary pulmonary and pulmonary involvement with other clinical types. With the ulceroglandular and typhoidal types, pulmonary involvement is common—single- or multiple-lobe infiltrates, often associated with pleural effusion on radiography. The observation of pneumonic tularemia in sheep shearers suggests inhalation associated with shearing. Half the patients experienced dry cough, retrosternal discomfort, pleural pain or dyspnea. One-fourth had sore throat. The most common radiographic findings were hilar adenopathy (36%) and pulmonary infiltrates (14%).

Laboratory Features. Laboratory findings are not helpful in a positive sense. Hematologic test values are usually normal. Leucocyte counts vary from 5,000 to 20,000 per ml (median 10,000). Urinalysis reveals sterile pyuria in 20 to 30% of patients. The basis and significance of this finding are unclear, but recognition of its occurrence may help avoid unnecessary diagnostic studies.

Diagnosis. The diagnosis is usually based on serologic tests rather than on culture. The *F tularensis* requires a medium containing cysteine for growth, and successful cultivation poses a laboratory hazard. Diagnosis is based on bacterial agglutination tests. A fourfold increase in titer is required to confirm the diagnosis. An acute-phase titer of 1:160 or greater is presumptive, but such levels seldom develop before the 11th day of illness and sometimes not until the third week.

Treatment

F tularensis are resistant to the natural penicillins and first-generation cephalosporins. Agents for which minimum inhibitory concentrations for 90% of strains (MIC_{90}) can be achieved include aminoglycosides, tetracycline, chloramphenicol, third-generation cephalosporins, erythromycin and rifampin. Data on the fluoroquinolones are not available. While streptomycin has been the drug of choice, it is no longer available for this indication. Gentamicin, 3 to 5 mg/kg per day IV for 10 to 14 days, has

2. On the Farm   45

been used successfully. Tetracycline is effective but requires a longer course of treatment; relapses are common after 1.0 gm daily for 15 days or 2.0 gm daily for 10 days. If tetracycline is used, the recommendation is 500 mg po four times daily for two weeks. It is reasonable to assume, although not proven in clinical studies, that doxycycline, 100 mg po twice daily for two or probably three weeks, would be equally efficacious.

Prognosis. The overall mortality for untreated tularemia was 8%. Today, with early diagnosis and appropriate treatment, the mortality is less than 1%.

Brucellosis

Brucellosis is another of the zoonoses which occur worldwide. It is primarily a disease of domesticated animals. Four species, *Brucella abortus* (cattle), *B suis* (swine), *melitensis* (goats) and *B canis* (dogs), are responsible for human disease.

Epidemiology. Brucella species infect a large number of animal species; however, cattle, goats and swine are epidemiologically most important in the United States. Brucella organisms are shed in the milk of infected animals. Brucella are transmitted to man by three routes: ingestion of contaminated milk or milk products such as cheese and ice cream, direct contact through skin breaks or the conjunctivae with infected tissues, blood or lymph, or inhalation of infectious aerosols. While brucellosis has been reported from all 50 states, in recent years more than one-half of the cases have been reported from Texas, California, Virginia and Florida. In the past five to 10 years, the majority of cases in Texas and California have been associated with the consumption of unpasteurized goat's milk cheese from Mexico (29). With this change in epidemiology, one-half of the patients are less than 20 years of age and one-half are women. Brucellosis acquired by direct contact occurs predominantly in men between the ages of 20 and 60 years as a result of occupational exposure. While brucella species are traditionally associated with specific hosts, i.e., *B abortus* with cattle, in recent years interhost spread has occurred, so that *B suis* or *B melitensis* may be encountered in cattle, etc.

Clinical Manifestations. Brucellosis in adults is a disease characterized by a multiplicity of symptoms and a paucity of physical findings (26). In countries where brucellosis is endemic, children account for 20 to 25% of cases. In children the disease is usually more mild. The incubation ranges from one week to several months, usually two to three weeks. The onset in two-thirds of patients is gradual over weeks. Fever, with or without chills, night sweats and weakness occur in over 90% of patients. Headache, malaise, anorexia and insomnia are also common. On physical examination, hepatomegaly, splenomegaly and lymphadenopathy are found in fewer than one-half of patients. Although a pattern of undulating fever has been considered characteristic, such is uncommon, occurring in one-third of patients with *B melitensis*, 10% with *B suis* and even less with *B abortus*. Specific clinical syndromes which may be seen include spondylitis and, interestingly, prepatellar bursitis.

Laboratory Findings. Routine laboratory tests are of little diagnostic value. Leucocyte counts are slightly decreased in one-third of patients, normal in one-third and slightly elevated (10,000 to 20,000 per μl) in one-third. Brucellosis is one of the infections in which the erythrocyte sedimentation rate is often normal; early in illness the Westergren sedimentation rate is 0 to 10 mm per hour in one-third of patients. Later in the course, most are elevated. Modest abnormalities in liver function tests, increased aspartate aminotransferase (SGOT), lactic dehydrogenase and alkaline phosphatase, occur in about one-half.

Diagnosis. The diagnosis is best based upon blood cultures. The laboratory should be notified that brucellosis is suspected since *B abortus* requires incubation under 5% CO_2 for primary isolation and growth is slow, often requiring 28 days. Also, brucella represent a significant laboratory hazard, hence precautions must be more carefully observed. With the more widespread use of automated radiometric and non-radiometric systems such as the Bactec systems, growth may be detected within 48 to 72 hours. Unfortunately, with the use of the API 2NE system for identification, isolates have been misidentified as *Moraxella phenylpyruvica* (16). The standard serological test is an agglutination test utilizing *B abortus* strain 456. Cross-agglutination enables detection of antibodies to *B abortus*, *B melitensis* and *B suis* with this antigen; hence, a single agglutination test can be utilized. A titer of 1:160 or greater is considered presumptive evidence of infection. The addition of 2-mercaptoethanol, which inactivates IgM antibodies, permits measurement of IgG antibodies, which are more suggestive of active infection. Antibodies to *B canis* will not be detected by the standard brucella agglutination test. Diagnosis depends upon isolation of the organism or referral of serum specimens to a reference laboratory.

Treatment. In the past, standard therapy has consisted of streptomycin (three weeks) and tetracycline (six weeks). More recently, the World Health Organization has recommended doxycycline 200 mg per day plus rifampin 600 mg per day for six weeks. In a recent controlled trial, the doxycycline-rifampin combination was as effective as the doxycycline-streptomycin regimen, with the possible exception of patients with spondylitis (1). In both groups, the relapse rate at 12 months was about 5%. An alternative regimen has been trimethoprim-sulfamethoxazole plus gentamicin. Ciprofloxacin is effective in vitro and in early responses; however, relapse rates have been high.

Prognosis. The prognosis is excellent, although a syndrome designated as chronic brucellosis, which closely resembles the chronic fatigue syndrome, has been described. This syndrome does not respond to antimicrobial therapy.

Campylobacteriosis

The reservoirs for most campylobacter species, *C fetus* and *C jejuni* are animals, especially poultry, cattle, swine and sheep.

Epidemiology. Up to one-half of poultry and 5% of beef and pork products sold in supermarkets are contaminated with campylobacter organisms. The organisms are highly susceptible to heating but may be acquired by ingestion of undercooked meat or cross-contamination of kitchen utensils. While persons working on farms or ranches would seem to be at increased risk of infection, such exposure does not seem to contribute significantly to the overall occurrence. Hence, except to mention it, campylobacteriosis will not be reviewed.

Listeriosis

Listeria monocytogenes is a well-recognized cause of septic abortion and a basilar meningoencephalitis in cattle and sheep. The organism can be recovered from animal feed, silage and a variety of foods. Cheese from unpasteurized milk, hot dogs and coleslaw have been implicated in out-breaks. Again, while the farm is the environment from which the organism arises, there is no epidemiologic evidence that occupational exposure on the farm constitutes a unique risk except for the occasional instance of infection being acquired by direct contact with an infected animal.

Pig Bites

For those interested in seeming trivia, the U.S. Census Bureau estimated that there were almost 330,000 pig farms with over 55 million pigs in the United States (11). Studies have shown that pigs exhibit characteristic aggressive behavior by biting, chewing and nosing. In Massachusetts, pig bites were the fifth most commonly reported type of animal bite. Yet the literature has been remarkably devoid of studies on the microbiology and management of pig bites. Recently several papers have appeared which address the subject. Swine bites appear to carry the widest variety of bacteria of any bite. Organisms have included coagulase-negative staphylococci, hemolytic streptococci, *Pasteurella multocida*, *Bacteroides* sp., *Proteus* sp., *Escherichia coli*, *Pasteurella aerogenes* and a more unusual Flavobacterium Group IIb-like isolate (11,28). From these reports, it is apparent that pig bites are not trivial; prompt cleansing and debridement are essential (28). Initial empirical therapy with an agent such as amoxicillin clavulanate would seem appropriate. All infections should be cultured and parenteral therapy may be required.

Fungal and Parasitic Organisms

By virtue of their presence in soil, fungi such as *Sporotrichum schenckii, Histoplasma capsulatum, Coccidioides immitis* and *Cryptococcus neoformans* might be encountered in the farm environment. Outbreaks have been associated with activities such as the cleaning of chicken houses and silos. However, as noted earlier, aside from the occasional point source outbreak, these infections are not peculiar to the farm environment. Parasites such as *Cryptosporidium parvum* and *Cryptosporidium muris* infect cattle. However, the epidemiology does not implicate the farm.

At this stage of review, I am reminded of the childhood song "Old MacDonald Had a Farm": ". . . with a pig, pig here, a pig, pig there, an oink, oink here, an oink, oink there", etc. If one is going to spend leisure time on the farm, it may be better to take the more passive approach of sitting on the porch rocking—but don't forget your insect repellent.

References

1. Ariza J, Gudiol F, Pallares R, et al. Treatment of brucellosis with doxycycline plus rifampin or doxycycline plus streptomycin. *Ann Int Med* 1992; 117:25–30.
2. Balfour HH Jr, Siem RA, Bauer H, et al. California arbovirus (LaCrosse) infection. I. Clinical and laboratory findings in 66 children with meningo-encephalitis. *Ped* 1973; 52:680–691.
3. Barnham M. Pig bite injuries and infection: report of seven human cases. *Epidem Inf* 1988; 101:641–645.
4. Centers for Disease Control. Rabies prevention—United States, 1991. *Morb Mort Wkly Rep* 1991; 40(RR-3):1–19.
5. Clark WH, Lennette EH, Railsback OC, et al. Q fever in California. VII. Clinical features in one hundred eighty cases. *Arch Int Med* 1951; 88:155–167.
6. Derrick EH. "Q" fever, new fever entity: clinical features, diagnosis and laboratory investigation. *Med J Aust* 1937; 2:281–299.
7. Eklund CM. Human encephalitis of the Western equine type in Minnesota in 1941: Clinical and epidemiological study of serologically positive cases. *Am J Hyg* 1946; 43:171–193.
8. Evans ME, Gregory DW, Schaffner W, et al. Tularemia: a 30 year experience with 88 cases. *Med* 1985; 64:251–269.
9. Fenner FM. Poxviruses, Chapter 75 in Fields BN (ed): *Virology*, 2nd ed, 1990, Raven Press, New York, pp. 2124–2128.
10. Fishbein DB. Rabies. *Inf Dis Clin NA* 1991; 5:53–71.

11. Goldstein EJC, Citron DM, Merkin TE, et al. Recovery of an unusual Flavobacterium Group IIb-like isolate from a hand infection following a pig bite. *J Clin Micro* 1990; 28:1079–1081.

12. Goodpasture NC, Poland JD, Franey DB, et al. Coloado tick fever: Clinical, epidemiologic and laboratory aspects of 228 cases in Colorado in 1973–1974. *Ann Int Med* 1978; 88:303–310.

13. Hughes LE, Casper EA, Clifford CM. Persistence of Colorado tick fever virus in red blood cells. *Am J Trop Med Hyg* 1973; 23:530–532.

14. Leedom JM: Q fever, an update, in Remington JS, Swartz MN (eds). *Current Clinical Topics in Infectious Diseases*, 1980, McGraw-Hill, Inc., New York, pp. 304–331.

15. Park SK, Lee SH, Rhee YK, et al. Leptospirosis in Chonbuk Province of Korea in 1987. A study of 93 patients. *Am J Trop Med Hyg* 1989: 41:345–351.

16. Peiris V, Fraser S, Fairhurst M, et al. Laboratory diagnosis of brucella infection: some pitfalls. *Lancet* 1992; 399:1415–1416.

17. Prezelomski MM, O'Rourke E, Grady GF, et al. Eastern equine encephalitis in Massachusetts: report of 16 cases, 1970–1984. *Neurol* 1988; 38:736–739.

18. Reid-Sanden FL, Dobbins JG, Smith JS, et al. Rabies surveillance in the United States during 1989. *J Am Vet Med Assoc* 1990; 197:1571–1583.

19. Sanders CV, Hahn R. Analysis of 106 cases of tularemia. *J La State Med Soc* 1968; 120:391–393.

20. Sanford JP. Tularemia, in Gorbach SL, Bartlett JG, Blacklow NR (eds). *Infectious Diseases*, 1992, W.B. Saunders Co., Philadelphia, pp. 1281–1285.

21. Sanford JP. Leptospirosis, in Wilson JD, Braunwald E, Isselbacher KT, et al. (eds): *Harrison's Principles of Internal Medicine*, 12th ed., 1991, McGraw Hill, Inc., New York, pp. 663–666.

22. Sawyer LA, Fishbein DB, McDade JE. Q fever: current concepts. *Rev Inf Dis* 1987; 9:935–946.

23. Silver HK, Meiklejohn G, Kempe CH. Colorado tick fever. *Am J Dis Child* 1961; 101:30–36.

24. Smith JS, Fishbein DB, Rupprecht CE, et al. Unexplained rabies in three immigrants in the United States: a virologic investigation. *N Eng J Med* 1991; 324:205–211.

25. Southern PM, Smith JW, Luby JP, et al. Clinical and laboratory features of epidemic St. Louis encephalitis. *Ann Int Med* 1969; 71:681–690.

26. Spink WW. The Nature of Brucellosis, 1956, University of Minnesota Press, Minneapolis.

27. Tsai TF. Arboviral infections in the United States. *Inf Dis Clin NA* 1991; 5:73–102.

28. Van Demark RE Sr, Van Demark RE Jr. Swine bites of the hand. *J Hand Surg* 1991; 16A:136–138.

29. Young EJ. Human brucellosis. *Rev Inf Dis* 1983; 5:821–842.

3
At the Shore

MARK A. CLEMENCE and RICHARD L. GUERRANT

Introduction

The numerous pleasures of recreation "at the shore" and the growing popularity of fish and seafood in gourmet diets have led to increased recognition and occurrence of a wide range of health hazards at the shore. As listed in Table 3.1, these syndromes vary from neurological, gastrointestinal, skin and ear diseases to meningitis, endocarditis, pneumonitis, osteomyelitis, and fatal septicemia. Fortunately, the severe syndromes are relatively rare and many can be avoided by taking appropriate precautions (such as avoiding red tides, avoiding ingesting undercooked seafood such as raw oysters, and prompt debridement and therapy of wounds). This chapter is divided into four Sections: fish and shellfish poisonings, vibrio infection, marine trauma and envenomation, and hepatitis and other viruses.

Section I: Fish and Shellfish Poisoning

Fish and Shellfish Intoxications

In the United States, the consumption of seafood in 1987 alone totaled more than 1.6 billion kg (3.5 billion lb), or 7 kg (15.4 lb) per person per year (1). An increase in the consumption of seafood is occurring with a resultant increase in the number of cases of fish- and shellfish-related food poisonings. In addition, improved reporting of cases due to a greater awareness by the public and health care personnel of the association between seafood consumption and illness had also contributed to this observed increase (2–4). Food-borne disease from fish and shellfish can be categorized into allergic, infectious, and toxin-mediated etiologies (4). The Centers for Disease Control and United States Department of Health and Human Services reported on all types of food-borne illness in the United States from 1978 to 1982. Bacterial causes were involved in

TABLE 3.1. Syndromes of health hazards "at the shore".

1. Neurological (fish and shellfish poisoning, see Table 3.2)
2. Gastrointestinal
    a. Noninflammatory
    b. Inflammatory
3. Skin/wound
4. Otitis (Swimmer's ear)
5. Meningoencephalitis
6. Endocarditis
7. Pulmonary
8. Osteomyelitis
9. Septicemia

more than 69% of confirmed outbreaks, whereas chemical poisonings from fish and shellfish toxins were responsible for 23.9% of the outbreaks (4).

Vertebrate fish intoxications can be divided into three groups: 1) ichthyosarcotoxic fish contain toxin in their viscera, mucous, skin, or musculature; 2) ichthyo-otoxic fish contain toxin in their gonads; and 3) ichthyohemotoxic fish contain toxin in their blood. At least nine types of ichthyosarcotoxism are known of which ciguatera, scombroid, and pufferfish poisoning are the most common (2).

The term "shellfish" includes crustaceans which are mobile animals that have a hard articulated exoskeleton, and mollusks which have hard shells and are sedentary or have limited locomotion. Crustacean species include lobsters, shrimp, crabs, scampi, and crawfish. Mollusks can be divided into the bivalves, which have two shells joined by a hinge, and the gastropods, which have a whorled snail-like shell. The bivalves include oysters, mussels, clams, and scallops. Gastropods of commercial importance include whelks and periwinkles. With the exception of scallops which reside in deeper waters, all mollusks grow in and are harvested from nearshore coastal waters (5). Ingestion of shellfish containing toxins produced by dinoflagellates may induce dramatic and sometimes fatal illness. (Table 3.2)

Dinoflagellates and Red Tides

Dinoflagellates, a form of plankton, are unicellular plant-like organisms with a worldwide distribution which serve as an important part of the marine food chain. During blooms, these organisms may achieve concentrations high enough to impart a reddish or yellowish discoloration to the sea due to the local production of neurotoxins and pigmented proteins, hence the name "red tide" (6). There are fifteen species of toxic dinoflagellates known to inhabit the waters surrounding the United States, of which four are related to human poisoning and six associated with the formation of red tides (4).

TABLE 3.2. Fish and shellfish poisoning.

Disease	Source	Toxin	Mech.	Epidem.	Clinical	Mortality	Treatment
Shellfish Poisoning:							
PSP Red Tide Dinoflagellates: *Gonyaulax cantella & tamarensis*	Alaskan butter clam (*Saxidomus*), mussels, oysters, scallops, cockles	Saxitoxin (heat stable)	like Tetrodotoxin, blocks Na^+ channels	Cold Temp. >30° N or S 10 outbreaks with 63 cases 1971–1977 in N. England, S.W., Alaska	½–3 hr. paresthesias dysesthesias mouth, extremities 14% with N/V/D	8%–9% die usually within 12–24 hrs.	Supportive
NSP Red Tide, unarmored Dinoflagellates *Ptychodiscus brevis* (old *Gymnodinium*) 13 × 30 μ	May be aerosolized in the surf	Brevetoxins (Heat, acid stable) A,B,C (polycyclic ethers)	Probably via altering Na conductance	Gulf coasts of Florida/Texas	<3 hr. paresthesias Temp. reversal; Cerebellar, GI symptoms	rare	Supportive B_2 agonists Cholinergic antagonists Ca^{2+} channel blockers
Amnesic Shellfish Poisoning: (Neurovisceral toxic syndrome)	*Nitzchia pungens* diatoms in mussels	Domoic Acid (heat stable)	Neuroexcitatory like glutamic acid. Causes hippocampal necrosis	Atlantic Pacific Indian Ocean	¼–38 h ($\bar{x}$ = 5½ hrs) Nausea, vomiting, GI bleeding Headache, Memory loss	3%	
Diarrhetic shellfish poisoning	Shellfish with dinoflagellate *Dinophysis fortii* or *acuminata*	Okadaic acid	blocks phosphatase that degrades A/G kinase products	Japan Netherlands	5–6 hrs. (½–30) Diarrhea N/V/abd. cramps		

Fish Poisoning (Ichthyosarcotoxic):

Pufferfish Poisoning (Tetraodontiae) Fugu Fugu	Pufferfish Shellfish Salamanders, frogs, newts	Tetrodotoxin (heat stable, nonprotein) blocks Na channels, axonal transmission	Japan N.J. Long Island	10–45 min (<3 hrs.) paresthesias weakness, paralysis, hypotension, bradycardia, respiratory paralysis	59% (in first 24 hrs.)	Supportive
Ciguatera Dinoflagellate *Gambierdiscus toxicus*	larger (>5#) carnivorous reef fish: Barracuda, herring, jacks, grouper, snapper, moray eels, etc.	Ciguatoxins maitotoxin heat stable tasteless polyether blocks Ca^{2+} regulation of Na^+ channels (opens voltage dep. Na^+ channels)	<35° N-S subtropical/ tropical Fla/ Hawaii S. Pacific Most common marine food poisoning in U.S.!	2–30 hr. ↑ or ↓ BP N/V/D/abd. pain Temp. reversal Teeth "loose"	<12% (rare)	Symptomatic (mannitol) (opiates are dangerous)
Scombroid fish poisoning	Tuna, mackerel, skipjack, bonito, albacore & bluefish Mahi-Mahi	Histamine (heat stable) from bacterial decarboxylation of histidine Histamine reaction	Common worldwide, esp. coastal U.S.	min-hrs ($\bar{x}$ 30 m) flush, HA dizzy burning	rare	antihistamine (IV cimetidine)

The association of red tides with human illness has been known since ancient times, the earliest description being from the Bible (Exodus 7:20–21): "And all the water that was in the Nile was turned to blood. And the fish that were in the Nile died, and the Nile became foul, so that the Egyptians could not drink water from the Nile." North American Indians were aware of red tides and their association with poisoning due to mussel ingestion (7). In 1793, Vancouver described what may be the first description of poisoning due to shellfish ingestion among sailors exploring passages off the mainland coast of what is now British Columbia; several men became ill after eating roasted mussels and death occurred in one of them within 5 hours (8). Walker, in 1884, described several people who became ill after eating oysters in Florida, possibly related to a red tide (9).

Red tides can be caused by nontoxigenic dinoflagellates, and shellfish may become poisonous even in the absence of a red tide (2). Vectors of shellfish poisoning are mainly filter-feeders that ingest large quantities of these dinoflagellates, many of which are toxigenic. The continuous filtration can result in the accumulation of large quantities of toxin within the digestive glands of the shellfish, or in the case of the Alaskan butter clam, the siphon (10).

Paralytic Fish Poisoning (PSP)

Paralytic shellfish poisoning (PSP) results fom the ingestion of marine mollusks containing potent neurotoxins, the best known being saxitoxin, named after the Alaskan butter clam, *Saxidomus*. Several other toxins are known, each of which shares the ability to invoke a variety of biological effects including, occasionally, severe and sometimes fatal impairment in sensory, cerebellar, and motor function.

During 1973 to 1987, state health departments reported 19 outbreaks of paralytic shellfish poisoning (mean: eight persons) to CDC's Foodborne Disease Outbreak Surveillance System (11), which accounted for 1.1% of all outbreaks of food-borne disease in the United States in 1972 to 1977 and 1.0% in 1978 to 1982 (6). The implicated mollusks included mussels, oysters, clams, scallops, and cockles. Worldwide, it was estimated that more than 1,600 cases occurred in 1974 alone, with more than 300 deaths (12). In 1990, two outbreaks occurred in the United States: one involving six people after ingesting mussels harvested off the Nantucket coast in Massachusetts, and another involving four people with one fatality in Alaska (11,13). The case fatality ratio is about 8% to 9%, usually secondary to respiratory failure (14). No deaths, however, were reported in 10 outbreaks involving 63 cases reported to the Centers for Disease Control from 1971 to 1977 (15).

The effects of paralytic shellfish poisoning are not only harmful to man but to fish, birds, and other wildlife as well that rely on aquatic sources of food. The ecological consequences can be devastating. One of the earliest signs of a toxic bloom is the sudden and unexplained death of large numbers of fish and wildlife in the vicinity. The American Indians were aware of these associations and avoided fish and shellfish ingestion during such times (7). These ecological effects may persist for months following the onset of an outbreak and require a year or more for affected shellfish to become safe for human consumption (10). Economic consequences can be equally devastating as the shellfish industry becomes paralyzed during this period. Widespread reporting by the news media and strict adherence to public safety measures leads not only to the significant depression of demand for fish and shellfish in affected areas but in unaffected regions as well. It is estimated that the cost of surveillance and enforcement during outbreaks of paralytic shellfish poisoning in the United States is about $1.2 million per year (10).

The dinoflagellates responsible for paralytic fish poisoning are widely distributed globally; however, actual outbreaks usually occur endemically in specific geographic areas. Such blooms are usually unpredictable and can occur with rapid accumulation of toxic concentrations. Most cases of paralytic shellfish poisoning occur in cold, temperate waters above $30°N$ and below $30°S$ (1,2); however, tropical cases have been reported in Thailand (16), Singapore (17), India (18), Guatemala (19), Malaysia (20), New Guinea (10), the Solomon Islands (21), Mexico (22), and El Salvador (22). Most North American cases occur along the Pacific coast from central California to Alaska and the Aleutian Islands and on the East coast in the New England coastal area as well as Nova Scotia, New Brunswick, and Quebec (10). The majority of outbreaks are reported in coastal areas; however, inland cases have occurred, occasionally remote from the seas (6).

Along the West coast, cases tend to occur from May to October and on the East coast from July to September (10). The Alaskan butter clam can be dangerous year-round (23). The period of toxicity usually lasts for a few days during each outbreak, but toxic levels may persist for many months. Factors favoring toxic blooms include warm water temperatures (usually when water temperatures reach $16°C$), periods of high solar radiation, the attainment of optimal concentrations of trace vitamins and minerals, and periods of turbulence such as during hurricanes, dredging, and the transplantation of shellfish (6,10). Afflicted shellfish can be found along open coasts, in bays, and in estuarine areas. The most important hydrographic factor is probably a thermocline imposed barrier; i.e., areas where water temperatures are greater than $16°C$ (10). Occasionally, red tides may be precipitated by the lowering of salinity such as at sites of river discharge or during periods of heavy rainfall.

Many types of molluscan shellfish may become toxic. The 19 outbreaks reported to the CDC during 1973 to 1987 were due to the ingestion of mussels, clams, oysters, scallops, and cockles. In Alaska, during 1976 through 1989, 55% of the 42 reported outbreaks were due to the ingestion of the Alaskan butter clam. Other shellfish implicated in Alaskan outbreaks included mussels, cockles, steamer clams, sea snails, and razor clams (11). In addition to the ingestion of shellfish, cases of paralytic shellfish poisoning have also been linked to the ingestion of mackerel, scad, and several species of crab (10).

Mollusks become toxic when they ingest toxic dinoflagellates. The toxins accumulate in the digestive glands and can remain there for a long time. This toxic accumulation can occur even in the absence of the build-up of sufficient numbers of dinoflagellates to discolor the water. If placed in dinoflagellate-free seawater, it can take up to 12 days for the shellfish to become nontoxic. In the case of the Alaskan butter clam, the toxins tend to accumulate in the siphon from which they are eliminated very slowly (10). Scallops, on the other hand, do not accumulate toxins in the adductor muscle which is the part usually by humans, although toxins may accumulate in the other tissues.

Several species of toxic dinoflagellates have been implicated in outbreaks of paralytic shellfish poisoning. In North America, *Protogonyaulaux catenella* is the principal dinoflagellate species responsible for outbreaks along the northwest Pacific coast of the continent, whereas *Protogonyaulaux tamerensis* is responsible for most outbreaks along the north Atlantic coast in addition to some outbreaks on the Pacific coast (4,10). In the tropics, *Pyrodinium bahamense* is responsible for most outbreaks (17–21). Each of these species is armored, ranges in size from 25 to 46 microns, and has a tendency to become highly bioluminescent during blooms (4). During the winter months, most toxic dinoflagellates exist as cysts in the sediment beneath the sea. Turbulent conditions can disperse these cysts; when water temperatures reach optimal conditions (16°C), blooming occurs by excystment and the formation of motile cells (6,10).

Saxitoxin is the primary toxin responsible for the biological effects of paralytic shellfish poisoning. Other toxins include neotoxin, and the gonyautoxins designated by Roman numerals in the order of their discovery (6,24). These toxins are pharmacologically similar to tetrodotoxin and are estimated to be 50 times more potent than curare (25). Saxitoxin is an alkaloid, nonprotein, low molecular weight, water soluble toxin, that is heat-stable (17). Cooking does not inactivate it, and it tends to become concentrated in broth (11). It bears some resemblance to guanine and may undergo trimethylation to form a toxic acetylcholine-like compound (24). The toxic effects result from binding of the toxin to either the cell membrane, a cation receptor, or both to inhibit sodium influx, thus blocking the action potential along neuronal axons or skeletal muscle (1,2,6,17,24). Higher concentrations may have a similar electrophysiological effect on cardiac and smooth muscle (26). Evidence exists that under acidic conditions, as in the stomach or in pickling containers, nontoxic products may become converted to toxins (18,27). Furthermore, shellfish may be capable of converting nontoxins to potent neurotoxins (27). Children may be more susceptible to the toxic effects (19). The lethal dose of saxitoxin has been estimated to be 0.3 to 1.0 mg; a single mussel may contain 30 to 50 mg (1). The safe level of toxin in shellfish has been defined as 80 micrograms/100 gram of shellfish (28).

The *symptoms* of paralytic shellfish poisoning usually begin within 30 minutes after the ingestion of toxic shellfish but can occur up to 3 hours later. The incubation period appears to be inversely related to the amount of toxin ingested. Initially there may be paresthesias and dysesthesias of the lips, tongue, and face which subsequently can progress to involve the neck, arms, fingertips, legs, and toes. Gastrointestinal symptoms, usually nausea, vomiting, and diarrhea, were seen in only 14% in one series (29). Many people have described a "feeling of floating" (30). Progression of symptoms is usually dependent on the dose of toxin ingested (6); more severe cases may be accompanied by weakness, ataxia, incoordination, and cranial nerve findings such as bulbar paresis, iridoplegia, dysphonia, and dysphagia (2,10,17,31). Other associated symptoms include headache, salivation, intense thirst, and temporary blindness (10). High toxin intake can result in muscular paralysis and respiratory failure which is the usual cause of death in fatal cases. The illness can be sufficiently severe to require hospitalization in 30% to 60% of affected patients (32). When it does occur, death usually ensues within 12 hours (2,17). If the patient survives 12 to 18 hours, the prognosis for recovery is good (33). Recovery usually occurs within a week without complications (4); however, several patients in one outbreak described persistent headaches, memory loss, and fatigue lasting for several weeks (19).

The *diagnosis* is based on a history of recent shellfish ingestion in the appropriate clinical setting. Routine laboratory tests are usually nonspecific and not helpful in establishing the diagnosis (1). The MB fraction of creatine kinase may be elevated in the absence of myocardial damage (34). Diagnosis can be confirmed by a standard mouse bioassay method in which toxin concentrations of the suspect shellfish are calculated by determining the dilution of a shellfish homogenate required to kill a 20 gram mouse in 5 to 7 minutes. The value can then be used to calculate an absolute concentration by comparison with a known control (10,27). Drawbacks include a precision of ±20%, interference from sodium chloride, and the need to keep a constant supply of mice (35). Other techniques have been developed such as a fluorimetric assay, an immunologic assay, a colorimetric assay, and high pressure liquid chromatography (35). Efforts to isolate the toxin from gastric contents have been limited (36).

Treatment is largely supportive. Attempts should be made to remove unabsorbed toxin through gastric lavage or the administration of a cathartic or enema (1,2,4,37). Mechanical ventilation may become necessary in the event of respiratory failure. Hemodialysis was used successfully in one patient (38). Atropine should be avoided because saxitoxin and its derivatives may be anticholinergic (4).

Neurotoxic Shellfish Poisoning (NSP)

Ptychodiscus brevis (formerly *Gymnodinium breve*) is the dinoflagellate responsible for neurotoxic shellfish poisoning, a syndrome similar to paralytic shellfish poisoning; however, symptoms are usually milder, and paralysis and respiratory failure do not occur (2). This dinoflagellate produces neurotoxins and is responsible for the formation of red tides off the Gulf coasts of Florida and Texas; occasionally, sea currents can carry the organism to Florida's Atlantic coast (2,39,40). In 1987, a red tide due *Ptychodiscus brevis* formed off the coast of North Carolina and was associated with an outbreak of neurotoxic shellfish poisoning involving 48 people (41). The source of this bloom was probably a red tide carried from Florida's southwest coast by Gulf Stream currents (42). Five cases were reported to the Centers for Disease Control from 1970 through 1974 (2).

Ptychodiscus brevis ranges in size from 20 to 40 µm in length and about 13 µm in width. It has been referred to as a "naked organism" because it lacks the shell of polysaccharide plates which characterizes *Protogonyaulax* species and other dinoflagellates (43). The neurotoxins produced by the dinoflagellate probably don't accumulate in fish, but will concentrate in filter-feeding shellfish in the vicinity of a bloom. Shellfish are not affected by the toxins; however, man becomes affected by ingestion of those shellfish containing high levels of neurotoxin. Shellfish which may become toxic include oysters, clams, coquinas, and other bivalve mollusca (44).

Five or more separate nonprotein toxins or toxin components are produced by *Ptychodiscus brevis*. These are termed "brevetoxins" and include brevetoxins A, B, C, and Gb-4. Brevetoxins A, B, and C are polycyclic ethers that have similar structures and may be convertible among each other (4,24). The toxins are lipid soluble, acid stable, and base labile; some are heat stable (45). They probably act by altering sodium conductance at or near sodium channels (46). Animal studies have demonstrated diverse biological effects including smooth muscle contraction through postganglionic parasympathetic acetylcholine release in dogs, inhibition of neuromuscular transmission in skeletal muscle, central nervous system stimulation with cardiovascular and respiratory impairment in dogs and cats, and norepinephrine release from nerve endings in rats (45,47–50). Brevetoxin B has been used as a model for a red tide pigment toxin (24).

Symptoms of neurotoxic shellfish poisoning usually begin within 3 hours after ingestion of contaminated shellfish and include circumoral paresthesias which progress to involve the pharynx, trunk, and extremities (2,4). Reversal of hot and cold temperature sensation as in ciguatera fish poisoning (24) can occur, as well as cerebellar symptoms such as vertigo, ataxia, and incoordination (2,4,44). Gastrointestinal symptoms are common and include nausea, diarrhea, abdominal and rectal pain. Bradycardia, headache, cramping of the lower extremities, and dilated pupils have been reported (44). Severe cases may be accompanied by convulsions with subsequent need for respiratory support (4). Paralysis and respiratory failure are not seen. No deaths are known to have been reported (1,4).

The *diagnosis* is based on clinical grounds in the appropriate setting. There is no known antidote, and treatment is supportive and symptomatic including airway management, intravenous fluids, atropine, and pressors if required. Symptoms are self-limiting and usually resolve completely without sequelae in a few days (1,2,4). One patient in North Carolina required admission to an intensive care unit for severe symptoms of bilateral carpopedal tremor and myalgia, total body paresthesia, ataxia, and vertigo after the ingestion of 45 oysters. Recovery was complete in approximately 9 hours (41).

The lack of an armored shell allows for aerosolization of the dinoflagellate during red tides by turbulent surf. This results in a unique syndrome seen along Florida's beaches characterized by respiratory and conjunctival irritation with the development of a nonproductive cough, shortness of breath, lacrimation, rhinorrhea, and sneezing. Asthmatics may develop wheezing. The syndrome is reversible upon leaving the beach (1,2). Beta-2 agonists, cholinergic antagonists, and calcium channel blockers may alleviate some of the respiratory symptoms (4).

Amnesic Shellfish Poisoning

In 1987, a previously unrecognized illness occurred among several hundred people who had ingested mussels harvested from cultivation beds located in three river estuaries on the eastern coast of Prince Edward Island (51,52). The affected individuals developed an acute illness characterized by severe nausea, gastrointestinal bleeding, and a severe and protracted neurological disorder which included disorientation, confusion, dizziness, seizures, coma, and a persistent memory loss. Many individuals required prolonged hospitalization and several deaths were reported. This syndrome, also known as "neurovisceral toxic syndrome", was subsequently linked to domoic acid, a toxin produced by the diatom *Nitzschia pungens* (53).

The implicated organism is widely distributed in the coastal waters of the Atlantic, Pacific, and Indian Oceans; however, not all strains have been shown to produce domoic acid. Mussels from the Canadian outbreak were shown to have high concentrations of this toxin in their digestive tracts. During the outbreak, a substantial bloom of *Nitzschia pungens* was noted by marine biologists patrolling the area (54). A possible reason for this is that freshwater runoff from record-breaking storms that year may have stratified the ocean layers of the estuaries, thereby enhancing the nutrients at just the right time in the diatom's lifecycle. Similar blooms have been recorded since the initial outbreak; however, proper surveillance measures enacted for domoic acid after the initial outbreak have effectively protected the public as well as the shellfish industry. Shellfish can clear the toxin from their tissues once exposed to clean seawater free of the toxic diatom (55).

Domoic acid is a heat-stable neuroexcitatory amine similar to glutamic and kainic acids. Its effects are about two to three times more potent than kainic acid and 30 to 100 times more potent than glutamic acid. Extracts of seaweed containing this toxin have been used in Japan as an ascaricidal agent for many years, although concentrations are significantly less than those causing illness and no adverse effects have been documented (51). In rats, domoic acid stimulates kainic acid receptors in the hippocampus and can produce limbic seizures, memory and gait abnormalities, and degeneration of the hippocampus (51). Autopsy reports of victims of the Canadian outbreak revealed neuronal necrosis and astrocytosis in several areas of the brain, particularly the hippocampus and amygdala (52).

At least 107 individuals were involved in the outbreak. Symptoms began 15 minutes to 38 hours (median, 5.5 hours) after the ingestion of mussels (51). In approximate order of appearance, they included nausea and vomiting (76% of the patients), abdominal cramps (50%), gastric bleeding, diarrhea (42%), incapacitating headache (43%), dizziness, confusion, loss of short-term memory (25%), weakness, lethargy, somnolence, coma, and seizures. Eighteen percent were hospitalized; death occurred in three (51,54). The memory loss was anterograde in all but the most severe cases and persisted for at least 2 years in a few individuals. Cognitive functioning remained intact. Cardiovascular instability was also noted, presumably due to the early excitatory effects of domoic acid. Alternating hemiparesis and ophthalmoplegia were noted in two patients (52). Evidence suggests that elderly individuals may be more susceptible to the neurological effects of domoic acid, possibly due to diminished renal function (57).

Pufferfish Poisoning

Ingestion of fish in the order *Tetraodontidae* which includes puffer fish, porcupine fish, and the ocean sunfish can result in an acute illness referre to as pufferfish poisoning or tetraodotoxication. This syndrome, although rare in the United States, is not all that uncommon in Japan where 6,386 cases were reported in a 78-year period with a mortality rate of 59% (58). Also known as "Fugu Fugu" in Japan, pufferfish there is considered a delicacy and is specially prepared by trained individuals who require licenses to serve this popular dish. In spite of these precautions, about 50 cases of "Fugu" poisoning occur annually in association with these specialty restaurants (23). Captain Cook, on his second voyage, ate a piece of pufferfish liver and became acutely ill, requiring 4 days to recover (37). Species of fish in this family are widespread and found in warm and temperate waters throughout the world; some species are eaten in New Jersey and Long Island (37).

Tetrodotoxin is a heat stable nonprotein toxin which is concentrated in the liver, ovaries, and intestine of infected fish. It is not unique in pufferfish and has been isolated from six different classes of animals including shellfish, salamanders, and a newt found on the campus of Stanford University (59). Certain frogs and newts in Central and South America harbor this toxin, and their skins are used to manufacture poison darts (37).

Tetrodotoxin has its own receptor located at or near the sodium channel of the external nerve axon cell membrane. Binding at this receptor inhibits nerve impulse propagation along preganglionic cholinergic, somatic motor, sensory, and sympathtic nerves in the central, peripheral, and autonomic nervous systems. Direct effects on the brainstem medulla can induce emesis or hyperemesis and respiratory depression. It is not a curare-like agent and doesn't act directly on the acetylcholine receptor at the motor endplate. Structurally it resembles morphine, which may explain some of its narcotic activity. Primary pharmacological effects include local anesthesia, hypotension, hypothermia, emesis, respiratory depression, and decreased systemic vascular resistance. High levels of toxin can inhibit impulse relay in skeletal or cardiac muscle (58).

Symptoms usually begin within 3 hours of ingestion of affected fish (usually 10 to 45 minutes). Symptoms include lethargy, weakness, paresthesias (including a numbness of the face and extremities), a floating sensation, emesis or hyperemesis, ataxia, salivation, and dysphagia (1). The extent of symptomatology varies with the amount of toxin ingested (23). Muscular weakness can progress to total paralysis, including respiratory paralysis. Hypotension, bradycardia, and fixed dilated pupils can occur in severe cases (1). Symptoms usually resolve over a period of days; the prognosis is good if the patient survives 18 to 24 hours (60). Death occurs in about 60% within the first 24 hours (23).

The diagnosis is based on clinical grounds. Treatment consists of airway support and volume expansion with intravascular fluids such as normal saline, and possibly pressors. Attempts should be made to remove unabsorbed toxins through gastric lavage and emesis (58). Some evidence exists that gastric lavage with 2% sodium bicarbonate is effective if used within the first hour of intoxication (61). Atropine is useful in the management of bradycardia. The anticholinesterases edrophonium, physostigmine, neostigmine, and galanthamine may have some benefits as might veratrine-like agents and cysteine, although none of these have been proven in large scale studies. Apomorphine currently appears to have the best antiemetic properties (58). Other potential treatment options include hyperbaric oxygen, the narcotic antagonist naloxone, and possibly monoclonal neutralizing antibodies (24).

Ciguatera Food Poisoning

Ciguatera is a distinct clinical syndrome that may follow the ingestion of certain tropical reef fishes which have acquired toxicity through the food chain. The name was given by Don Antonio Parra in Cuba in 1787 from the Spanish "cigua" which refers to the poisonous turban shellfish *Turbindae* (62). Sailors with Captain Cook suffered from this malady during his voyages (63). Outbreaks of ciguatera occur in tropical and subtropical regions between 35°N and 35°S latitudes (64). Ciguatera is the most commonly reported food-borne illness of marine origin in the United States; overall, it accounted for 5.8% of all disease-related food-borne outbreaks from 1972 to 1977, and 7.4% of outbreaks from 1978 to 1982 (6). The Centers for Disease Control has reported that 90% of cases in the United States occur in Florida and Hawaill (2). In Miami alone, there were 43 outbreaks reported involving 129 cases from 1974 to 1976, which probably represents less than 10% of the actual cases due to the inability of the public and medical profession to recognize the illness—the actual incidence during this period has been estimated to be 50 cases/100,000 population/year (45). In 1987, an outbreak occurred in North Carolina involving 10 persons in what is probably the first case of ciguatera associated with consumption of fish harvested from mainland U.S. coastal waters outside of Florida (66). A number of cases have been reported in nontropical areas such as Vermont and Iowa due to the transport and retail of affected fish from Florida (67). In some areas of the world, the disease is so prevalent that only the largest outbreaks are reported. An epidemiological analysis reported on more than 3,000 cases in the South Pacific (68). On one Pacific atoll, a 43% annual incidence was found during a routine survey of households in one such epidemic (6).

Gambierdiscus toxicus is the primary dinoflagellate responsible for the production of a number of closely related but distinct toxins responsible for the complex symptomatology of ciguatera (66). Other dinoflagellates may also be toxigenic, including *Procentrum lima* (69,70). These dinoflagellates adhere to dead coral, bottom-associated marine algae, and seaweed (6). Herbivorous fishes ingest the dinoflagellates, and the toxins are subsequently passed up the food chain to the larger carnivorous reef fishes which concentrate the toxins in their tissues; when eaten this results in human poisoning. Toxins are ultimately accumulated in viscera, although muscle tissue may also contain lethal amounts. Contamination of reef fishes is more likely to occur during storms or other periods of water turbulence (6). Larger fish are more likely to be contaminated (71,72).

Fish are unaffected by the toxins (23). More than 400 species of fish have been implicated in ciguatera including anchovy, barracuda, filefish, herring, jacks, moray eles, oceanic bonito, parrotfish, porgie, seabass, grouper, red snapper, squirrelfish, surgeonfish, triggerfish, trunkfish, and wrasse (23). In Miami, a high incidence of ciguatera due to the ingestion of barracuda has resulted in a ban on the sale of this fish (50).

The toxins recovered from fish implicated in ciguatera include ciguatoxin(s), maitotoxin, lysophosphatidylcholine (maitotoxin-associated hemolysin), scaritoxin(s), palytoxin, and ciguatoxin-associated ATPase inhibitor (24,73). The toxins are lipid soluble, colorless, odorless, and heat stable; thus, affected fish lack any unusual taste, odor, or appearance; Cooking does not inactivate the toxins (72). Ciguatoxin is a polyether compound which probably acts by competitive inhibition of calcium regulation of the sodium channel (72,74). For this reason, calcium gluconate has been advocated in the treatment of ciguatera, although its efficancy has not been proven (6,24). The toxin appears to act by opening voltage-dependent sodium channels in all cell membranes, with initial neural stimulation followed by conduction block primarily in skeletal muscle and neuronal membranes and less so in cardiac muscle. Higher doses can result in phrenic nerve paralysis and respiratory arrest (72). Maitotoxin is cardiotoxic and is also the most potent marine toxin known. Its cardiotoxic effects are due to enhanced calcium influx through the cardiac membrane with a resultant calcium overloaded state. These effects are abolished by verapamil in a rat model (75). In ciguatera, maitotoxin can reslut in hypotension, whereas ciguatoxin has hypertensive effects; the former may be responsible for ciguatera shock, whereas the latter may play a role in the chronic hypertension occasionally seen in chronic ciguatera (24). Immune sensitization to polycyclic ethers occurs in ciguatera by a T-cell dependent mechanism which results in serotonin release via abnormally released IgE. Subsequently, hypotension can ensue in response to certain medications (e.g., paraldehyde), foods, and factors generated in shock (e.g., thromboxane A_2). Morphine may form polycyclic ethers on epoxidation or endoperoxidation of the olefin moiety; this may account for the dramatic hypotension seen in some victims of ciguatera when administered opiates (24).

The symptoms of ciguatera have an ethnic variation which may be due to differences in diet; persons of Philippine or Chinese extraction are more severely affected, Hawaiians least affected, and other groups interposed between (24). Overall, 175 symptoms have been noted (24). The incubation period has been reported to be from 2 to 30 hours (65,66,68). Gastrointestinal symptoms such as watery diarrhea, nausea and vomiting, and abdominal pain tend to predominate early followed by neurological symptoms, although great variation exists (4,66). Virtually all experience gastrointestinal symptoms during the course of their illness, which usually resolve in 24 to 48 hours (1,4). Myalgias and weakness, particularly of the lower extremities, may occur at any time. Intense generalized pruritus may occur, and women may complain of pruritus of the vaginal vault (23). Bradycardia with hypotension occurs in 10% to 15% of cases (10); higher doses of toxin(s) may elicit a biphasic response where the bradycardia and hypotension are followed by tachycardia and hypertension (76). Shock and respiratory failure may occur within minutes. Skin lesions and a distinct erythematous desquamative rash have occasionally been reported (51). Fever, lacrimation, severe muscle spasms, and dysuria may also occur (4,73).

Initial neurological symptoms usually consist of circumormal and distal paresthesias. Vertigo and ataxia are common and are accompanied by a wide variation of other neurological manifestations such as cranial nerve palsies, motor paralysis, blurred vision, and coma (4). Pregnant women may complain of bizarre seizure-like fetal activity (1). Temperature reversal is an unusual characteristic commonly seen in ciguatera which occurs in 2 to 5 days (24). Hot objects may seem cold and cold objects can elicit an electric shock-like sensation. Serious thermal injury has been reported due to the individual's failure to recognize extreme heat as such (6). In the Bahamas, natives may be seen holding beer cans wrapped in towels to keep their fingers from touching the cold metal (23). Teeth may seem painful or loose. Nightmares are quite common, whereas some patients may complain of auditory hallucinations and zoopsia (1,69). All food may taste metallic (23).

Symptoms may wax and wane during any 24-hour period and give a "pseudodiurnal periodicity" (72). Alcohol may exacerbate or induce the recurrence of symptoms in up to 28% of recovered patients (72). Other conditions that increase blood flow such as increased temperature or physical exertion can also exacerbate symptomatology (65,66). Whereas gastrointestinal symptoms usually resolve in 24 to 48 hours, neurological, musculoskeletal, and cardiovascular symptoms may persist for months to years (1,4,72). Furthermore, recurrence of symptoms may intermittently appear for several months after recovery. Total duration of symptoms is usually several days to months with neurological symptoms and pruritus being the slowest to resolve (6). Sensitization is common, and immunity does not occur (1). Some individuals may never eat fish again, as exposure to even miniscule amounts of ciguatera toxins may reproduce dramatic symptoms (6,23). Malignancy has developed in a few individuals (24). Death is rare and occurs in up to 12% of reported cases; no deaths occurred in 184 cases reported to the Centers for Disease Control from 1970 to 1974 (2).

The diagnosis is based on clinical grounds. Laboratory abnormalities, if present, are usually due to fluid and electrolyte disturbances secondary to gastrointestinal manifestations. Elevated serum ammonia levels with abnormal prothrombin and partial thromboplastin times may reflect liver toxcity (24). When severe muscle spasms are present, there may be marked elevations of creatinine phosphokinase, serum glutamic oxaloacetic acid, and lactic acid dehydrogenase (73). Reversible T-wave changes on electrocardiograms have been reported (77). The toxins may be detected by a mouse bioassay which is subject to the same limitations as detection of saxitoxin and its derivatives in paralytic shellfish poisoning (see above). Radioimmunoassay, often referred to as a "poke" or "stick" test, and chromatography have also been utilized to detect ciguatera toxins, though they are expensive and subject to limitations as well (6,73).

Treatment is primarily symptomatic and supportive. Attempts to remove toxin through emesis or gastric lavage with activated charcoal should be made if vomiting has not occurred A cathartic may be administered to remove toxin from the lower intestinal tract (1,2). Intravenous mannitol provided rapid and dramatic relief in 24 patients with ciguatera in one study, with rapid recovery from shock and coma in two patients. The effect of mannitol on the course of ciguatera is unknown but may be due to competitive inhibition of the toxin(s) on the sodium channels or the neutralization of toxin(s) (78). Atropine may be used to control symptomatic bradycardia (24). Calcium gluconate and dopamine infusions have been effective in the treatment of hypotension (24). Amitriptylline has been used successfully to alleviate the paresthesias (79). Pruritus has responded to antihistamines. Affected individuals should avoid alcohol, excessive exercise or other activities which may result in high ambient temperatures (6,24). Myalgias may respond to acetaminophen or indomethacin. Opiates and barbiturates should be avoided as they may aggravate hypotension (24).

A ciguatera diet has been devised to be used in the treatment of affected patients (24). It consists of a diet high in protein, carbohydrates, and vitamins and the avoidance of fish, shellfish, seeds, nuts, mayonnaise, and their products. In addition alcohol, marijuana, solvents, herbicides, insecticides, glues, epoxies, ethers, resins, and cosmetics should be avoided as well. These restrictions should be maintained for at least 3 to 6 months after complete resolution of symptoms, and probably 12 months in those severely afflicted. Ingestion of fish weighing more than 2.3 kg (5 pounds) or fish caught during red tides should be avioded by the general public as these are more likely to contain ciguatera toxins (80).

Scombroid-Fish Poisoning

Scombroid-fish poisoning is an acute clinical syndrome characterized by symptoms of histamine toxicity resulting from the ingestion of spoiled fish (81). It represents the most common form of icthyosarcotoxism in the world (82). In the United States, 30 to 153 cases of scombroid-fish poisoning were reported annually to the Centers for Disease Control from 1978 to 1982 in a total of 73 outbreaks; this accounted for 7.2% of all food-borne disease outbreaks (1,6,83). Among 697 outbreaks of food-borne disease cuased by chemical agents from 1973 through 1987, scombroid-fish poisoning was responsible for 29% of the outbreaks and 27% of the cases (3). One-half of the 18 outbreaks reported to the Centers for Disease Control in 1982 occurred in fish served in restaurants and cafeterias (6). Most cases in the United States are reported from coastal states and Hawaii, although cases have occurred in the Midwest (1,6).

The disease is associated with ingestion of fish which belong to the families *Scombridae* and *Scomberesocidae* including tuna, mackerel, skipjack, bonito, and albacore. Nonscombroid fish, such as mahi-mahi, bluefish, amberjack, herring, sardines, and anchovies, as well as cheese, have also been implicated (84,85). Scombroid fish are distributed worldwide throughout temperate and tropical waters and have occasionally been found in polar waters (2).

Histamine has been identified as the toxin responsible for the symptoms of scombroid-fish poisoning (81). The affected fish do not contain high levels of histamine in their flesh at the time of capture; instead, they contain histidine. Histamine is produced during the process of spoilage by the enzymatic decarboxylation of histidine by certain marine bacteria, particularly *Proteus morganii, Klebsiella pneumonia, Escherichia coli, clostridia,* and *Achromobacter histamineum* which are common surface bacteria on fish (84–87). This occurs optimally at temperatures between 20° C and 30° C (2). Typically, this takes place when previously refrigerated fish is allowed to warm for a period of time before it is prepared. Histamine is heat stable and not destroyed by cooking. It is also stable at freezing temperatures. Oral histamine administered in large doses is rapidly metabolized in the liver and intestinal mucosa, and symptoms, if present, are generally mild. For this reason the presence of an unknown synergistic substance(s) has been proposed to account for the high levels of histamine noted in individuals afflicted with scombroid-fish poisoning (81,85).

Symptoms generally appear within several minutes to several hours of ingestion (median of 30 minutes) with a median duration of 4 hours (2). Symptoms may persist for 12 to 24 hours (1). The fish taste occasionally has been described as being sharp, peppery, or bitter but usually not unpleasant (6). Symptoms initially appear as flushing and a hot sensation of the skin, dizziness, headache, a burning sensation in the mouth and throat, shortness of breath in the absence of bronchospasm, itching with or without urticaria, and palpitations. Gastrointestinal symptoms appear as diarrhea, nausea, and rarely vomiting. A sunburned-appearing skin rash with sharply demarcated borders may develop, as well as conjunctival injection. More severe symptoms include difficulty swallowing, respiratory distress with bronchospasm, hypotension, tachycardia, and blurred vision (1,2,6,85). People receiving isoniazid and other inhibitors of endogenous histaminase may have more severe symptoms (6). Deaths have occurred but are very rare.

The diagnosis is made on clinical grounds and is usually fairly evident, as the incubation period is relatively short and several people are usually affected at once. Many people are erroneously diagnosed as having a "fish allergy" and are told to abstain from eating fish for the rest of their lives which is not necessary in cases of scombroid (1). Laboratory data are usually not helpful. Levels of histamine and its metabolite N-methylhistamine are elevated in urine samples at the time of onset of symptoms and may persist for more than 24 hours, although this is not routinely performed (81). Laboratory confirmation of scombroid-fish poisoning is accomplished by measurement of histamine in suspect fish. The concentration may vary from one portion of the fish to another so several areas must be sampled. The Food and Drug Administration has established the maximum safe level of histamine in tuna to be 450 micromoles per 100 grams of fresh tuna; fresh tuna contains levels less than 9 micromoles per 100 grams (81,85). In one recent outbreak in Tennessee, marlin, which was the implicated fish, was found to contain levels of histamine greater than 2,500 micromoles per 100 grams (81).

Treatment is supportive and symptomatic. If the gastrointestinal symptoms are not severe, gastric lavage or catharsis may be employed to remove unabsorbed histamine (88). Depending on the severity of symptoms, management can best be accomplished by the use of any one or combination of agents such as epinephrine, oxygen, diphenhydramine, hydroxyzine, and corticosteroids (24). Aminophylline may be used for the rare case of severe respiratory distress due to bronchospasm (1). Intravenous cimetidine has been reported to provide rapid and complete resolution of symptoms in severe cases not responding to antihistamines (88). Caution must be exercised in the simultaneous use of H_1 and H_2 blockers to aviod hypotension (24).

Diarrhetic Shellfish Poisoning

This clinical syndrome has not been reported in the United States to date but has been implicated in a number of short-lived outbreaks of acute onset of diarrhea following shellfish ingestion in other parts of the world, particularly Japan and the Netherlands. It is caused by the ingestion of okadoic acid and other toxins concentrated in shellfish that feed on the dinoflagellates that produce the toxins. During the period 1976 to 1982, more than 1,300 cases were diagnosed in Japan, while sporadic cases occurred in the Netherlands and Chile (89). In 1989, 150 people on the Adriatic Coast of Italy were afflicted by this illness after ingesting contaminated mussels. This was the first reported case of diarrhetic shellfish poisoning in the Mediterranean area (90).

Dinophysis fortii is the responsible toxin-producing dinoflagellate in Japan, whereas *Dinophysyis acuminata* produces the toxin in outbreaks occurring in the Netherlands (10,91). Mussels, clams, and scallops are the usual implicated shellfish which cause human outbreaks (90). Outbreaks are associated with dinoflagellate blooms (91).

Symptoms usually begin about 5 to 6 hours after shellfish ingestion with a range of 30 minutes to 12 hours (90,91). Although usually mild, the severity of the illness is dependent on the amount of toxin ingested (91). Symptoms consist of diarrhea, abdominal cramps, nausea, and vomiting. No fatalities have been reported and recovery generally occurs within 2 days. Treatment is supportive as the symptoms are self-limited (91,92).

Section II: *Vibrio* Infection

The Vibrios

Prior to the 1960s, the focus of *Vibrios* as pathogens of human disease focused primarily on *Vibrio cholerae*, the etiological agent of cholera. First described in 1854 by Pacini (93), *Vibrio cholerae* was the only currently recognized *Vibrio* known to cause human disease until 1951 when Fujino described a bacterium resembling *Vibrio cholerae* which was responsible for an epidemic of acute gastroenteritis in Japan involving 272 people with 20 deaths. He named this organism *Pasteurella parahemolyticus*, which was subsequently placed in the genus *Vibrio* in 1983. Two distinct biotypes were recognized at that time which were found to be separate species. In 1968, biotype 1 became known as *Vibrio parahemolyticus*, whereas biotype 2 became known as *Vibrio alginolyticus* (94). Since then, 34 species of *Vibrio* have been recognized of which at least 13 are known to be pathogenic to man (Table 3.3). Furthermore, several unnamed species recently have been identified so the list is likely to grow (95).

Pathogenic members of the genus *Vibrio* are gram negative, curved, rod-shaped facultative anaerobes capable of both fermentative and respiratory metabolism. They are motile organisms that measure 1.5 to 3.0 μm in length and 0.5 to 0.8 μm in width. They contain a single, sheathed polar flagellum in liquid media and occasionally may display shorter lateral flagella on solid media. They are anaerogenic (with the exception of *V furnisii* and some strains of *V damsela*), oxidase positive (except *V metschnikovii*), and have the ability to reduce nitrate to nitrite. Most are susceptible to the vibriostatic effects of the compound O/129 (96).

The pathogenic *Vibrios* can be divided into two groups based on their ability to grow in a saline environment (97). Nonhalophilic *Vibrios* will grow in the presence or absence of sodium chloride, and include *V*

TABLE 3.3. Clinical presentations of pathogenic *vibrio* infections in humans.*

	Diarrhea Watery/dysentery	Wound	Otitis	Sepsis
Nonhalophilic				
V cholerae 01	+	±		
V cholerae-non-01 ●	+/+	+	+	±
V mimicus ●	+/+		+	
Halophilic				
V parahemolyticus	+/+	+	±	±
V hollisae (EF13) ●	+/±			±
V fluvialis (EF6)	+/+			
V furnissii	+			
V alginolyticus		+	+	
V vulnificus (L+) ●	±			++
V damsella (EF5)		+		
V metchnikovii (gp16)		+		±

● Especially associated with oyster consumption
* Single cases of *V cincinnatiensis* and *V carchariae* have been reported with sepsis and shark bite wound infections, respectively

cholerae, *V cholerae*-non-O1, and *V mimicus*. Halophilic *Vibrios*, on the other hand, require sodium chloride to support growth and survival and will reach very high concentrations in waters of 5% to 8% salinity (95).

Isolated *Vibrios* can occasionally be confused with other bacteria of medical importance such as *Enterobacteriaceae*, *Pseudomonas*, *Aeromonas*, and *Plesiomonas*. The *Enterobacteriaceae* are straight rather than curved and are oxidase-negative with peritrichous or circumferential flagellae. *Pseudomonas* species, although oxidase-positive, have an oxidative rather than fermentative metabolism. Species of *Aeromonas* and *Plesiomonas* do not require sodium chloride for growth and are able to grow in the presence of vibriostatic O/129 (93).

Most standard laboratory media used for biochemical testing contain 0.5% sodium chloride and will therefore support the growth of both halopilic and nonhalophilic *Vibrios*. Isolation is usually accomplished through selective or enrichment media. Alkaline peptone broth is the most suitable general enrichment media for all pathogenic *Vibrio* species (98). A modified two-step method has been successfully utilized to prevent bacterial overgrowth by other bacteria in the peptone broth (99). Thiosulphate-Citrate-Bilesalt-Sucrose (TCBS) agar is the most widely used selective agar medium for isolation of pathogenic *Vibrio* species; however, several newly described pathogens may fail to grow on this agar medium (100). Furthermore, individual variations of commercially available TCBS agar may affect recovery of the organism (101).

Vibrios are aquatic organisms that can be found in a wide variety of environmental water sources such as oceans, estuaries, lakes, and ponds.

The highest concentrations are generally achieved in the marine waters along the East and Gulf Coasts primarily in the summer months; lower concentrations exist along the West Coast. Their numbers fluctuate widely with marked variation due to such variables as temperature, salinity, sediments, and the presence of certain marine organisms, particularly the copepods and other plankton in which *Vibrios* may play a role in salt retention by these species (102).

Water temperature appears to be the single most important variable affecting the growth and survival of the *Vibrios*. Pathogenic *Vibrios* are usually isolated from waters where temperatures exceed 10°C for at least several consecutive weeks (103,104). They are less frequently found in waters where temperatures exceed 30°C (105,106). Variation occurs worldwide and among different species, *V cholerae*, for example, prefers temperatures between 20°C and 35°C (95).

Individual *Vibrio* species have different optimal sodium chloride requirements, with a range of 5% to 30% which accounts for the primary isolation of these organisms from marine and estuarine waters (101, 103,106,107). Although *V cholerae*, *V cholerae*-non-O1, and *V mimicus* do not require sodium chloride for growth, they achieve higher numbers in its presence. *V cholerae* has an optimal requirement of 2% to 20% salinity, whereas halophilic *Vibrios* usually achieve optimal concentrations in sodium chloride concentrations of 5% to 8% (95). Pathogenic *Vibrios* may be isolated from freshwater where salinity is less than 5%, probably due to a complex interaction between high water temperatures and increased organic content which may compensate for the detrimental effects of low to absent salinity (104,108–110). Evaporation of fresh and brackish waters during summer months may increase the sodium chloride content (99).

As temperatures drop below 10°C, *Vibrios* characteristically disappear rapidly from the water but can persist throughout the winter in the sediment. This has been shown for *V parahemolyticus*, *V cholerae*, and *V alginolyticus*, and may well hold true for all pathogenic *Vibrios* (101,105,111,112). As water temperatures increase during the spring and summer months, the organisms can then re-emerge once again to reach high water concentrations, accounting for as much as 26% to 40% of the total bacterial population in some areas (113).

By associating themselves with higher organisms such as shellfish, plankton, and fish, *Vibrios* may maintain high numbers and prolong their existence. Adsorption onto the chitinous component of plankton has been shown to significantly prolong the survival of some pathogenic *Vibrios*, and it is possible that this may represent a major means of prolonging survival for all pathogenic species (110,112–116). Bivalve molluscan shellfish that filter feed on zooplankton may themselves become rapidly contaminated during periods of high bacterial counts. Improper storage of the shellfish may then allow proliferation of the pathogenic bacteria with resultant outbreaks of food-poisoning (117–120). Crustacean shell-fish and fish can also become contaminated during such periods of abundant *Vibrio* growth (110,114,121,122). *Vibrio* species have also been cultured from the teeth, skin, the gum lines of sharks (123,124).

The spectrum of human disease due to the pathogenic *Vibrios* is mainly dependent on the causative species and ranges from mild self-limiting gastroenteritis and soft tissue infections to severe necrotizing would infections and fulminant bacteremia primarily in patients with underlying diseases. Illness can result from a variety of means such as ingestion of contaminated shellfish or exposure of open wounds to contaminated seawater. Raw oyster eaters, particularly those with liver disease, have been shown to be at risk of developing severe illness with *Vibrios*, particularly *V vulnificus* (125). An increasing incidence of *Vibrio*-related illness is occurring for a variety of reasons including an increased awareness by the public and medical profession of *Vibrio* infections, improved biochemical and serologic means for the detection of *Vibrios*, increased recreational exposure to coastal regions, increased foreign travel, increased seafood ingestion, and increasing numbers of susceptible immunocompromised individuals (95,125).

Vibrio species have been isolated from virtually every geographic region within the United States, although most cases occur along coastal areas. Of 713 isolates reported to the Centers for Disease Control from various human anatomical sites, 75% belong to one of three species: *V cholerae*, *V parahemolyticus*, and *V vulnificus*, with gastrointestinal symptoms predominating (126). Between 1974 and 1978 in a Chesapeake Bay community, 40 *Vibrio* isolates were recovered from 32 patients with *V parahemolyticus*, *V vulnificus*, and *V cholerae*-non-O1, accounting for 33 of the total isolates. Illnesses were mild and self-limiting with no mortalities reported (127). Over a 10-year period in a Gulf Coast community, 23 cases of *Vibrios* infections were reported with *V vulnificus*, *V parahemolyticus*, and *V cholerae*-non-O1 accounting for all but two cases, and included gastroenteritis in three patients, wound infection in 14 patients, and bacteremia in 12 patients (128).

Vibrio cholerae

Seven cholera pandemics have been recorded since 1817, six of which began before the twentieth century (129). The current seventh, one began in Sulawesi, Indonesia in 1961 and then spread to Asia, Africa, the Middle East, Oceania, and part of Europe, while sparing the Western Hemisphere (130,131). No cases of domestically-acquired cholera were reported in the United States after 1911, until 1973 when it was diagnosed in a resident of the Gulf Coast of Texas (132). In 1978, 11 people were involved in an outbreak of cholera following the ingestion of crabs gathered from a Louisiana coastal marsh (130), and in 1981, 16 oil workers were involved in a cholera outbreak on a Texas oil rig after eating rice cooked in water which had been contaminated by canal water containing sewage discharged from the rig (133). These and other similar cases account for a total of 65 cases of domestically-acquired cholera reported to the Centers for Disease Control, most of which have been only isolated incidents (134). Almost all of these cases have been reported in the Gulf of Mexico region; however, there has been at least one such case acquired from the Cheasapeake Bay (135). All of the Gulf Coast isolates were of the EI Tor biotype, serotype Inaba, which strongly suggested that this organism is endemic along the Gulf Coast of Mexico. Since then, *Vibrios cholerae* serogroup O1, including toxin-producing strains, have been isolated from U.S. coastal waters of the Gulf of Mexico and Chesapeake Bay throughout the year (136,137). Numbers tend to be highest in the warmer summer months, and they are frequently associated with plankton and shellfish. Toxigenic and nontoxigenic strains of *V cholerae* O1 have been cultured from shellfish harvested from commercial U.S. waters (138–141). Pollution does not appear to be a necessary factor, as the organism can be found in waters with no evidence of human waste (140). Case-controlled studies of localized outbreaks of *V cholerae* O1 in the United States have shown that the recent ingestion of raw or partially cooked seafood or contact with contaminated water is a significant risk factor (130,133,142).

In January of 1991, toxin-producing strains of *V cholerae* O1, biotype EI Tor, serotype Inaba, appeared in several cities in Peru, which marked the first time this century that cholera has been reported in South America (143,144). As of January, 1992, over 300,000 cases of cholera have been reported in 14 countries in North and South America, with almost 4,000 deaths. United States citizens accounted for 17 of these cases; six associated with travel to South America and eleven with the ingestion of crabs imported illegally from Ecuador. Between January 1 and February 29, 1992, 42 cases were identified in the United States among travellers to and from South America; 40 of these cases, including one death, were reported among passengers on the same airline flight from South America to the United States (134). The Latin American strain is different from the endemic U.S. Gulf Coast isolates (which are hemolytic) and is similar to the pandemic, nonhemolytic EI Tor Inaba isolates in Asia and Africa (145).

Over 70 different serotypes of *Vibrio cholerae* exist based on a somatic "O" antigen (146). These strains are phenotypically indistinguishable and share a common flagellar "H" antigen. *Vibrio cholerae* serotype O1 is the strain associated with cholera. All others are referred to as noncholera *Vibrios* (NCV), *Vibrios cholerae*-non-O1, or nonagglutinable *Vibrios* (NAG, due to their inability to agglutinate in O1 antiserum). Most strains of *Vibrio cholerae* O1 produce an enterotoxin (cholera toxin) which is responsible for the severe fluid losses seen in cholera. Non-O1 *V cholerae* strains often do not produce cholera toxin but may produce toxins capable of eliciting an illness identical to cholera (147–149). *V cholerae* can be divided into two biovars, Classical and EI Tor. Classical strains tend to be more virulent than the EI Tor biotypes. EI Tor strains were originally detected by their ability to lyse sheep erythrocytes; however this trait has not been shown to be consistent. They will agglutinate chicken erythrocytes, are not sensitive to polymyxin B, and are Voges-Proskauer positive. Classical strains fail to lyse sheep erythrocytes or agglutinate chicken erythrocytes, are VP-negative, and are sensitive to polymyxin B. Biotypes may also be distinguished by phage susceptibility, a tool mainly used for epidemiological purposes. Additionally, both biotypes can be further classified into one of three serotypes; Inaba, Ogawa, or Hikojima (150). The EI Tor biotype initially appeared in endemic cholera regions in the Ganges Delta in 1969 and quickly became the dominant biotype for most of the world (151). The more severe Classical strain has since reappeared in Bangladesh in 1982 and has once again become the dominant strain in that region (152). At the time of this writing, all biotypes in the Western hemisphere have been of the EI Tor biotype. Reasons for the persistence of EI Tor strains include its greater ability to survive in the environment and a larger ratio of symptomatic cases to asymptomatic carriers (1:30–100 for EI Tor and 1:2–4 for Classical biotypes) (153).

Under adverse environmental conditions, *V cholerae* O1 can enter a state of dormancy in which the organism remains viable and potentially pathogenic, yet fails to grow on conventional culture media. The presence of the organism under such conditions has clearly been demonstrated by fluorescent and immunologic techniques in the absence of a positive culture. It has been proposed that, in this way, *V cholerae* O1 may persist indefinitely and go undetected in waters such as the Gulf Coast, only to emerge periodically under more favorable conditions and cause disease. This may also explain the periods between epidemics in endemic cholera areas. This phenomenon has been referred to as "viable but nonculturable" (146).

In the United States, cases of cholera have usually occurred in the summer or fall months following the ingestion of raw or undercooked shellfish (154). Once in the intestinal tract, the organism may become adherent to the intestinal cell wall by means of a specialized pilus where it may grow and produce enterotoxin (155,156). Factors slowing transit time, such as the ingestion of solid foods rather than liquids, may increase the chances of colonization and development of cholera (157). Furthermore, because the organism is less likely to survive in an acidic environment, the use of antacids or previous gastrectomy will increase the chance of developing disease (158). Adherence of the organism to chitin particles in shellfish may also enchance survival in acidic environments (142). Perhaps related to specific glycosidated mucus proteins, persons with blood type O have been noted to be at a higher risk for cholera (159).

Cholera toxin is a heat-labile protein produced by most strains of *V choleraee* O1. The molecule is composed of five B subunits arranged in a circle around and A_1 and an A_2 subunit. The B subunits are responsible for binding the toxin to the receptor, ganglioside GM1, on cell membranes. The A_1 subunit, bound to the complex by the A_2 subunit, stimulates adenylate cyclase activity causing increased levels of cyclic AMP and hypersecretion of chloride with the result of massive losses of salt and water (160,161). Cholera victims may lose over one liter of fluid per hour and up to 100% of their body weight in 4 to 7 days of diarrhea as a result of the toxin (98,162). Cholera toxin is not the only factor capable of causing the severe diarrhea in cholera victims; an identical illness has been noted in individuals infected with nontoxigenic variants of *V cholerae* O1 (163,164). Factors other than cholera toxin which have been proposed to play a role in producing illness include a heat-stable toxin similar to a toxin produced by *Vibrio parahaemolyticus* or *E coli* (161,165), lecithinase (166), phospholipase (167), and prostaglandin E (168). *Escherichia coli*, may produce a plasmid-mediated toxin that is very similar in structure and mode of action to cholera toxin (160).

The incubation period in cholera varies between 6 hours to 5 days. The average is 2 days in endemic areas (138). Initial symptoms may include anorexia, abdominal cramping, and mild diarrhea. Vomiting without nausea typically begins within hours of the onset of diarrhea. Fever is usually absent or low-grade. Stools are initially brown in color and loose, but within hours become watery and pale grey in appearance, and lose all odor except for perhaps a "fishy" smell. Scattered flecks of mucous give the stools a "rice water" appearance. A feeling of relief, rather than tenesmus, accompanies each bowel movement. Peak stool loss occurs at around 24 hours of illness. Shock may occur within 12 hours in untreated cases, with death ensuing in 18 hours to 5 days. Gallbladder disease associated with *V cholerae* O1 has been reported, including one case of acute cholecystitis in Alabama in which the organism was isolated from the gallbladder and bile. Serum vibriocidal antibodies were present as well (169). Chronic, asymptomatic gallbladder carriage has also been documented, especially in endemic areas of the world where the risk of exposure is great (170,171). Extraintest inal infections are rare, nontoxigenic strains may be isolated from wound infections on occasion (142,172).

Cholera is fatal in less than 1% of properly recognized and treated cases, although fatality can be as high as 50% if untreated (138,142,173). The mainstay of therapy consists of rapid and effective fluid and electrolyte replacement. Oral rehydration is effective for most patients who are able to tolerate this mode of therapy. Currently, oral rehydration salt packets are available as are a variety of other premixed rehydration solutions that have been shown to be effective in the treatment of cholera. In the event that vomiting is severe enough or the patient is too obtunded to tolerate enteral hydration, intravenous infusion of lactated ringers solution has been effective in initial rehydration, with oral therapy being initiated as soon as the patient is able to tolerate it. Normal saline is less effective because it lacks bicarbonate and potassium. The amount of fluids administered should be determined on the basis of dehydration at presentation as well as the rate of ongoing losses (134).

Antibiotics may decrease the duration of illness, the period of *Vibrio* excretion, and the amount of fluid needed for rehydration (173). Tetracycline and doxycycline are currently the drugs of choice in the treatment of cholera. Doxycycline may be administered as a single dose of 300 mg. The dose of tetracycline is 500 mg four times a day for 3 days. Resistant strains may be treated with erythromycin or the combination of trimethoprim and sulfamethoxazole (134). Treatment with furazolidine may be preferable in children and pregnant women (67). Norfloxacin recently has been shown to be effective (174). Antispasmodics, antidiarrheal agents, and corticosteroids are not indicated in the treatment of cholera (134). Although a parenteral vaccine is currently available within the United States, it is not likely to be of benefit because of the low risk of infection in international travellers and the small number of cases acquired to date in the United States (175).

Non-O1 *Vibrio cholerae*

Strains of *Vibrio cholerae* that do not agglutinate in O1 antiserum, or non-O1 *V cholerae*, are common inhabitants of both sewage-contaminated and sewage-free waters of bays, estuaries, brackish inland lakes, and seafood. Besides being environmental contaminants, the organism has been isolated from domestic animals, waterfowl, and a variety of wildlife (120). Non-O1 species have even been implicated in enteric infections of horses, lambs, and bison in western Colorado (176). Most disease-associated isolates have been obtained from the coastal waters of Florida, the Gulf of Mexico, and the Chesapeake Bay, although isolates may be found all along the East Coast (177). Fewer isolates are noted along the West Coast, possibly due to colder water temperatures. Infections due to non-O1 strains have also been acquired from freshwater lakes distant from the sea (178,179). Infections are more common during the warmer water months of summer and fall.

The first reported case of human disease due to non-O1 strains of *V cholerae* acquired in the United States occurred in 1972 in Louisiana in an individual who developed profuse and prolonged diarrhea following the ingestion of raw oysters (180). Since then, this organism has been increasingly recognized as a cause of human illness in this country, usually occurring as cases of sporadic illness (154). In a Chesapeake Bay hospital over a 15-year period, 40 *Vibrio* isolates were obtained of which 10 were strains of non-O1 *V cholerae* (127). Similarly, in a Gulf Coast community over a 10-year period, 4 of 23 *Vibrio* isolates were non-O1 *V cholerae* (128). Although diarrheal illness is the most common manifestation of disease due to non-O1 *V cholerae* strains, 10% of the cases are wound infections and an additional 10% are ear infections (173). Unlike the strain which causes cholera, non-O1 species are rarely linked to epidemic disease (148). Isolated outbreaks of illness have occurred, usually in association with a common contaminated food source. Three previous outbreaks of diarrheal illness linked to non-O1 *V cholerae* in Czechoslovakia, the Sudan, and Australia were linked to food sources in two (potatoes and an asparagus salad), and polluted well water in the other (181–183).

More than half of the non-O1 *V cholerae* isolates received by the Centers for Disease Control are from stool samples (173). Gastroenteritis is the most common manifestation of illness in the United States and is almost always due to the ingestion of raw oysters (50,125,148,184). In the U.S., the incubation period has generally been less than 48 hours; however, it has been as long as 4 days in at least one foreign outbreak (142). The following symptoms were noted in one review of U.S. cases: diarrhea (100%), abdominal cramps (93%), fever (71%), and nausea and vomiting (21%) (148). Another review reported nausea and vomiting occurring more frequently (77% and 69%, respectively) (185). The diarrhea can be severe, with up to 30 watery stools per day, and up to 25% will have bloody diarrhea (173). In some cases fluid losses may equal that see in cholera (130). Illness lasts an average of 6.4 days in the cases reported in the U.S. (range, 2 to 12 days) but has been less than 2 days in some overseas outbreaks (148,181,183).

Non-O1 strains of *V cholerae* exert their pathogenic effects through a variety of extracellular toxins and hemolysins. Enterotoxins identical or nearly identical to cholera toxin have been detected (186). Although rare in the United States (148), up to 40% of isolates in India and Bangladesh may produce this toxin (130,187). In fact, severity of diarrheal illness seems to correlate with production of this toxin (95,187). The lack of this cholera-like toxin in United States isolates indicates that other mechanisms are involved in their pathogenicity. Other factors which may be produced include enterotoxins other than the cholera-like toxin, including a heat stable enterotoxin that is also produced by *V mimicus* and *V fluvialis* (173,188–190), several hemolysins (186) including a hemolysin similar to the Kanagawa hemolysin produced by *Vibrio parahemolyticus* (191), and a Shiga-like toxin which may be responsible for the occasional bloody diarrhea (192).

Septicemia due to non-O1 strains of *V cholerae* is a less frequent complication of infection. During 1977 through 1979 there were 70 isolates of *V cholerae* reported to the Centers for Disease Control, of which 12 were obtained from the blood (177). The case fatality for septicemia has been estimated at 61.5% based on previously reported cases in the

United States (177). Predisposing factors include alcohol abuse, previous gastric surgery, advanced age, and chronic underlying conditions such as hematologic malignancy, liver disease, immune deficiency, diabetes mellitus, peripheral vascular disease, and achlorhydria (95,125,173,177, 193,194). The source of the *Vibrio* in many cases is raw oyster ingestion (125). In addition to septicemia and gastroenteritis, non-O1 *V cholerae* has also been implicated in cases of wound infections (95,173,177), otitis media and externa (173,195,196), prostatic abscess (177), cholecystitis (197), pneumonia (198), and meningitis (199,200), including one case of neonatal meningitis in an infant who drank milk from a bottle stored near live crabs (201). Extraintestinal infections are usually the result of contact with seawater (173).

Most cases of non-O1 *V cholerae* are relatively mild cases of gastro-enteritis which are usually self-limiting in nature; only a minority will require hospitalization (148,183). Treatment should consist of supportive care with intravenous hydration in severe cases of gastroenteritis (97). Septicemic cases and severe localized infections such as meningitis should be treated with intravenous antibiotics. In cases of gastroenteritis, antibi-otics may decrease the severity of illness and shorten its duration (97). Non-O1 *V cholerae* strains are susceptible in vitro to a wide range of antibiotics including tetracycline, trimethoprim-sulfamethoxazole, chlo-ramphenicol, and nalidixic acid (173). Susceptibilities to ampicillin and gentamicin are variable (173).

Vibrio parahaemolyticus

Virbrio parahaemolyticus has a worldwide distribution in both tropical and temperate inshore coastal and estuarine waters. Isolates have been obtained from water, sediment, suspended particulates, plankton, fish, and shellfish in marine environments (173). Although halophilic, the organism can occasionally be isolated from freshwater areas, possibly through association with the chitin of plankton and shellfish or sediments which may allow it to survive in areas of low salinity (94). Most cases of illness occur in summer when warmer water temperatures favor growth of the organism. During winter, the organism can be isolated from sediment (146). *Vibrio parahaemolyticus* has been isolated from nearly every coastal state in the United States and is frequently found in Canadian waters as well (94). Outbreaks of diarrheal illness are the most common form of disease caused by this organism, which usually follows the inges-tion of raw or improperly cooked seafood particularly crabs, shrimp, lobsters, and raw oysters. Most United States outbreaks have been caused by gross mishandling of the seafood, such as improper refrigera-tion, insufficient cooking, cross-contamination, with other seafood and recontamination (140). Incubation of the organism in seafood can reduce the generation time to as little as 12 minutes (202). Previously thought to be a rare strain of *Vibrio parahaemolyticus* and not described in the United States until 1982 (147,203), a urease-positive strain of *Vibrio parahaemolyticus* representing a new serovar has been established as the predominant cause of *Vibrio parahaemolyticus*-associated gastroenteritis on the West Coast of the United States and Mexico (204,205).

In Japan, over 70% of food-borne diarrheal illness is caused by *V parahaemolyticus* (140). First described as a pathogen in the United States in 1971 following the ingestion of improperly cooked crabs in Maryland (206), the organism has been increasingly recognized as a cause of sporadic cases of diarrheal illness, usually in association with food-borne outbreaks (207). In a Chesapeake Bay hospital over a 15-year period, *Vribrio parahaemolyticus* was the most common *Vibrio* species identified and accounted for 16 of 40 isolates obtained from 32 (127) patients. During an outbreak of *Vibrio* gastroenteritis among attendees at a scientific congress in New Orleans, *Vibrio parahaemolyticus* accounted for 35 of the 51 stool specimens yielding a *Vibrio* species (208). Extraintestinal manifestations may also occur, including sometimes fatal septicemia.

The incubation period has ranged from 4 to 96 hours (209). In a review of eight *V parahaemolyticus* outbreaks in the United States (209), the clinical manifestations included diarrhea (98%), abdominal cramps (82%), nausea (71%), vomiting (52%), headache (42%), fever (27%), and chills (24%). The illness was self-limited in most cases, with a median duration of 3 days. Fever rarely exceeds 38.9°C. Abdominal pain can be severe (202). The diarrhea is acute in onset and usually watery and mild, although it can, rarely, be severe enough to cause dehydration, hypotension, and acidosis (210,211). A dysentery-like illness with fecal leukocytes, superficial ulcerations of the colonic mucosa, and blood and mucous in the stool has been described in India and Bangladesh (207,212,213). This form of disease has rarely been encountered in the United States (173,213). The incubation period in dysentery-like disease is shorter (as short as 2.5 hours), although the duration of illness approximates that of the more common form of illness (142).

The ability to cause human disease has been associated with a heat-stable enterotoxin capable of lysing erythrocytes on Wagatsuma agar (94). Strains producing this thermostable direct hemolysin (TDH) are known as "Kanagawa positive," named after the prefecture in Japan where it was first studied (173,214). The observation that over 95% of clinical isolates and less than 1% of environmental isolates are Kanagawa positive has suggested that TDH is the toxin associated with pathogenicity (94,173). In several studies involving animal models, purified TDH was able to produce clinical and histopathological effects similar to those seen in disease due to *Vibrio parahaemolyticus* (215–217). In one report from the Pacific Northwest, only 6 of 13 clinical isolates from patients with diarrhea or wound infections due to *Vibrio parahaemolyticus* were

Kanagawa positive (205). The ability of Kanagawa-negative strains lacking TDH to produce diarrheal illness has led to the discovery of other enterotoxins (150,218). In addition to several hemolysins with unclarified or potential roles in pathogenicity including a Shiga-like toxin (94,218), a TDH-related hemolysin has been suggested to be an important virulence factor in TDH-negative clinical isolates (219). The presence of specific intestinal adherence factors may contribute to the pathogenicity of some strains (220).

In rare instances *Vibrio parahaemolyticus* can result in extraintestinal infections. A history of trauma or insult to the infected anatomical site can be elicited in the majority of cases (95). Wound infections or cellulitis can develop as a primary focus of infection or can result from secondary hematogenous seeding (221). Although less common than stool isolates, wound isolates can constitute a significant number of *Vibrio parahaemolyticus* isolates. Five of sixteen *V parahaemolyticus* isolates collected over a 15-year period in the Chesapeake Bay region were acquired from wounds (127). Vascular thrombosis and gangrene have been reported (222). In some instances, *Vibrio parahaemolyticus* and another *vibrio* species may be isolated concurrently (223). Ocular (224,225) and ear infections (127,173) can occur, as well as pneumonia (226), and osteomyelitis (227).

Most cases of *Vibrio parahaemolyticus* gastroenteritis are self-limited and resolve in a matter of days. Rarely are cases severe enough to require vigorous fluid support. Mortality is unusual and has been estimated to be 0.04% in Japan (130). From 1981 to 1988, there were four fatalities due to *Vibrio parahaemolyticus* in Florida. All patients were bacteremic and had either cirrhosis or an underlying malignancy (198). In view of the fact that most cases of infection due to *Vibrio parahaemolyticus* are gastroenteritis, methods to avoid such illness include proper handling of seafood. Heating at 60° C for 15 minutes will kill *V parahaemolyticus*. In addition, storing at temperatures at or below 4° C will inhibit growth of the organism (77). Persons susceptible to septicemia, such as those with liver disease or any other immunosuppressive condition, should probably avoid raw seafood ingestion (125,127).

Vibrio vulnificus

Beginning in 1964, the Centers for Disease Control began receiving extraintestinal isolates that were throught to be variants of *Vibrio parahaemolyticus* but were shown to be different by means of a variety of biochemical tests, including the ability to ferment lactose (130). Referred to initially as the "halophilic lactose-positive marine *Vibrio*," the name *Beneckea vulnifica* was initially proposed, although not widely accepted (150,228). The virulence of this particular species was first recognized in 1976 by a review of clinical isolates reported to the Centers for Disease Control which revealed that 53% of these isolates were recovered from blood (229). The name *"Vibrio vulnificus"* was formally recognized in 1979 (230). This organism has been found in seawater, sediments, zooplankton, and shellfish (97). In two separate studies, over 50% of oysters sampled during selected months (231) and 11% of crabs harvested during summer months (232) yielded *V vulnificus*. Water temperature seems to be an important factor; organisms are rarely isolated from waters with temperatures lower than 17°C (154). Almost all cases of infection have been reported between the months of May through October (140). Cases have been reported along both the Pacific and Atlantic coasts (as far north as Cape Cod), Hawaii, the Gulf of Mexico, and occasionally in such inland areas as New Mexico, Oklahoma, Kentucky, and the Great Salt Lake (36,127,128,233–236). In a Gulf Coast community over a 10-year period, 12 of 23 *Vibrio* isolates obtained were *Vibrio vulnificus*, of which 9 were wound isolates (128). Similarly, in a Chesapeake Bay hospital over a 15-year period, 10 of 40 *Vibrio* isolates were *Vibrio vulnificus*, of which 7 were obtained from wounds (127). The organism can proliferate in seafood at room temperature but is killed by storing at or near freezing temperatures or by cooking seafood at boiling temperatures (237). *V vulnificus* has been isolated in oysters that have been refrigerated for 4 days (238).

Vibrio vulnificus is one of the most invasive and rapidly lethal human pathogens ever described. Two major syndromes can result from infection with this organism (239). Primary septicemia typically follows the ingestion of raw oysters by individuals with liver disease. This syndrome can have a rapidly fatal course in up to 60% of cases (240). The other major presentation is that of wound infections which may occur by either primary inoculation or secondary hematogenous spread in a bacteremic individual. Antibiotics, vigorous debridement, and occasionally amputation are necessary to control the massive necrosis and systemic spread which can occur (241). Unlike other vibrioses, gastroenteritis is not a major hallmark of infection with this species and, although gastrointestinal symptoms may accompany other forms of illness, the relationship is unclear (95,242). In one epidemiological study of *V vulnificus* infections in Florida from 1981 to 1987, seven patients out of a total of 62 (11%) had gastrointestinal symptoms as their only manifestation of disease (243). Stool specimens from these patients yielded *V vulnificus* and blood cultures were negative. The diarrhea was described as watery, profuse, and accompanied by vomiting and abdominal pain. Six patients (86%) were hospitalized for a median of 6 days. Medications that reduce gastric acidity may be a factor in the development of gastroenteritis (242). Of 62 cases reported in Florida between 1981 and 1987, 38 were primary septicemia (62%), 17 were wound infections (27%), and the remaining 7 were gastrointestinal illness referred to above (11%) (243). Other infections due to *Vibrio vulnificus* include pneumonia (244,245), endocarditis (246), osteomyelitis (247), ocular infections (248), and meningitis

(229). One reported case of endometritis due to *Vibrio vulnificus* occurred in a female who had engaged in sexual intercourse in seawater (150).

The severity of intections due to *Vibrio vulnificus* is dependent on host as well as bacterial factors. The presence of an acidic polysaccharide capsule correlates strongly with virulence (249). This capsule may confer resistance to phagocytosis and bactericidal activity of human serum (250,252). Strains may shift between encapsulated and unencapsulated forms at a very low frequency by poorly understood mechanisms. Growth of both encapsulated and unencapsulated phenotypes is enhanced significantly by the presence of iron (249). The organism is able to use transferrin-bound iron for growth if the transferrin is 100% iron-saturated (normal uman serum is 30% saturated). Iron in hemoglobin and hemoglobin-haptoglobin complexes may also be utilized (251). *Vibrio vulnificus* also produces siderophores which are low molecular weight chelators capable of binding available iron (253). Mouse studies have shown that passage of the organism through the animal may enhance virulence significantly, suggesting that the reintroduction of strains shed by infected individuals may increase the potential pathogenicity of environmental or food-borne strains if reintroduced to the environment by infected individuals (254). Various toxins and enzymes may be produced by the organism. They include mucinase, protease, lipase, DNAse, chondroitin sulfatase, hyaluronidase, cytolysin, and collagenase (113,255,256). The contribution to virulence by each of these factors has not yet been fully determined. Anticytolysin-directed antibody has been detected in the serum of individuals with invasive disease suggesting that this toxin may play a major role in invasive forms of disease (257).

Individuals susceptible to primary septicemia are most commonly those with liver disease, particularly alcoholic cirrhosis. This is due in part to shunting of blood around the liver, thereby bypassing the hepatic reticuloendothelial system and subsequent clearing by hepatic macrophages. Additionally, these individuals may also have deficiencies in leukocyte chemotaxis and complement that can impair host defenses (97). Patients with hepatic disease commonly have high serum iron levels due to liberation of iron stores from damaged hepatocytes (258). In addition, other conditions leading to increased serum levels of iron, such as thalassemia major and hemochromatosis, can also contribute to primary septicemia (95). Alcoholics without liver disease are at risk for primary septicemia, probably due in part to saturated transferrin levels (259). Other conditions predisposing to primary septicemia include hematopoietic disorders, chronic renal insufficiency, dyspeptic disease or a history of gastric resection, the use of immunosuppressive drugs, and diabetes mellitus (260). Primary septicemia occasionally occurs in previously healthy persons (243).

There is little doubt that the gastrointestinal tract is the portal of entry in primary septicemia. The organism can survive between pH 3.6 and

12.5 when incubated at 37° C for 1 hour and grows best between pH 7 and 9 (261). Therefore, the organism is capable of surviving passage through the stomach. Most commonly, this occurs following the ingestion of raw oysters. An epidemiological study in Florida of oyster eaters between 1981 and 1988 estimated the age-standardized annual incidence of any *Vibrio* illness per million as 95.4 for raw oyster eaters with liver disease, 9.2 for raw oyster eaters without liver disease, and 2.2 for nonraw oyster eaters (125). Although these estimates were based on the chances of developing any *Vibrio* illness, the risk was shown to be greatest for *vibrio vulnificus*. Other types of raw fish or shellfish may cause septicemia and, on occasion, illness has followed ingestion of deep-fried fish, grilled crab, boiled shrimp, and broiled grouper (243,262). *Vibrio vulnificus* invades the gastrointestinal mucosa at the level of the proximal small bowel into the systemic circulation to produce sepsis (263,264). On occasion, the organism may penetrate the intestinal wall into the ascitic fluid of cirrhotics to produce peritonitis (264).

The mean incubation period is 16 hours, although it has been as long as 2 weeks (240,265). Chief symptoms associated with septicemia include fever (94%), chills (91%), and nausea (58%) (95). Diarrhea occurs in less than half of the patients with primary septicemia (239,243). Approximately one-third become hypotensive within 12 hours of admission (266). Signs and symptoms of disseminated intravascular coagulation and septic shock may appear (266). Thrombocytopenia and leukopenia are common, although leukocytosis can appear less frequently (173). Arthritis and arthralgias may develop, and the organism has been cultured from affected joints (239,265). Other associated clinical characteristics may include the rapid development of anemia, adult respiratory distress syndrome, and heart block (97).

Over 70% of patients with primary septicemia develop skin lesions, usually within the first 36 hours of illness (36,173). Lesions are common on the trunk and extremities and frequently begin as tender erythematous or ecchymotic areas which may progress to bullae or vesicles that develop into necrotic ulcers (93,267). They may occasionally appear as ecthyma gangrenosa-like lesions, erythema multiforme, cellulitis, and papular or maculopapular eruptions (95,169). Similar lesions have been reported in individuals who had bacteremia due to *Pseudomonas aeruginosa*, *Aeromonas hydrophilia*, and *Yersinia enterocolitica* (36). Gangrene of a limb can develop as a result of major vessel occlusion (267). Histological examination reveals cellulitis with subcutaneous tissue necrosis and septal panniculitis characterized by paucity of an inflammatory infiltrate in the dermis (267). Necrotizing vasculitis and subepidermal bullae can be seen as well as gram negative coccobacilli. Gram stain and culture of vesicular or bullous fluid may yield the organisms which have been described as resembling "seagulls" (262).

Localized wound infections with *Vibrio vulnificus* may occur in otherwise healthy people after an open wound comes in contact with seawater or seafood contaminated with the organism. A typical scenario is the development of a wound infection following injuries sustained while peeling shrimp, cleaning crabs, or shucking oysters (97,173,243). Infection may also follow exposure of a pre-existing wound with seawater. Approximately one-third to one-half of cases of wound infections due to *V vulnificus* occur in patients who have underlying illnesses such as alcohol abuse, congestive heart failure, stasis ulcers, arthritis, liver disease, diabetes mellitus, and malignancy (239,240,265). Initially, the wound may appear trivial; however in a matter of hours, it characteristically becomes edematous and erythematous with development of lymphadenopathy and lymphangitis. Intense pain may develop at the wound site. Patients are frequently ill with fever and chills (240,265). Anorexia, nausea, and vomiting may occur, although less frequently than in primary septicemia (239,265). Occasionally, more than one *Vibrio* may be isolated from the wound (223). Unlike primary septicemia, wound infections usually remain localized; however bacteremia with secondary development of cutaneous intections can occasionally occur (260). Approximately one-third of individuals with localized wound infections will have positive blood cultures (173). Individuals with underlying diseases (rarely healthy persons) may develop progressive cellulitis, myositis, or fasciitis (97). Leukocytosis is usually noted; thrombocytopenia and disseminated intravascular coagulation generally do not occur (260). Severe necrotizing fasciitis can occasionally occur with gross purulence and easy separation of fascial planes. Findings of fascial necrosis separates this entity from cellulitis (268). The histopathology of wound infections is similar to that which occurs in primary septicemia, although it is generally not as severe. Mortality ranges from 7% to 22% of cases, being higher in those individuals with underlying diseases who are more likely to develop progressive soft tissue involvement and bacteremia (97).

Treatment of *Vibrio vulnificus* infections consists of rapid recognition with prompt institution of antibiotics and supportive measures along with management of adult respiratory distress syndrome, disseminated intravascular coagulation, and shock if present (97,173,264). Surgical debridement of all necrotic tissue is recommended (269). Proximal amputation of infected limbs may be necessary in severe cases of wound infection (97). Tetracycline has been shown to be highly effective against *Vibrio vulnificus* in a mouse model (270). Low efficacy was noted for ampicillin, cefotaxime, and cefazolin. Carbenbicillin, and gentamicin were not effective. The quinolones may be an effective alternative; ciprofloxacin has been used effectively in the treatment of one case of infection due to *Vibrio vulnificus*; however, conclusive clinical studies are lacking (271,272). Auerbach (273) has recommended oral ciprofloxacin the combination of trimethoprim and sulfamethoxazole for coastal wound infections in patients with immunologic impairment, liver disease, or elevated serum iron levels. Initial therapy should probably consist of a tetracycline, usually doxycycline, possibly in combination with an aminoglycoside or possibly chloramphenicol (164,272,274).

Vibrio mimicus

In 1981, a new *Vibrio* species was detected by virtue of DNA and biochemical analysis. Previously thought to be a biochemical variant of *Vibrio cholerae*, the new species differed in its inability to ferment sucrose and its negative Voges-Proskauer reaction. The name *Vibrio mimicus* was proposed because of its similarity to *Vibrio cholerae* (275). The organism is nonhalophilic and has been isolated from both saltwater and freshwater (276). A high percentage of strains (49%) are able to grow in 6% sodium chloride (126). Brackish water with an average salinity of 4.0% was found to be suitable for *V mimicus*. It has been isolated from fish and shellfish (usually oysters), as well as freshwater prawns (277–279). Unlike, *V cholerae*, it probably does not adhere to plankton samples in the environment (276). Over the period 1977 through 1981, the Centers for Disease Conrtol received 21 clinical isolates of this organism, although the true incidence is unknown (278), Nineteen of the isolates were obtained from stool samples and the other two were obtained from human ears. Clinical isolates have been obtained from the waters of the Gulf of Mexico, the mid-Atlantic Coast, and the Chesapeake Bay (278). Among 40 *Vibrio* isolates collected over a 15-year period in a Chesapeake Bay hospital, 3 were identified as *Vibrio mimicus*; all were isolated from stool samples (127). The organism has also been implicated along with *Vibrio fluvialis* in a case of terminal ileitis (280).

Gastrointestinal illness is the predominant manifestation of disease, and this typically follows the ingestion of seafood, primarily raw oysters (278). In the largest reported review of illness due to *Vibrio mimcus* in the United States, involving 21 cases, the median incubation perild was shown to be 24 hours with a range of 3 to 72 hours (278). Symptoms included diarrhea (94%); nausea, vomiting, and abdominal cramps (67%); mild fever (44%); and headache (39%). Three of the 17 patients with diarrhea had bloody diarrhea (18%). The median leukocyte count was 13,400, with a median differential of 73% polymorphonuclear cells, 7% bands, 16% lymphocytes, and 4% monocytes. Electrolytes were all within normal limits. Diarrheal illness lasted a median of 6 days. Two cases were ear infections acquired from contact with seawater. Outbreaks of seafood-associated gastroenteritis caused by *Vibrio mimicus* have been described in Japan (276).

Approximately 10% of clinical strains and 16% of all strains produce a heat-labile toxin that appears to be identical to cholera toxin (173).

An enterotoxin similar to that described for non-O1 *V cholerae* and *V fluvialis* has been described (190).

Antimicrobial testing has shown that *V mimcus* is susceptible to tetracycline, which may be the drug of choice in severe infections (278). The combination of trimethoprim and sulfamethoxazole, aminoglycosides, chloramphenicol, and ampicillin have been shown to be effective in vitro. Eighty-three percent of environmental isolates in one study were shown to be resistant to ampicillin, with intermediate sensitivity and no resistance to tetracycline in 17% (276).

Vibrio fluvialis

Vibrio fluvialis was first isolated in 1975 from the stool of a patient in Bahrain with diarrhea (281). In 1976 to 1977, it was responsible for an outbreak of diarrheal illness involving over 500 persons in Bangladesh (282). About one-half of the patients were children under 5 years of age. Originally referred to as Group F or Enteric Group EF-6, it was later named *Vibrio fluvialis* (from the latin "river") in 1980 on the basis of its original isolation from river and estuarine waters (142,283). This organism has marked biochemical similarities to *Aeromonas* species and can be distinguished by its ability to grow in 6% to 7% sodium chloride (in which *Aeromonas* species will not grow) and its inability to grow in the presence of the vibriostatic agent O/129 (in which *Aeromonas* species will grow) (142). Based on these similarities, it is probable that many clinical isolates previously reported as *Aeromonas* species may have in actuality been *V fluvialis* (106). One-third of organisms labelled as *Aeromonas* in the past by the British Public Health Laboratories were actually found to be *V fluvialis* on reexamination (283). In the United States, the organism has been isolated from water and sediment in New York (106), shellfish in Louisiana, and water and shellfish in the pacific Northwest and Hawaii (284). Almost all cases of infection due to *Vibrio fluvialis* in the United States have been gastrointestinal illness. A history of seafood ingestion prior to the onset of illness is reported in most cases (198). In Florida between 1982 and 1988, 12 clinical isolates of *V fluvialis* were recovered of which 10 were obtained from stool samples, one was obtained from the drainage of a colostomy bag, and one was recovered from a wound (198). One isolate was recovered from a stool sample in a Chesapeake Bay hospital over a 15-year period (127). A fatality occurring in the United States due to *V fluvialis*-related illness has been reported in the case of a Texas man who developed profuse diarrhea with electrolyte imbalance (284). Outbreaks of gastroenteritis linked to a common food source have been reported (285). Occasionally, wound infections can occur in association with injuries sustained near seawater (198,284). The organism was recovered from the purulent bile of one patient in Japan with acute suppurative cholangitis (286).

The median incubation period for gastrointestinal illness has been reported as 39 hours (range, 16 to 60) with a median duration of illness of 6 days (range, 1 to 60 days) (198). In the Bangladesh outbreak, reported clinical features included diarrhea (100%), vomiting (97%), abdominal pain (75%), moderate to severe dehydration (67%), and fever (35%) (282). Invasive disease probably occurs, as 75% of the patients in that outbreak had fecal leukocytes and blood in the stools. Secondary infection occurs rarely (287).

Vibrio fluvialis is capable of stimulating fluid accumulation in rabbit ileal loops (106). An enterotoxin similar to that described for non-O1 *Vibrio cholerae* and *Vibrio mimicus* has been described (190). Other factors associated with toxicity may also be produced with a variety of effects including cytolytic activity against mammalian erythrocytes, lethal activity in mice, and nonhemolytic cytotoxicity (94,288).

Severe cases of gastroenteritis should be treated with intravenous fluid and electrolyte replacement and antibiotics (93). *Vibrio fluvialis* is sensitive to tetracycline, ampicillin, chloramphenicol, gentamiacin, and the combination of trimethoprim and sulfamethoxazole (287).

Vibrio hollisae

This organism was previously known as Enteric Group EF-13 until 1982 when it was shown to be a separate species by DNA hybridization studies (100). It was named after the researcher at the Centers for Disease Control who first identified it *V hollisae* grows inconsistently on TCBS agar and so may not be isolated routinely (289). Isolation may rely on recovery of colonies on blood agar plates (289). There are few ecological studies on *V hollisae* however, it has been isolated from deep sea invertebrates and healthy coastal fish (290,291). Fifteen clinical isolates were received by the Centers for Disease Control from 1971 to 1981 of which fourteen were stool isolates and one was a blood isolate (289). Cases occurred in states along the Atlantic and Gulf Coasts, with three cases in Florida, four in Maryland, and one each in Virginia and Louisiana. In Florida in the years 1981 to 1988,34 isolates of *V hollisae* were identified from clinical cases, of which 28 were obtained from individuals with gastrointestinal illness, 4 were from individuals with septicemia, and 2 were isolated from wounds (125). The risk of infection is most often associated with raw seafood ingestion, particularly raw oysters, although cases of illness have followed ingestion of fried fish and fish preserved by drying and salting, which suggests that this organism may be resistant to some methods of cooking and preservation (125,289,292,293).

In nine selected cases of gastrointestinal illness reported to the Centers for Disease Control, all had diarrhea and abdominal pain, five had vomiting, and five had fever (289). Diarrhea was bloody in one case. The median white blood cell count was 11,200 cells per microliter. The median duration of illness was 1 day (range, 4 hours to 13 days). Reported cases of septicemia include one fatal case occurring in an individual with hepatic cirrhsis (289) and another case occurring in a 65-year-old man who developed septicemia following consumption of a freshwater catfish and who was successfully treated with tobramycin, cefamandole, and tetracycline (292).

Several toxins may be produced including a hemolysin with potential virulence activity (294) and a heat sensitive enterotoxin which has been associated with some virulent strains (295). *Vibrio hollisae* possesses gene sequences homologous with those coding for the thermostable direct hemolysin in *V parahaemolyticus* (296).

Vibrio damsela

Vibrio damsela, previously known as Enteric Group EF-5, was renamed in 1981 after the damselfish, for which it is an important pathogen (297). This organism is known to cause skin ulcerations and death in fish, and has been isolated from seawater (297). Between 1971 and 1981, eight clinical isolates were reported to the Centers for Disease Control, of which seven were obtained from wounds (one was a urine isolate) (289). Cases occurred on the Atlantic, Pacific, and Gulf coasts and were reported in Florida, Louisiana, Hawaii, and the Bahamas. Typically, infection is the result of injuries sustained to the foot or leg while swimming or as is handling fish (298). Infection is uaually seasonal and probably dependent on water temperature and, possibly, its interaction with certain fish species (289,298,299).

Lesions usually began as erythematous indurated areas which may later exhibit a purulent discharge (289,300). Immunocompetent patients usually require little more than local wound care; however, severe necrotizing infections have been described (289,298). One fatal case involved a diabetic, alcoholic patient who had sustained a small laceration to his hand while cleaning catfish (298). The initial superficial wound evolved into an edematous and necrotizing process with bulla formation. He subsequently died of medical complications including disseminated intravascular coagulation. Tissue damage may be toxin mediated (272,300). *Vibrio damsela* may produce an extracellular hemolytic toxin which has been shown to be lethal in mice (301). Of five *V damsela* isolates tested, all were sensitive to gentamicin and chloramphenicol, four were sensitive to tetracycline and cephalothin, and none were sensitive to sulfonamides, ampicillin, or penicillin (289).

Vibrio alginolyticus

Originally classified as biotype 2 of *V parahaemolyticus*, this organism was found to be a separate and distinct species on the basis of several fermentative and biochemical properties. It was renamed *Vibrio alginolyticus* in 1968 (302). This organism was not known to be pathogenic in man until 1973 when six isolates from tissue specimens collected in 1969 thought to be *V parahaemolyticus* were in actuality found to be *V alginolyticus* (207). The ecological niche of this organism is probably similar to *V parahaemolyticus*, and it has been isolated from seawater, fish, shrimp, crabs, oysters, and clams (133). Numbers of this organism in seawater are generally higher than *V parahaemolyticus* and are associated with warm water temperatures (133,146). This organism fails to grow at temperatures less than 8°C (207). In the United States, clinical isolates of *V alginolyticus* have been obtained from waters along the Atlantic, Pacific, and Gulf coasts, as well as in Hawaii and the Chesapeake Bay (127,128,207).

Clinically, wound and ear infections represent the majority of cases of illness due to this organism (95,207). Wound infections almost always follow exposure of open wounds to seawater (150). Frequently, a number of different organisms may be isolated, making the pathogenic role of *V alginolyticus* uncertain (95). In one study in Western Australia, 56% of infected wounds contaminated with seawater yielded *V alginolyticus* (303). In a similar study in Hawaii, the organism was isolated from 11% of traumatic marine injuries (304). In Florida between the years 1981 to 1988, 14 clinical isolates of *V alginolyticus* had been reported, of which 11 were wound isolates (79%) (125). The incubation period is about 24 hours (207,303). Most wound infections are self-limiting and consist of mild cases of cellulitis with varying amounts of a seropurulent exudate; however, more severe cases with bacteremia may be noted in immunocompromised individuals (128,207,305,306). One fatal case of bacteremia involved a 37-year-old woman who was doused in seawater after an explosion on a recreational boat (307). The organism was isolated from burn wounds as well as blood. The organism may produce extracellular protease and collagenase, although the role of these factors in the virulence of this organism has not yet been established (173,308). Local wound care is probably sufficient for superficial wounds in immunocompetent individuals; however, patients with impaired host defenses or severe, complicated infections should be treated with antibiotics. In vitro, *V alginolyticus* is susceptible to tetracycline, the combination of trimethoprim and sulfamethoxazole, aminoglycosides, and chloramphenicol (309).

Vibrio alginolyticus has a predisposition towards individuals with ear disorders (146). These infections are generally associated with swimming in seawater. Both otitis media and externa have been reported (207,305). This organism has rarely been associated with gastrointestinal illness, although cases have been reported (125,310,311). Conjunctivitis, pneumonia, osteomyelitis, and a case of an epidural abcess due to *V alginolyticus* have been reported (94,305,312,313). Peritonitis has been reported in an individual undergoing peritoneal dialysis who had changed his peritoneal dialysis fluid bag on the beach without taking adequate precautions (314).

Vibrio furnissii

This organism was originally classified as biovar II of *Vibrio fluvialis*. This species differs from *Vibrio fluvialis* in its aerogenicity (produces gas from glucose). In 1983 if was renamed *Vibrio furnissii* in honor of a researcher at the British Public Health Laboratories in Maidstone, England (315). The organism has been recovered from the marine environment (283). Most clinical isolates have been from Japan and other parts of the Orient (173). Illness related to this species consists of gastroenteritis, most likely due to ingestion of raw or undercooked seafood (315). Occasional outbreaks of gastroenteritis have been recorded including one such episode on board a flight from Tokyo to Seattle involving 23 passengers (316,317). Symptoms included diarrhea (91%), abdominal cramps (79%), nausea (65%), and vomiting (39%). Two patients required hospitalization, and one died. The organism has been recovered from the feces (along with *V fluvialis*) of an infant with diarrhea, and has also been isolated from the stool of asymptomatic individuals (318,319). *Vibrio furnissii* is capable of producing an enterotoxin similar to that described for *V fluvialis* and *V mimicus* (189).

Vibrio metschnikovii

Previously known as Enteric Group 16, this organism was first described in 1888 (301). In 1987 it was redefined on the basis of DNA homology studies (150,320). Freshwater and marine isolates of this organism have been obtained from rivers, estuaries, sewage, cockles, lobsters, oysters, clams, and a bird that died of a cholera-like illness (320). Human disease involving this organism was not recognized until 1978 when it was recovered from the blood of an 82-year-old diabetic female in Chicago who presented to a hospital with septicemia due to an inflamed gallbladder (321). She was treated successfully with a cholecystectomy and antibiotic treatment with clindamycin and tobramycin. Although the organism has been isolated from the stool of asymptomatic individuals (150), diarrheal illness has been described in at least one instance (322). An extracellular cytolysin has been characterized, although its role in virulence is uncertain (323).

Vibrio cincinnatiensis

Only one case of human disease involving this organism has been reported to date (324). A 70-year-old man with a history of alcohol abuse developed disorientation and questionable nuchal rigidity upon admission to a hospital. A spinal tap was performed which revealed a gram-negative bacillus; an identical isolate was obtained from his blood. Genetic and biochemical analysis revealed that this was a new *Vibrio* species which was subsequently named *Vibrio cincinnatiensis* (325). The patient was treated successfully with 9 days of moxalactam. There was no history of exposure to saltwater or ingestion of seafood.

Vibrio carchariae

First isolated from a brown shark that died in captivity in 1984, this organism has been known to be a pathogen of fish (326). Named *Vibrio carchariae* (from the Greek "carcharias," meaning shark), this species had not been implicated as a human pathogen until a single report described the case of a wound infection occurring in an 11-year-old girl who was attacked by a shark off the South Carolina coast (327). She suffered extensive trauma to her left calf, requiring plastic surgery. A swab of the leg obtained on the day of the shark bite revealed *V carchariae*. Minimal drainage occurred from the wound which subsequently healed well. Antimicrobial testing showed it to be susceptible to cephalothin, cefamandole, cefoxitin, gentamicin, and the combination of trimethoprim and sulfamethoxazole. Resistance was noted to ampicillin and carbenicillin; amikacin sensitivity was intermediate.

Section III: Marine Trauma and Envenomation

Mycobacterium marinum

Mycobacterium marinum was first isolated by Aronson in 1926 from saltwater fish that died in a Philadelphia aquarium (328). In 1942, Baker and Hagan isolated this mycobacterium from freshwater platyfish in Mexico; they named it *Mycobacterium platypoecilus* (329). Human disease attributed to this organism was not recognized until 1951 when an epidemic of self-limiting skin granulomas occurred involving 80 individuals in a town in Sweden; 75 were children and lesions were mostly on the elbows (330). All five adult patients were avid swimmers which suggested that a common swimming pool may have been involved. Tissue specimens from patients and cultures of the swimming pool yielded an atypical *Mycobacterium* which the investigators termed *Mycobacterium balnei* (Latin, meaning "of the bath"). In order to affirm the association between the organism and the clinical findings, the investigators inoculated themselves with the *Mycobacterium* and were able to produce the lesions. In 1959, the previously reported mycobacterial isolates were found to represent the same species (331). *Mycobacterium marinum* became the officially recognized name, as this was the earliest term proposed by Aronson. The first association of this organism with tropical fish tanks was made in 1962 (332). Since then, *M marinum* has become a well-recognized cutaneous pathogen with a strong association with aquatic environments and water-related activities. The organism has been called a "leisure-time pathogen" and the disease referred to as a "hobby hazard" (333,334). Manifestations of disease have also been referred to as "fish fancier's finger" and "swimming pool granuloma."

Mycobacterium marinum belongs to Runyon group I (the photochromogens) of atypical *Mycobacteria* along with *M kansasii* and *M simiae*. These organisms are capable of producing a yellow carotene pigment when exposed to a strong light. *M marinum* grows optimally on Lowenstein-Jensen medium and, unlike other *Mycobacteria*, growth occurs at 28° to 32° C rather than 37° C. This is an important distinction which may be responsible for the fact that most *M marinum* infections do not invade beyond the superficial cooler regions of the skin (335). Colonies may be visible in as early as 7 days, although rarely may take up to 2 months (331,336). Growth also occurs on blood agar, though not on MacConkey agar. The organisms are acid-fast and appear as long, slender, occasionally beaded rods; however, they may appear short and compact. Biochemical reactions include a negative response to niacin, neutral red, and arylsulfatase, and a positive response to Tween 80 hydrolysis in 10 days (331,337).

M marinum is a pathogen of salt water and freshwater fish. It is widely distributed in the environment and may be isolated from contaminated water, the walls of swimming pools or aquariums, and dead or diseased fish (338). Affected fish may be cachectic and frequently show skin changes consisting of pigment changes, loss of scales, blood spots with eventual formation of ulcers, and fin and tail rot (339). Microscopically, miliary tubercles may be found in virtually every organ system. The disease is thought to spread among fish by the ingestion of infective material. In humans, the organism most commonly causes benign superficial cutaneous illness, although destructive tenosynovitis, osteomyelitis, septic arthritis, sclerokeratitis, and, rarely, disseminated systemic illness have been reported (34,335,340–347). The organism is usually acquired through abrasions, lacerations, or punctures sustained in an aquatic environment. Commonly associated activities include swimming, boating, fishing, handling of fish and shellfish, and the keeping of tropical fish tanks. Occasional nonaquatic exposures have been documented from an asphalt school yard, school desks, an electrical installation, rose thorns, and even a laboratory (331,333,340,348). Cases have been reported along the Gulf, Pacific, and Atlantic coasts as far north as Oregon and Long Island (349). Inland cases also occur. An epidemic in Colorado involving 290 individuals was linked to community swimming pools (350).

The incubation period ranges from 2 weeks to 2 months (351). Superficial lesions appear which usually range in number from one to six and appear as chronic, dusky, erythematous plaques or verrucoid papules or nodules in areas subject to trauma (352). More than 75% of reported cases involved the hand and upper extremity, usually the dominant right hand (349,351). The lesions can appear as solitary granulomas or verrucous papules 1 to 2.5 cm in diameter which may ulcerate and drain purulent material. Most lesions are asymptomatic and cause only cosmetic inconvenience. Symptoms, if present, are mainly slight tenderness and discharge. Limitation in movement of the affected extremity may be noted. Lymphadenopathy occurs rarely (351). Occasionally, spread in a sporotrichoid fashion may occur. Rarely, disseminated cutaneous spread develops (345,353). One such case involved a 16-month-old child who developed disseminated lesions after being bathed in a bathtub which her father had previously used to clean his fish tanks (345). The time lag between appearance of the lesion and its correct diagnosis ranges from a few weeks to a few years. Left untreated, 80% of the lesions may resolve completely in an average of 14 months, the longest being 45 years (341,354). Truncal cutaneous dissemination has been described in an AIDS patient who kept tropical fish as a hobby (355).

Histologically, the lesions of *M marinum* change their appearance according to the age of the infection (353). Early lesions (2 to 3 months' duration) show nonspecific inflammatory infiltrates in the upper corium. Multinucleated giant cells and epithelioid cell granulomas generally appear at 4 to 6 months and typical tuberculoid structures appear in older lesions. All stages can be observed simultaneously. Staining of tissue specimens reveals the organism in only about 10% of cases. Ten or more slides of thick smears from homogenized tissues are often required for examination after preparation with auramine-rhodamine fluorochrome stain (356).

Deep tissue infections were first recognized in 1973 (357). Superficial lesions may invade deeper tissues by attempted self-excision, by intralesional cortisone injections, or by incomplete surgical excision that is not combined with appropriate antibiotics (349). Unlike superficial lesions, these infections are more destructive and more resistant to treatment. Tendon and synovial structures of the wrist and hand are affected in most cases. Diffuse edema at the site of infection is the most common finding (352). A slight fullness may be palpated at the site of the affected tendon sheath. Unlike pyogenic infections, the dorsum of the hand does not swell and a throbbing pain does not occur. Joint limitation with subsequent development of draining sinus tracts may occur. Up to one-half of the deep infections involving the hand and wrist may be associated with the carpal tunnel syndrome (336). Systemic complaints, fever, and lymphadenopathy are usually absent. The erythrocyte sedimentation rate is usually normal and x-ray findings are nonspecific (352). Factors associated with a poor prognosis include persistent pain, the presence of a draining sinus tract, and previous local injection of cortcosteroids (356).

Diagnosis relies primarily on isolation of the organism by staining or culture. A thorough history should be obtained to include information such as hobbies and recreational interests. *M marinum* rarely grows at temperatures utilized for the incubation of most other *Mycobacteria*. If *M narinum* is suspected, specimens should be incubated at 30°C on Lowenstein-Jensen medium (in addition to 37°C for the isolation of other *Mycobacteria*) (331). Specific mycobacterial skin testing has been utilized, although with inconsistent results (340,351). The differential diagnosis of *M marinum* infections includes sporotrichosis, tularemia, nocardia, yaws, syphilis, leishmaniasis, common warts, coccidioidomycosis, blastomycosis, histoplasmosis, tuberculosis verrucosa cutis, sarcoidosis, gout, rheumatoid arthritis, iodine or bromine granuloma, and benign or malignant tumors (352). Although usually self-limiting, superficial infections should probably be treated with antimicrobial agents. Minocycline has been considered to be the drug of choice (358–360). *M marinum* does not respond to many of the antimycobacterial agents. It is usually susceptible to rifampin, ethambutol, the combination of trimethoprim and sulfamethoxazole, the tetracyclines, and amikacin (361). Resistance to doxycycline has been described (362). Ciprofloxacin and other quinolones show good in vitro activity against *M marinum* (363). Treatment should probably be continued for at least 6 to 12 weeks (361). Patients should be instructed not to "pick at" their lesions to reduce the risk of deeper tissue involvement (349). Deeper tissue involvement usually requires surgical intervention which may include excision, tenosynovectomy, synovectomy, arthrodesis, or incision and drainage of infected bone or joints (349). Superficial lesions should not be excised or biopsied without the addition of appropriate drug therapy in order to decrease the risk of deeper tissue spread (349).

Marine Trauma

Sharks

Shark attacks have been a popular focus of many books and movies which often depict these creatures as ruthless, savage predators randomly attacking swimmers or divers along beaches or other aquatic recreational areas. In actuality, only 68 proven shark attacks and seven deaths have been reported in the United States since 1926 (364). Of the 350 known species of sharks, only 32 have been implicated in the 30 to 100 shark attacks reported annually worldwide (365). In the United States, the most common offenders are the great white, grey reef, blue, and mako sharks. Most shark attacks occur in temperate waters between 46°N latitude to 47°S latitude. Associated risk factors include murky, warm water (70°F), sewer outlets, late afternoon and early evening hours, recreational areas, deep channels or drop-offs, movement, and bright objects (365). The victim does not see the shark in most cases, although skin abrasions from "bumping" (due to the shark's skin denticles) may precede the bite. In more than 70% of reported attacks, the victim was bitten one to two times (364).

Sharks can range in length from 9 inches to 50 feet (the whale shark). The largest great white shark verified was 19.5 feet long (364). They are extremely well adapted as predators in their environment with exceptional sensory systems enabling them to detect electrical fields and motion which may compensate for their poor color vision. Specialized telereceptors known as the "ampullae of Lorenzini" are exquisitely sensitive to vibration and low-frequency sound waves which allow these animals to detect struggling creatures (365). Keen olfactory and gustatory chemoreceptors allow them to sense body fluids.

The shark's jaws consist of mutirowed crescentshaped sets of rip-saw teeth which are replaced every few months. The biting force has been estimated at 18 tons per square inch! The jaw opening of some sharks may be large enough to accommodate a horse's head (365).

Sharks usually feed slowly and purposefully; however, they will occasionally become frenzied, usually by an inciting event, snapping at anything in sight. Humans are usually mistaken for food (seals). Recent shark attacks in northern California have been focused on surfers who had entered migratory habitats of the elephant seal which the shark feeds on (365). Possible explanations for the precipitation of a shark attack include anomalous behavior by the shark, the violation of courtship patterns, or territorial invasion (366).

Initial management of the shark attack victim consists of basic trauma management: airway, breathing, bleeding control, and the management of hemorrhagic blood loss (364,365). The immediate life threat is hypovolemic shock and, occasionally, primary pulmonary or cardiac injury. Bleeding is controlled with compression and occasionally ligation of vessels. Wounds should be irrigated and debrided and packed open with primary closure. Tetanus toxoid, 0.5 cc IM, tetanus immune globulin, 250 to 400 units IM, and prophylactic penicillin, imipenem-cilastatin, a third generation cephalosporin, chloramphenicol, or an aminoglycoside have been indicated (273,364,365) (Table 4). Wounds are susceptible to contamination by both aerobes and anaerobes, including *Aeromonas, Vibrio*, and *Clostridium* (364). Buck and his colleagues cultured the teeth of a great white shark caught off Long Island and isolated the following organisms: *V alginolyticus, V parahaemolyticus, V fluvialis, Pseudomonas putrefaciens*, and *Staphylococcus* species (124). *Vibrio carchariae*, a newly recognized human pathogen, was responsible for a wound infection following a shark bite off the South Carolina coast (327).

Measures to be taken to avoid a confrontation with a shark include avoidance of shark infested waters or waters near sewage outlets or deep channels (especially at night or dusk), never swimming with open

TABLE 3.4. Microorganisms associated with marine wound infections and antimicrobial therapy.*

	First Choice	Alternative
Aeromonas hydrophila	TMP-SMX	Gentamicin, Tetracycline
Bacteroides fragilis	Metronidazole	Clindamycin
Chromobacterium violaceum	Treatment should be guided by clinical presentation and in vitro susceptibility testing (Mezlocillin and aminoglycoside have been used in a case report)	
Citrobacter diversus	Imipenem	Ciprofloxacin (or others if susceptible in vitro)
Clostridium perfringens	Penicillin G	Clindamycin, Metronidazole
Enterobacter cloacae	Cefotaxime, ceftriaxone or ceftizoxime + aminoglycoside	Imipenem, Aminoglycoside, Sulfa-trimethoprim, Ciprofloxacin
Erysipelothrix rhusopathiae	Penicillin G or Ampicillin	Cephalosporins (1st generation)
Escherichia coli	TMP-SMX	Cephalosporin, Ampicillin, Quinolones, Aminoglycoside
Mycobacterium marinum	Minocycline	Rifampin + Ethambutol Rifampin + TMP-SMZ
Providencia stuartii	Cefotaxime, ceftriaxone or ceftizoxime + aminoglycoside	Imipenem, Aminoglycoside, Sulfa-trimethoprim, Ciprofloxacin
Pseudomonas aeruginosa	Aminoglycoside + antipseudomonal penicillin	Aminoglycoside + ceftazidime
Salmonella enteritidis	Ceftriaxone	Ampicillin, Ciprofloxacin, TMP-SMX
Staphylococcus aureus methacillin-sensitive: methacillin resistant	Penicillin resistant synthetic Penicillin Vancomycin	Vancomycin ?TMP-SMX
Streptococcus species	Penicillin G	Erythromycin, Clindamycin
Vibrio species (see text)	Tetracycline ± aminoglycoside (if systemic spread is suspected)	TMP-SMZ (possibly quinolones if susceptible in vitro)

*With rapid emergence of antimicrobial resistence, these empiric recommendations should be confirmed by in vitro susceptibility testing.

wounds or in isolated waters, and storing captured fish away from divers (364,365). If confronted by a shark, the swimmer should leave the water with slow, purposeful movements, facing the shark and avoiding the urge to flee rapidly. In deeper waters, the diver should seek refuge near a wall or other object offering protection from behind or find a confined area which the shark would have difficulty accessing. The shark may desist with blows applied to its snout, gills, or eyes.

Barracuda

Sphyraena barracuda, or the great barracuda, is the only species implicated in human attacks (364,365). These fish may grow to 10 feet in length and weigh 100 pounds. They can be found in tropical and semitropical waters of the Atlantic (Brazil to Florida), and the Pacific (Hawaii). Barracudas involved in attacks are usually solitary, although attacks have occurred by schools. (Their attacks are swift and ferocious and usually occur out of confusion in turbid waters or when they are attracted by shiny objects. Their teeth are canine-like and sharp. The bite produces a V-shaped or straight laceration, often in rows. Treatment is analagous to shark bites.

Moray eels

Moray eels are found in tropical, semitropical, and some temperate waters (365). They are fierce, muscular bottom dwellers that hide in crevices and under rocks and coral. Some species may grow up to 15 feet in length. Divers usually confront these creatures while probing around rocks and coral with their hands. Most smaller species will flee when confronted. If provoked or cornered, an eel may inflict a serious laceration with its vise-like jaws and fang-like teeth.

Occasionally an eel will not release its grip. Attempts to disarticulate the jaw or kill the animal may be necessary. An eel's skin is leathery and may not be easily cut. Treatment is similar to that for shark bites (365).

Other

Needlefish are long, streamlined surface fish found in tropical waters that may attain lengths up to 2 meters (365). They have a long sharp snout which occasionally has been reported to impale people, as this fish frequently jumps out of the water. Injuries have involved the chest, abdomen, neck, and head with one case of a fatal brain injury (367). Sea lions, may be aggressive, especially mating males or females and their pups (364). AAs seals are mammals, rabies prophylaxis should be considered for their bites (364).

Envenomations

Stingrays

Eleven species of stingrays are found in United States' waters, of which seven are found in the waters of the Atlantic Ocean and four in the Pacific Ocean (273). Stingrays are frequently implicated in cases of human envenomation, with at least 2,000 stingray injuries recorded in the United States annually (364). They may be subdivided into four categories which are (in ascending order of toxicity): the butterfly rays (gymnurid type), the eagle and bat rays (myliobatid type), the stingrays and whiprays (dasyatid type), and the round rays (urolophid type) (273). Stingrays are found in tropical, subtropical, and warm temperate waters in shallow intertidal areas such as bays, lagoons, river mouths, and sandy areas between reefs. These marine animals, which may reach up to 50 to 60 "square" feet in size, are round, diamond, or kite shaped objects with wide wing-like pectoral fins. They often lie on the surface bottom covered by sand with only their eyes, spiracles, or parts of their elongated, whip-like tail exposed. Stingrays have one to four venomous stingers arranged on the dorsum of the tail. The stingers consist of dentine spines which are tapered and retroserrated so they may enter the skin easily but are extracted with difficulty and worsening of the laceration (273). Each spine is covered by an integumentary sheath which houses a venom gland in the ventrolateral groove along either side. The spine is covered by a layer of venom and mucus. The venom is a highly unstable and a very heat-labile protein consisting of at least 10 amino acids with toxic components such as serotonin, 5'-nucleotidase, and phosphodiesterase (273,368). Envenomation usually occurs when an unwary swimmer steps on the stingray while wading in shallow waters. The stingray in turn strikes the individual by lashing its tail upward forcing its spines into the victim. The lower extremities are involved in most cases, although any part of the body is susceptible.

Initial manifestations consist of intense localized pain with soft tissue edema and bleeding (273,369). The pain may intensify and spread over a period of 30 to 90 minutes and then gradually diminish over the next 6 to 48 hours. Minor wounds resemble cellulitis; however, more severe wounds may appear dusky and cyanotic with progression to rapid hemmorhage and necrosis of fat and muscle. Secondary infection is common (364).

The venom affects the cardiovascular system and can cause peripheral vasoconstriction or dilatation and cardiac arrhythmias (369). Respiratory depression (via the medullary centers) and convulsions may also occur. Other symptoms include nausea, vomiting, generalized edema (with truncal wounds), limb paralysis, and hypotension (273).

Initial treatment should consist of irrigation with cool water cool water or saline to produce local vasoconstriction and debridement with exploration to remove any sheath contents left in the wound (273,364). X-rays should be obtained to identify any missed fragments. The wound should be soaked in hot water (113 °F) for 30 to 90 minutes. The benefit of this probably has to do with the thermolabile nature of the protein. Narcotics and infiltration with 1% to 2% lidocaine without epinephrine may provide pain control. Regional nerve anesthesia with 0.5% bupivicaine may be necessary (273). The wound should be packed open for delayed primary closure or sutured loosely. Antibiotic prophylaxis is recommended as noted above for shark bites. Steroids and antihistamines are without documented efficacy (364).

Scorpionfish

Scorpionfish can be found in the shallow reef waters of the Gulf of Mexico, the Florida Keys, and coastlines of California and Hawaii (365). Members of this group are responsible for about 300 envenomations annually in the United States (370). Several hundred species are known to exist which can be divided into three genera based on the structure of the venom glands: *Synanceja* (stonefish); *Scorpaena* (sculpin, scorpionfish, and bullrout); and *Pterois* (zebrafish, lionfish, and butterfly cod) (273,364). Scorpionfish often hide under rocks, in coral crevices, or buried in the mud blending in excellently with their surroundings due to their colorful and ornate camouflage. Stonefish aré unattractive bottom dwellers which are regarded as the most lethal of these poisonous marine denizens. The potency of their venom is comparable to cobra venom. A small number of domestic envenomations occur in tropical fish hobbyists who carelessly handle illegally obtained scorpionfish (371). The venom organs consist of 12 to 13 dorsal, 2 pelvic, and 3 anal spines. The ornate pectoral spines are not venomous. Paired glands exist at the base of the anterolateral spines and venom flows along grooves in these spines. Approximately 5 to 10 mg of venom may be found in each paired gland (273). When threatened, these fish erect the dorsal spines, flare out the armed gill covers, and protrude the pectoral and anal fins (372). Venom is injected in a manner analagous to a stingray envenomation. The potency of the venom varies according to the species. The pharmacology of scorpionfish venom is poorly understood (373). Wounds inflicted by lionfish are mild compared to scorpionfish, with stonefish wounds being the most severe (273).

Intense pain occurs immediately after the injury and radiates up the extremity (273,364). If untreated, the pain peaks in 60 to 90 minutes, often lasting 6 to 12 hours or perhaps days. Stonefish envenomation may produce pain severe enough to precipitate delusions (372). The wounds initially appear ischemic and cyanotic with surrounding areas of erythema, edema, and warmth (273). Progressive cellulitis and local induration may follow, occasionally with vesicle formation. Tissue necrosis with sloughing may occur within 48 hours. Wounds may take months to heal, with occasional soft tissue fibrous defects or cutaneous granulomata persisting. Secondary infection or deep abscesses may occur. Systemic effects include paresthesias, skin rash, nausea, vomiting, arthralgias, fever, diarrhea, delirium, seizures, abdominal pain, hypertension, arryhthmias, limb paralysis, congestive heart failure, hypotension, and death. In the case of stonefish envenomation, dyspnea and circulatory collapse may occur within 1 hour, with death ensuing within 6 hours (364).

Initial treatment of scorpionfish injuries is analogous to stingray injuries with proper irrigation and debridement to ensure removal of any persistent source of venom (273,364). Inadequate debridement may predispose to ulceration with tissue extension. Immersion in hot water (113 °F) for 30 to 90 minutes may alleviate the pain, possibly secondary to toxin inactivation; longer durations may be needed for persistent pain. Wounds should be packed open for delayed primary closure or sutured loosely to allow drainage. Antibiotic therapy is recommended for deep puncture wounds of the hand or foot because of the high incidence of tissue complications (273). Recommended antibiotics include third generation cephalosporins, trimethoprim-sulfamethoxazole, chloramphenicol, tetracycline, aminoglycosides, or imipenem-cilastatin (273). Severe systemic reactions due to *Synanceja* species (and less rarely from other scorpionfish) necessitates the use of intravenous stonefish equine antivenin. It is supplied in 2 mL ampules, with 1 mL capable of neutralizing 10 mg of dried venom. Antivenins are produced in Australia and India and may be acquired in the United States from the Health Services Department; Sea World in San Diego; Sea World in Aurora, Ohio; and the Steinhart Aquarium in San Francisco. Physicians may alternatively locate antivenin by contacting an accredited regional poison center (273).

Sea Snakes

Sea snakes are probably the most abundant reptile in the world. Fifty-two species are known and all are venomous (372). At least seven species have been implicated in fatal envenomations (1). The sea snake is a marine adapted serpent belonging to the family Hydrophidae and is closely relatied to the cobra and krait. They are widely distributed in tropical and subtropical waters along the coasts of the Indian and Pacific Oceans and the Gulf of California. There are no sea snakes in the Atlantic Ocean or Caribbean Sea (1). These reptiles have a flat tail which assists them in propulsion. They can travel with ease in both a forward and reverse direction. Some species may attain lengths of up to 10 feet. These creatures can remain submerged in the water for hours utilizing an air retention system to control buoyancy. Although usually docile, they may attack when provoked, especially during the mating season (372). Sea snakes have two to four maxillary fangs, each of which is associated with a pair of venom glands. Fangs of most species are too short to penetrate a diver's wet suit (372). Many envenomations are avoided by the fact that the fangs are easily dislodged. The venom is more potent than terrestial snake venom and its toxicity is derived primarily from potent neurotoxins (373). Neurotoxins may exert their effects through the inhibition of cholinesterase or by blocking presynaptic or postsynaptic impulses. Most sea snake venom contains only postsynaptic neurotoxin which strongly binds to the acetylcholine receptor at the neuromuscular junction. The venom may contain other toxins including hyaluronidase, phosphodiesterase, phospholipase A, and proteases (373). Phospholipase A and other myotoxins may cause muscle necrosis with myoglobin release (374). These myotoxic, hemolytic, neurotoxic, and vasoactive components constitute a serious medical emergency if envenomation occurs.

The bites are extremely small and characterized by multiple (usually 1 to 20) pinhead, hypodermic-like puncture wounds (372). Initially, the pain is only minimal without any local reaction. Neurological symptoms occur within 2 to 3 hours in most cases and always within 8 hours of the bite. If no symptoms develop within 8 hours, significant envenomation did not occur. Typical signs and symptoms include painful muscle movement, myoglobinuria, euphoria, trismus, malaise, anxiety, ascending paralysis, slurred speech, dysphagia, ptosis, and ophthalmoplegia. Death is rare and is usually due to more severe reactions including myonecrosis, respiratory insufficiency, bulbar paralysis, and hepatic, cardiac, or renal failure (273,375).

Diagnosis is based on several factors such as location (sea snake bites occur only in the water), absence of pain (initial pain is unusual), the typical appearance of the fang bites (usually 1 to 4), identification of the snake (it should be caught if possible), and the development of characteristic symptoms within 8 hours (occasionally as early as 5 minutes) (365).

Treatment is similar to that for most terrestrial snake bites (273). Local suction without incision can be performed if used immediately with a plunger device. Incision and drainage are of no value if delayed for several minutes after the bite, and cryotherapy is contraindicated. The affected limb should be immobilized with application of a proximal venous and lymphatic occlusive band or use of the pressure immobiliztion technique (a cloth pad is pressed directly over the wound by a circumferential elastic wrap at a pressure of ≤70 mmHg) to minimize systemic toxicity. Antivenin is effective if used within 24 to 36 hours and should be used quickly (376). The minimum initial dose of sea snake antivenin is 1 to 3 vials; up to 10 vials may be required. Polyvalent equine antivenin to *Enhydrina schistosa* (beaked sea snake) and *Notechis scutatus* (terrestrial tiger snake) will neutralize the bites of most sea snakes. Anaphylaxis and serum sickness may occur and intradermal sensitivity testing with 0.02 ml of a 1:10 antivenin dilution should be done. *N scutatus* antivenin is a second choice alternative (273). Antivenin in the United States may be obtained from the sources listed in the section on scorpionfish.

Weeverfish

These fish, also referred to as sea cat, sea dragon, adderpike, and stang are found in the temperate waters of the Atlantic Ocean, Mediterranean Sea, and European coastal waters (375). Weeverfish are one of the most venomous fish found in these waters. They are small fish (<50 cm) which can be found buried in the mud or soft bottom which only their head exposed. They produce a venom located in glands associated with dorsal and opercular dentine spines which are capable of piercing a leather boot. Weeverfish are generally docile yet, if provoked, they may become extremely aggressive and strike. Victims are usually professional fishermen or wading swimmers.

The venom is a heat-labile protein substance which also contains 5-hydroxytryptamine, histamine, epinephrine, and norepinephrine (373). An intense burning pain is felt immediately following the sting (375). The pain often spreads throughout the entire limb and generally peaks in intensity within the first hour and usually subsides within 24 hours, although it may persist for days. The initial wound is pale and edematous and becomes erythematous, warm, and ecchymotic with increasing edema. It may take months to heal. Headache, delirium, fever, dyspnea, diaphoresis, nausea, vomiting, seizures, hypotension, and cardiac arrhythmias may occur (365).

Treatment is similar to stingray envenomations. The pain is often poorly controlled even with the liberal use of narcotics (365). An antivenin may be available soon (364). Weeverfish should never be handled when alive; they may survive for hours out of water (375).

Catfish

More than 1,000 species of freshwater and saltwater catfish exist (364). These fish are named for the sensory barbels surrounding the mouth. Catfish have long thin venom glands covered by an integumentary sheath located on lateral ridges along the dorsal and pectoral spines (315). Catfish may lock these fins in an extended position when excited, thereby inflicting a dramatic sting if mishandled. Fragments of tissue and spine may remain in the wound. The venom contains dermatonecrotic, vasoconstrictive, and other bioactive agents (364). Immediate severe pain, throbbing, and weakness occur. The pain usually radiates locally and proximally and generally resolves in 30 to 60 minutes, occasionally lasting 48 hours. Nausea, vomiting, respiratory distress, and mild hypotension may occur. Muscle fasciculations and local muscle spasms are common. The wound site may appear pale and bleed longer than expected. Cyanosis at the puncture site may occur followed by local tissue necrosis or skin sloughing. Swelling of the extremity, a serous discharge, slow wound healing, and local lymphadenopathy may persist for weeks to months

(377). Secondary infections are common and gangrene has been reported. Envenomation by the oriental catfish(*Plotosus lineatus*)may produce more marked systemic symptoms (311).

Treatment is similar to that for stingray envenomations, although the venom is not as potent (365). X-rays should be obtained, as the radiopaque spines are frequently left in place. The wound should be thoroughly irrigated and debrided. Irrigation with permanganate, bicarbonate, acetic acid, or papain have not been shown to be of benefit. Tourniquets have no value (365). Updating of tetanus immunization, as in other marine puncture wounds, is essential. Antibiotics should be administered if the wound is dirty or complicated. Local wound care alone is probably adequate for properly treated clean wounds in healthy individuals (377).

Invertebrate Envenomations

Coelenterates

The phylum Cnidaria (formerly Coelenterata) is a massive group of marine invertebrates consisting of more than 9,000 species, of which at least 100 are hazardous to humans (273). Classes are Scyphozoa (true jelly fish), Hydrozoa (Fire coral, Portuguese man-of-war, Pacific blue bottle), and Anthozoa (sea anenomes, soft coral) (378). These species may contain millions of nematocysts (also known as "stinging capsules" or "nettle cells") which are microscopic toxin-containing organs capable of injecting venom into their prey when triggered. Nematocysts are found along the outside of long, streaming tentacles and near the mouth of the animal. Each nematocyst consists of a minute capsule (cnidoblast) that contains a spiral-coiled thread with a barbed end. Specialized triggers (cnidocil) on the capsule are capable of forcefully ejecting the venomous barbs at pressures up to 2 to 5 psi, enough to penetrate a surgical glove (364). This produces a severe "sting." The size of the barb and the potency of the venom varies among the different species. The cnidocil may be triggered by abrasion or freshwater contact. A single man-of-war envenomation may involve several hundred thousand nematocysts (365).

The human reactions to jellyfish toxin may be classified as systemic, local, chronic, or fatal (379). Local reactions include persistent or recurrent eruptions, eruptions distant to the site of envenomation, exaggerated local angioedema, papular urticaria, and contact dermatitis. Chronic reactions include keloid formation, pigmentation, fat atrophy, mononeuritis, autonomic nerve paralysis, gangrene, vascular spasm, and ataxia. Systemic reactions may include muscle cramps, nausea, vomiting, tachycardia, abdominal pain, and hypertension. Death may occur through cardiotoxic, central respiratory, or renal mechanisms. Anaphylaxis has been reported (380).

The potency and composition of the toxin varies among different species. After injection of large doses of toxin into human skin, a perivascular mononuclear cell infiltrate appears within the dermis. A cell-mediated and humoral immune response then occurs. Lymphokines and prostaglandins account for some of the cutaneous manifestations of jellyfish envenomation (342). Serotonin, histamine, or histamine-releasing agents are responsible for much of the burning pain and urticaria. High molecular weight toxins may inhibit nerve activity through altered ionic permeability. These protein and tetramine fractions have direct and indirect effects on the autonomic nervous system and end organs, particularly the vascular, cardiac, and central nervous systems. A destabilizing effect on the cell membrane appears to be mediated by the calcium channel. Verapamil may block this effect (364).

Fire corals (*Millepora*) are not true corals. They are branching bottom dwellers which may attain heights of 1 to 2 meters. They develop upright, clavate, bladelike, or branching calcareous growths that form encrustations over rocks, shellfish, other coral, and man-made objects. The white to yellow-green lime carbonate exoskeleton may become razor sharp. The nematocyst-bearing tentacles protrude from numerous minute surface gastropores (372). These stings account for the majority of coelenterate envenomations. An intense burning pain, with central radiation and reactive regional lymphadenopathy follows envenomation (273).

The Portuguese man-of-war (*Physalia physalis*) and the Pacific blue bottle (*Physalis utriculus*) are not true jellyfish, they are colonial hydroids (378). These open sea surface creatures are widely distributed in the Atlantic (*Physalia physalis*) and Pacific (*Physalia utriculus*) Oceans and are most commonly found in the semitropical Atlantic Ocean. They are composed of a large nitrogen and carbon monoxide-filled sail which may achieve lengths up to 30 cm across. Numerous nematocyst-laden tentacles (up to 750,000 nematocysts per tentacle) stream downward from the sail, attaining lengths of up to 30 meters (*Physalia physalis*). The animal is carried along by wind and ocean currents. Fish and other objects may become entangled in the tentacles which contract rhythmically in search of prey. Broken-off tentacle fragments may retain their potency for months (365).

Chironex fleckeri (Box-Jellyfish or Sea Wasp) is the most venomous sea creature known (365). Death may occur within 1 minute of envenomation and the overall mortality is 15% to 20%. These creatures are found in the protected waters off the northern Australian coast. A less lethal variety is found in the waters of the Chesapeake Bay (364). Up to 10 mL of venom may be injected during a "sting." Sea wasps are small creatures (2 to 10 cm in diameter) capable of attaining speeds up to 2 knots in steady winds with swift currents. Factors determining the severity of envenomation include the length and width of the wheal, the length of the contact, the thickness of the skin, the percentage of nematocysts discharged, and the "venom load" which is related to recent feeding (381). A sheep-derived antivenin is available and is given intravenously or intamuscularly (20,000 units, or one vial, IV over 5 minutes or three vials IM) (381).

Sea anenomes are sessile, multicolored, flower-like Anthozoans which may attain diameters of up to one-half meter (365). They have finger-like projections containing numerous modified nematocysts referred to as sporocysts. They are usually encountered by skin divers and waders.

The Irukundji syndrome may follow stings by the Cuboza class jellyfish (*Carukia barnesi*) (379). A small but transient sting initiates this reaction. A severe, boring pain may develop in the abdomen or sacrum with gradual spread to the thighs and chest where the sensation is described as cramping. Severe, excruciation myalgias persist over the next 24 to 48 hours. Other symptoms include tremor, anxiety, piloerection, hyperpnea, headache, nausea, vomiting, sweating, restlessness, tachycardia, blood-streaked sputum, and oliguria. A rapidly developing pulmonary edema leading to acute respiratory failure may develop (382). This syndrome, similar to excess catecholamine release, is assumed to represent a toxic reaction to the venom of this small jellyfish. (379).

The person who has endured a coelenterate sting should immediately soak the area in 5% acetic acid (vinegar) (273). Isopropyl alcohol (40% to 70%) is a reasonable alternative, although some argue that this may cause further venom release. Other detoxicants of possible benefit include dilute ammonium hydroxide, sodium bicarbonate, olive oil, sugar, urine, and papain (unseasoned meat tenderizer). Fresh water should never be applied to the area as this may trigger further nematocyst release. The area should be soaked for at least 30 minutes or until the pain disappears. The area should not be abraded or scrubbed. Any large tentacles or remaining fragments should be removed by a forceps with doubly-gloved hands. Once cleaned, shaving cream should be applied and the area shaved gently.

Anaphylaxis should always be anticipated. After decontamination, corticosteroids or topical anesthetics can be used. Antibiotics are usually not needed; however, large open lesions should be cleaned daily and covered with a thin layer of nonsensitizing antiseptic ointment. Tetanus immunization should be current. Wounds should be checked by a physician for signs of infection 3 and 7 days after the injury.

Echinoderms

Sea urchins and star fish are found in this group of marine animals. The venom contains many toxic substances including steroid glycosides, serotonin, and acetylcholine-like substances. Certain sea urchins may produce potent neurotoxins (365).

Sea urchins are globular or flattened animals with a hard shell enclosing their vital organs (372). Regularly arranged spines and a triple-jawed seizing organ (pedicellariae) cover this shell. Spines may be venom-bearing or nonvenom-bearing. The pedicellariae are dispersed among the spines and may grab hold of prey with their pincer-like jaws. They also contain venom glands that release toxic material when they contract. The venom inflicts intense burning stings which may progress to muscular paralysis, respiratory distress, and occasionally death if numerous spines are involved. Hot water may provide relief. The pedicellariae and embedded spines should be removed with care because they are easily fractured. Residual spines may form granulomas (273).

Starfish are simple, free-living, stellate echinoderms covered with simple thorny spines of calcium carbonate crystals held erect by muscle tissue (372). Glandular tissue interspersed throughout or located beneath the integument produces a slimy, venomous substance that causes a contact dermatitis. Envenomation occurs when the victim contacts the thorny spines, some of which may grow to 6 cm in length. Envenomation rarely induces systemic symptoms such as paresthesias, vomiting, and muscular paralysis. The dermatitis may be treated with hot water and topical calamine with 0.5% menthol.

Mollusks

Cone shells are potentially lethal gastropods that possess a sophisticated venom apparatus (365). At least 18 to 400 species have been implicated in human fatalities. They are nocturnal feeders located in the Indo-Pacific area. A set of minute harpoon-like radular teeth may contain venom which is injected from an extensible proboscis. The venom interferes with neuromuscular transmission in a manner analogous to curare. Initial symptoms include local ischemia, cyanosis, and numbness. More severe envenomations may induce parasthesias and generalized muscular paralysis with respiratory failure. Other symptoms include dysphagia, aphonia, weakness, diplopia, blurred vision, cerebral edema, disseminated intravascular coagulation, coma, and cardiovascular collapse. Death may occur in as little as 2 hours. Therapy is largely supportive. Hot water immersions may alleviate some of the pain.

Octopi are cephalopods found in the warm waters of the intertidal zon (365). The Australian spotted (*O maculosus*) and blue-ringed (*O lunulatus*) octopi have been implicated in human fatalities. The blue-ringed octopus is covered with poorly visible blue rings which become iridescent peacock blue when the octopus is angered. Parrot-like and powerful chitinous jaws are capable of penetrating through the dermis of the skin and into the muscle tissue. Venom is injected into the victim who is usually a naive swimmer playing with what seems to be a harmless creature. The toxin blocks nerve conduction, most likely by altering sodium conductance. Myocardial and respiratory depression are observed in animal models. Following the initial bite, an intense burning or throbbing with central radiation occurs. Within 30 minutes marked local erythema, swelling, pruritis, and pain may occur. Severe envenomations include nausea, vomiting, paresthesias, blurred vision, aphonia, dysphagia, ataxia, myoclonus, flaccid paralysis, hypotension, and respiratory failure. Treatment is supportive with wide excision of the involved area down to deep fascia. Closure may be primary or by a full-thickness skin graft. There is no effective antivenin available.

Dermatitis

Most cases of dermatitis in swimmers and beachgoers are the result of contact with the Coelenterata. In 1991, an outbreak of cercarial dermatitis was noted among 37 students frequenting a Delaware beach. Cercarial dermatitis, or "swimmer's itch," is a cutaneous inflammation due to penetration of the skin by cercariae, which are the free-living larval stages of bird schistosomes (383). Hosts include migratory waterbirds, including shorebirds, ducks, and geese. Adult worms are carried in the bloodstream and produce eggs that are passed in the feces. Once exposed to the water, the eggs hatch to produce miracidiae which infect mollusks. The parasite develops in the snail to produce cercariae which penetrate the skin of birds to complete the cycle. Humans are accidental hosts. The cercariae are able to penetrate the skin but do not develop further.

This dermatological entity has a worldwide distribution. Symptoms include reddening and itching of exposed skin in the water or immediately after emerging, and delayed onset of pruritic raised papules which may form vesicles. Previous exposure may elicit a more severe response upon reexposure. Treatment consists of antihistamines and topical antipruritic medications.

Cutaneous larva migrans is a dermatitis caused by invasion of the skin by larval nematodes (384). Most infections are due to the filariform larvae of the dog and cat hookworm, *Ancyclostoma braziliense*, although several other larval nematodes may cause the disease including *A caninum*, *A duodenale*, and Necatur americanus. Adult *A braziliense* inhabit the intestines of dogs and cats. They produce eggs which pass in the feces to hatch in the soil in 1 to 2 days. Within a week, they become infective filariform larvae. Humans are inadvertent hosts when the larvae penetrate the skin, although they usually don't penetrate further than the epidermis. The disease has a worldwide distribution and is much more common in tropical and semitropical areas. People who frequent beaches are at increased risk (hence, the synonym "sandworm").

Symptoms develop within a few hours of penetration into the skin. A pruritic red papule develops which may form a serpiginous tract. The surrounding tissues become edematous and acutely inflamed. The tracts may become encrusted and secondarily infected. The pruritus may become extremely intense. Untreated, the larvae may persist in the skin for months. Treatment consists of thiabendazole administered orally or topically.

Swimmer's Ear

Swimmer's ear, or acute external otitis media, is the most common medical problem faced by swimmers (385). It begins initially not as an infection, but as an eczema of the ear canal caused by retention of water in the ear following bathing, showering, or swimming (386). By the time medical attention is sought, the ear is usually secondarily infected. The normal external auditory canal is sterile bacteriologically in up to 30% of the population, with the remainder harboring mixed flora including *Staphylococcus albus*, *Staphylococcus epidermidis*, diphtheroids, and to a lesser extent, *Staphylococcus aureus* and *Streptococcus viridans* (387,388). In external otitis media, cultures usually reveal mixed flora with gram-negative bacteria predominating in up to three-quarters of affected individuals under the age of 21. *Pseudomonas* species, the most common offending organisms, are isolated in up to one-half of the cases (389). Other species include *Proteus vulgaris*, *Escherichia coli*, *Staphylococcus aureus*, *Staphylococcus epidermidis*, *Streptococci*, diphtheroids, *Enterobacter aerogenes, Klebsiella pneumoniae*, and *Citrobacter*. Approximately 40% of infected ears yield fungal isolates, with *Aspergillus* species representing the majority of such cases (385).

The pathogenesis of swimmer's ear is multifactorial, with cerumen playing a major role. Cerumen imparts an acid reaction to the external canal lowering its pH to 5 and thereby inhibiting bacterial and fungal growth. In addition, its lipid content provides a protective surface to the squamous epithelium and pilosebaceous elements of the canal. Cerumen, therefore, provides a chemical and mechanical barrier to infection. Excessive moisture in the external canal, which can occur during swimming, bathing, or excessive sweating, can lead to mechanical disruption of this barrier with subsequent desquamation and maceration. In addition, the decrease in cerumen results in a raising of the pH to 7 which allows bacterial species to proliferate. As inflammation occurs, a purulent exudate forms which mixes with dry skin providing a wet environment suitable for bacterial prowth.

The earliest symptom is usually itching which often leads to manipulation. Trauma from cotton swabs or mechanical objects inserted into the canal can exacerbate the condition. A purulent discharge develops accompanied by progressive tenderness and pain. Hearing loss may result from canal skin edema and accumulation of debris. The diagnosis can be confirmed by manipulation of the tragus and pinna which elicits a severe painful reaction. Attempts at otoscopic visualization may be hampered by the pain as well as the accumulation of debris. Regional lymphadenopathy and cellulitis of the external auricle can occasionally occur. Fungal otitis externa may be accompanied only by itching and a feeling of fullness. In thses cases, hyphae may be visualized on microscopic examination, or in the case of *Aspergillus niger*, a greyish membrane may be noted in the external canal.

Initial treatment should begin with the recognition and elimination of specific precipitating factors, such as swimming or manipulation of the ear, until the disorder is corrected (385). Pain control may be necessary during the first 24 to 48 hours of treatment (390). Severe cases may require narcotic analgesics or even hospitalization for intramuscular analgesics and intravenous antibiotics. Thorough irrigation and cleaning is essential to remove the purulent debris and allow penetration by topical antibiotics. Various cleansing solutions have been utilized including 3% acetic acid, 70% alcohol, 3% boric acid-70% alcohol solution, and Burrow's solution (385). Cleansing and irrigating may be required on a daily basis. In cases where the debris is too thick, an expanding cellulose wick may be implanted within the canal to allow antibiotic penetration.

Topical antibiotics are usually adequate in all but the most severe cases which may require systemic agents. The most widely prescribed otic solutions contain the antibiotics neomycin and polymyxin which are effective against most of the usual pathogens. Neomycin is effective against *Proteus* and *Staphylococcus* species; polymyxin is usually effective against *Pseudomonas* Chloromycetin otic drops are available for less commonly encountered anaerobic infections. In the event of otitis externa due to *Aspergillus niger*, local application of amphotericin B, oxytetracycline and polymyxin, iodochlorhydroxyquin, and nystatin may be effective (385). Candidal infections may be treated with topical nystatin. Most otic preparations also contain an acidifying agent(s) and a topical steroid to reduce the inflammation.

Individuals prone to otitis externa who are frequently exposed to water may benefit from any of several commercially available ear plugs and other devices which prevent water from entering the canal. A recent comparison of seven different ear protectors used by a group of swimmers found the most effective plugs to be cotton wool coated in paraffin jelly (391). Prevention may be further enhanced by the use of acidifying drops and/or drying ear drops before and after swimming. Domeboro, Swim Ear, Aqua Ear, Ear Magic, and VoSol Otic drops are several such commercial agents (385). Alternatively, the user may make his or her own preparation by mixing white vinegar with 70% alcohol. Controversy exists with regard to swimming with tympanostomy tubes in place (392–394). While some experts advocate the use of protective ear plugs or avoidance of water immersion, others have recommended pre- and postexposure antibiotic otic drops. A third group utilizing data revealing that the incidence of otitis media is no greater in swimmers with tympanostomy tubes in place who swam without protection than those without tympanostomy tubes has recommended that no ear protection or instillation of pre- and postexposure antibitic drops are necessary (393–395). Until this matter is clarified, it may be prudent to advocate some means of protection against infection in susceptible individuals who are frequently exposed to water (385).

Section IV: Hepatitis and Other Viruses

Marine samples of water have been estimated to yield between 5×10^6 and 15×10^6 total viruses per mL (396). Even though the majority of these viruses are nonpathogenic in man, viral agents associated with hepatitis and gastroenteritis are known to be present in and capable of producing disease through contaminated water (397). Samples of water taken off the Texas Gulf Coast have revealed the presence of enteroviruses such as coxsackievirus, echovirus, poliovirus, and hepatitis A (398). These enteroviruses were detected in over 40% of waters deemed safe for recreational use by fecal coliform standards. Thirty five percent of waters approved for shellfish harvesting yielded enteroviruses (398). Enteroviruses have been reported to survive 2 to 130 days in seawater in laboratory studies (399) and possibly up to 18 months (400). Temperature seems to be the most important factor, with many enteroviruses able to survive for months at temperatures below 10° C (401). Marine sediments also protect against virus inactivation, probably by reducing the rate of thermal inactivation (401).

Although controversy exists, swimming areas have been suggested to be involved in the spread of some common viral illnesses (402,403). In Wisconsin, a statistically significant increase was noted in the use of public beaches by children with documented enteroviral illness as compared to children without enteroviral illness (404). Several other reports have similarly suggested increased enteroviral infections in swimmers using public swimming areas (402,403,405–407). A survey of oysters contaminated by enteroviruses in Japan found nearly identical viruses in sick children in the immediate area. The authors suggested that water and oyster contamination ultimately depend on the prevalence of enteric viral infections in local inhabitants (408). In addition to more common and less severe enteroviral illnesses, an outbreak of hepatitis A involving 20 campers in Louisiana was associated with swimming in a contaminated swimming pool (409).

Shellfish harvested from contaminated waters have been implicated in numerous outbreaks of food-borne illness (410). They spread disease by virtue of their ability to filter large amounts of water, retain filtered products in the gills and alimentary tract, and accumulate them in the liver. Shellfish have the ability to concentrate hepatitis A virus up to 15 times the level in the immediate water (411). Commercially harvested waters are monitored for contamination through the use of bacterial counts. Although this method effectively decreases the incidence of illness related to contaminated shellfish, there is not a reliable correlation between bacterial counts and the presence of pathogenic viruses (398). Several methods of detecting viruses or viral particles have been investigated, although the use of any one method of testing may not be sufficient enough to provide accurate measurements (408). Furthermore, viral testing has proven to be costly and time consuming (412). Control measures have included the regulation of drainage effluent into monitored areas, supervision of drainage from commercial fishing boats, frequent testing of water and shellfish from harvest areas for fecal coliforms and other bacteria, closing of contaminated waters, and removal of contaminated shellfish from markets (412). Depuration measures in which bacteria and viruses are removed by bathing in rapidly circulating salt water treated continuously by ultraviolet radiation for up to 72 hours have decreased the incidence of food-borne outbreaks, although this process is not infallible (413,414). Outbreaks of viral diseases have been attributed to depurated shellfish (415). Prevention of illness additionally relies on public education, particularly in regard to proper cooking of shellfish. It has been shown that it takes up to 6 minutes of steaming for the internal temperature of clams to reach that of the immediate seurrounding (416). Clams will open their shells in less than 1 minute. Hepatitis A virus has been shown to be inactivated by heating at 85°C for 1 minute, and partially inactivated by heating at 85°C for 1 minute, and partially inactivated at 60°C for 60 minutes (417,418). Recent evidence suggests that microwaving may be beneficial in inactivating hepatitis A, however further studies are needed (419).

Hepatitis A Virus

Hepatitis A was first linked to the ingestion of raw shellfish in Sweden in 1956; 629 oyster-associated cases were documented (420). The first cases of hepatitis A linked to raw shellfish consumption in the United States occurred in 1961; both clams and oysters were involved (421). Hepatitis A caused less than 7% of the 224 recorded outbreaks of water-borne disease in the United States between 1971 and 1978; it caused none of the outbreaks recorded in 1981 (422,423). During 1983 to 1988, the incidence of reported cases of hepatitis A increased from 9.2 to 10.9 cases per 100,000 population, which represented the first increase in hepatitis A in more than a decade (424–426). In 1988, 26,600 cases of hepatitis A were reported in the United States, 7.3% of which were associated with food-borne or water-borne outbreaks (425,427). In August of 1988, 61 persons developed hepatitis A after having ingested oysters illegally harvested from coastal waters off Bay County, Florida (428,429). That same year, the largest documented epidemic to date occurred in Shanghai, China in which more than 288,000 people developed hepatitis A after ingesting raw or improperly cooked clams (412,430).

Shellfish implicated in cases of hepatitis A include oysters, clams, cockles, and mussels (431). In addition, the illness had been traced to contaminated lettuce, raspberries, ice-slush beverages, and community water sources (410,428,432,433). Sporadic cases also occur; disease is probably underreported. Restaurant-related outbreaks due to poor personal hygiene by infected food preparers has also been noted (419,431). In many cases, a source for outbreaks is never determined (419,428).

The incubation period ranges from 3 to 6 weeks. Presentation consists of a prodrome of fatigue, malaise, anorexia, nausea, and right upper quadrant discomfort. Dark urine subsequently develops, with liver enlargement and biochemical evidence of hepatitis. Icteric disease may be prolonged in adults, lasting 4 to 6 weeks; fulminant hepatic failure is rare and chronic disease or a carrier state does not develop. Secondary cases in families may be seen. Attack rates vary ranging from 10% to 97%, with higher rates associated with increasing dose and age (410,434).

Norwalk Virus

Norwalk virus is the most common infectious cause of acute gastroenteritis following shellfish ingestion (434). Named after the town in Ohio in which an outbreak of acute gastroenteritis occurred in 1968, it wasn't until 1972 that this virus was first identified by immune electron microscopy of bacteria-free stool isolates from the 1968 outbreak (435). The particles measured 27 nanometers and were noted to be more visible when present in clusters covered with antibody. They were also noted to aggregate with convalescent but not acute serum from patients with the gastroenteritis. A serum radioimmunoassay (RIA) for IgM antibody to the Norwalk virus or the demonstration of a fourfold rise in titers utilizing paired acute and convalescent sera is more sensitive and specific than electron microscopy (434,436,437). Using similar methods, the Norwalk virus was identified as the cause of 42% of the 74 outbreaks of acute, nonbacterial gastroenteritis investigated by the Centers for Disease Control between 1976 and 1980 (422,437,438). Six additional outbreaks involving more than 820 persons were noted between 1981 and 1983 (438). Drinking water and recreational water used for swimming were the vehicle of transmission in most of these earlier outbreaks. Contamination by human sewage was the most likely explanation, although this was never proven. Shellfish-associated Norwalk viral illness was first recognized in Australia in 1978 when 2,000 people developed acute gastroenteritis following raw oyster ingestion (439). Immune electron microscopy of 93 stool specimens revealed the 27 nanometer viral particle in 39% of those examined. An additional, as yet unclarified 22 nanometer viral particle was also identified in 50% of the specimens examined. In 1982, 103 well-documented outbreaks of oyster- and clam-associated illness involving 1,017 persons were attributed to the Norwalk virus in New York state in 1982 (440). Seroconversion to Norwalk virus antibody or a positive response for IgM antibody to the virus (or both) were noted in 5 of 7 outbreaks; clams and oysters revealed Norwalk virus antibody by radioimmunoassay in 4 of 6 specimens examined, including clams and oysters from two of the outbreaks. Coliform testing of the waters from which the shellfish were harvested were well within acceptable limits.

Incubation times have ranged from 24 to 48 hours in most recorded outbreaks, with a duration of illness ranging from 2 to 60 hours (mean, 12 to 60 hours). Symptoms have consisted of nausea, vomiting, diarrhea, abdominal cramps, and headache, with vomiting being more prominent than diarrhea in children and diarrhea being more common than vomiting in adults. Fever, myalgias, chills, and upper respiratory complaints such as a sore throat, cough, and runny nose, were also noted on occasion. The disease is rarely severe enough to require hospitalization and no fatalities have been recorded. Secondary spread is quite common.

The antibody response is not entirely understood. Antibody prevalence appears to peak within the first 5 decades of life, reaching a prevalence in the United States of 50%. Children tend to acquire antibody earlier in less developed countries. Individuals exposed to the Norwalk agent in volunteer studies who do not become ill have been shown not to develop an antibody response. When immunity develops, it is specific towards the Norwalk virus and short-lived, lasting from 6 weeks to 2 months (435).

The mechanism by which the Norwalk virus causes diarrhea is not known. Related agents include the Hawaii, Snow Mountain, and Taunton agents, each named after the place they were first described. Only the Snow Mountain agent has been associated with water-borne transmission. Illnesses caused by these Norwalk-like agents are indistinguishable from that due to the Norwalk agent. These other agents are antigenically distinct and antibodies are not cross-protective (410).

Hepatitis E Virus

Hepatitis E virus is the only known cause of enterically transmitted non-A, non-B hepatitis. Hepatitis E is largely water-borne and has been responsible for epidemics of infectious hepatitis in parts of Asia, Indonesia, Africa, and Mexico (441). Previously known as enterically transmitted non-A, non-B hepatitis (ET-NANBH), illness due to hepatitis E was first documented in New Delhi, India in 1955 when 29,000 cases of icteric hepatitis were identified following fecal contamination of the city's water supply (442). A similar epidemic occurred in 1975 in Ahmedabad, India when that city's water supply became fecally contaminated as well (443). Both epidemics were thought to be due to hepatitis A virus until retrospectively analyzed paired serum samples from documented cases revealed in 1980 that neither hepatitis A or B were responsible for the epidemics (444). It now appears that in developing countries more than 50% of acute viral hepatitis appears to be caused by agents other than hepatitis A or B viruses (445). Numerous epidemics of hepatitis E have been reported in Pakistan, Bangladesh, Nepal, Burma, Borneo, Algeria, Somalia, Sudan, Ivory Coast, Mexico, China, Egypt, Ethiopia, and the former Soviet Union (441,446). Imported cases have been reported in the United States (447).

The incubation period appears to be 2 to 9 weeks, with an average of 6 weeks (445). Attack rates have been variable, with the highest rates noted in young to middle-aged adults (15 to 40 years old). The clinical presentation is that of a self-limiting disease resembling infection due to hepatitis A virus. Chronic liver disease or persistent viremia has not been reported. Mortality has been reported to be between 0.5% to 3.0% in the general population. Pregnant women in the third trimester of Pregnancy have an unusually high mortality of up to 20%, for unknown reasons. In contrast, pregnant women infected with hepatitis A infection have a mortality ranging from 3% to 8%.

The diagnosis of infection due to hepatitis E virus has primarily been based on the identification of the virus in stool samples by immune electron microscopy. Hepatitis E is a spherical, nonenveloped virus 32 to 34 nanometers in size with a genome consisting of a single strand of polyadenylated RNA (445,448). Identification of viral particles in clinical samples has been inconsistent, possibly due to proteolytic degradation or susceptibility to freezing and pelleting (445). Cynomolgus monkeys and, more recently, owl monkeys, have been shown to be promising animal models of the serologic response of infection by the hepatitis E virus (449). Radioimmunoassay (RIA) or enzyme-linked immunoassay (EIA) for hepatitis E antigen using acute-phase or convalescent-phase IgM or IgG have previously met with little success, possibly due to the lability of the virus (445). More recently, an enzyme-linked immunosorbent assay (ELISA) based on clonal recombinant hepatitis E antigen has been developed to detect hepatitis E IgG and IgM antibodies (441). Preliminary results are encouraging.

Rotavirus and Small Round Virus

Rotavirus is a common viral pathogen responsible for a large percentage of childhood diarrheal illness. Rotavirus may be responsible for up to 50% of all cases of diarrhea in hospitalized children and 10% to 20% of diarrhea in the community. By the third year of life, 90% of children will have been exposed to rotavirus and develop antibody. Seventy percent of adults have antibody to rotavirus (450). Adult epidemics of diarrheal illness due to rotavirus in the absence of contact with children have been reported (451,452). Water-borne transmission of rotavirus occurs and was first described in Africa in 1978 (423). In 1981, an outbreak of gastroenteritis due to water-borne transmission of rotavirus involving 1,761 cases occurred in Colorado (422).

Small round viruses are poorly understood, unculturable viruses which have been linked to shellfish-related epidemics of gastroenteritis (453, 454). They are morphologically distinct from other gastroenteritis viruses by electron microscopy and antigenically distinct from the Norwalk and Norwalk-like viruses. Asymptomatic individuals have been shown to shed the virus in some instances.

Conclusion

In conclusion, a wide array of seafood and seacoast injuries involve infections or intoxications that warrant precautions and alert, prompt consideration in the appropriate clinical setting. It clearly behooves the astute physician as well as those who visit or work at the sea or seacoast to be aware of the shellfish and fish poisonings, marine microbial infections, and potential intoxication and envenomations from the vast and challenging world of life in and around the sea.

References

1. Eastaugh J, Shepherd S. Infectious and toxic syndromes from fish and shellfish consumption. A review. *Arch Intern Med* 1989; 149:1735–1740.
2. Hughes JM, Merson MH. Fish and shellfish poisoning. *N Engl J Med* 1976; 295:1117–1120.
3. Hughes JM, Potter ME. Scombroid-fish poisoning. From pathogenesis to prevention. *N Engl J Med* 1991; 324:766–768.
4. Sakamoto Y, Lockey RF, Krzanowski JJ. Shellfish and fish poisoning related to the toxic dinoflagellates. *South Med J* 1987; 80:866–872.
5. West PA, Wood PC, Jacob M. Control of food poisoning risks associated with shellfish. *J R Soc Health* 1985; 105(1):15–21.
6. Sanders WE Jr. Intoxications from the seas: ciguatera, scombroid, and paralytic shellfish poisoning. *Infect Dis Clin N Am* 1987; 1:665–676.
7. Carson RL. The changing year. In: Carson RL (ed): *The Sea Around Us.* New York, Oxford University Press, 1961: 28–36.
8. Vancouver G. A Voyage of Discovery to the North Pacific Ocean and Round the World. London, Robinson, 1798.
9. Walker ST. Fish mortality in the Gulf of Mexico. *Proc US Nat Museum* 1984; 6:105–109.
10. Halstead BW, Schantz EJ. Paralytic shellfish poisoning. *WHO Offset Publ* 1984; 79:1–59.
11. Centers for Disease Control. Paralytic shellfish poisoning—Massachusettes and Alaska, 1990 (published erratum appears in MMWR 1991, Apr. 12, 40[4]242). *MMWR* 1991; 40(10):157–161.
12. Prakash A. An overview. *Proceedings of the First International Conference on Toxic Dinoflagellate Blooms* 1975; 1–6.
13. Food safety. Paralytic shellfish poisoning. *WHO Wkly Epidem Rec* 1991; 66:185–187.
14. McGuigan M. Shellfish poisoning. *Clin Toxicol Rev* 1981; 3:12.

15. Adams WN, Miescier JJ. Commentary on AOAC method for paralytic shellfish poisoning. *J Assoc Off Anal Chem* 1980; 63:1336–1343.

16. Kodama M, Ogata T, Fukuyo Y, et al. *Protogonyaulax cohorticula*, a toxic dinoflagellate found in the Gulf of Thailand. *Toxicon* 1988; 26:707–712.

17. Tan CTT, Lee JD. Paralytic shellfish poisoning in Singapore. *Ann Acad Med Singapore* 1986; 15:77–79.

18. Karunasagar I, Oshima Y, Yasumoto T. A toxin profile for shellfish involved in an outbreak of paralytic shellfish poisoning in India. *Toxicon* 1990; 28:868–870.

19. Rodrigue DC, Etzel RA, Hall S, et al. Lethal paralytic shellfish poisoning in Guatemala. *Am J Trop Med Hyg* 1990; 42:267–281.

20. Kan SKP, Singh N, Chan MKC. *Oliva vidua fulminans*, a marine mollusc, responsible for five fatal cases of neurotoxic food poisoning in Sabah, Malaysia. *Trans R Soc Trop Med Hyg* 1986; 80:64–65.

21. Eason RJ, Harding E. Neurotoxic fish poisoning in the Solomon Islands. *P N G Med J* 1987; 30:49–52.

22. Paralytic shellfish poisoning (Red tide). *Epid Bull PAHO* 1990; 11:9.

23. Harrison LJ. Poisonous marine morsels. *J Florida M A* 1991; 78:219–221.

24. Sims JK. A theoretical discourse on the pharmacology of toxic marine ingenstions. *Ann Emerg Med* 1987; 16:1006–1015.

25. Yasumoto J. Recent progress in the chemistry of dinoflagellate toxins. In: Anderson, White, Baden (eds): *Toxic Dinoflagellates*. New York, Elsevier, 1985:259–270.

26. The red tide (editorial). *Med J Aust* 1981; 2:2.

27. Anderson DM, Sullivan JJ, Reguera B. Paralytic shellfish poisoning in Northwest Spain: the toxicity of the dinoflagellate *Gymnodinium catenatumQ. Toxicon* 1989; 27:665–674.

28. Centers for Disease Control. Annual mussel quarantine—California. *MMWR* 1983; 32:281.

29. Blanc MH, Zwahlen A, Robert M. Symptoms of shellfish poisoning. *N Engl J Med* 1977; 196:287–288.

30. McCollum JPK, Pearson RCM, Ingham HR. An epidemic of mussel poisoning in Northeast England. *Lancet* 1968; 2:767–770.

31. Long RR, Sargent JC, Hammer K. Paralytic shellfish poisoning: a case report and serial electrophysiologic observations. *Neurology* 1990; 40: 1310–1312.

32. Hughes JM. Epidemiology of shellfish poisoning in the United States, 1971–1977. In: Taylor, Seliger (eds): *Toxic Dinoflagellate Blooms*. New York, Elsevier/North Holland, 1979:23–28.

33. Centers for Disease Control. Paralytic shellfish poisoning—Washington. *MMWR* 1978; 27:416–417.

34. Cheng H-S, Chua SO, Hung J-S, et al. Creatine kinase MB elevation in paralytic shellfish poisoning. *Chest* 1991; 99:1032–1033.

35. Sullivan JJ, Iwaoka WT. High pressure liquid chromatographic detrmination of toxins associated with paralytic shellfish poisoning. *J Assoc Off Anal Chem* 1983; 66:297–303.

36. Stahr B, Threadgill ST, Overman TL, et al. *Vibrio vulnificus* sepsis after eating raw oysters. *J Ky Med Assoc* 1989;87:219–222.

37. Mills AR, Passmore R. Pelagic paralysis. *Lancet* 1988; 331(8578):161–164.

38. Bagnis R, Chanteau S, Chungue S. Origins of ciguatera fish poisoning: a new dinoflagellate, *Gambierdicus toxicus adachi* and *fukoyo*, definitely involved as a causal agent. *Toxicon* 1980; 18:199–208.
39. Hemmert WH. The public health implicaitons of *Gymnodinium breve* red tides, a review of the literature and recent events. In: Locicero (ed): *Proceedings of the First International Conference on Toxic Dinoflagellate Blooms.* Boston, Massachusetts Science and Technology Foundation, 1975:489–497.
40. Murphy EB, Steidinger KA, Roberts BS, et al. An explanation for the Florida East Coast *Gymnodinium breve* red tide of November 1972. *Limnol Oceanog* 1975; 20:481–486.
41. Morris PD, Campbell DS, Taylor TJ, et al. Clinical and epidemiological fetures of neurotoxic shellfish poisoning in North Carolina. *Am J Pub Health* 1991; 81:471–474.
42. Tester PA, Fowler PK, Turner JT. Gulf stream transport of the toxic red tide dinoflagellate *Ptychodiscus brevis* from Florida to North Carolina. In: Cosper, Carpenter, Bricelj (eds): *Novel Phytoplankton Blooms: Causes and Impact of Recurrent Brown Tides and Other Unusual Blooms.* Berlin, Springer-Verlag, 1990:349–358.
43. Steidinger KA. Collection, enumeration, and identification of free-living marine dinoflagellates. In: Taylor, Seliger (eds): *Toxic Dinoflagellate Blooms.* New York, Elsevier/North Holland, 1979:435–442.
44. Baden DG. Marine food-borne dinoflagellate toxins. *Int Rev Cytol* 1983; 82:99–150.
45. Baden DG, Mende TJ. Toxicity of two toxins from the Florida red tide marine dinoflagellate *Ptychodiscus brevis. Toxicon* 1982; 20:457–461.
46. Risk M, Werrbach-Perez K, Perez-Polo JR, et al. Mechanism of action of the major toxin from *Gymnodinium breve davis.* In: Taylor, Seliger (eds): *Toxic Dinoflagellate Blooms.* New York, Elsevier/Holland, 1979:367–372.
47. Asai S, Krzanowski JJ, Anderson WH, et al. Effects of the toxin of red tide, *Ptychodiscus brevis*, on canine tracheal smooth muscle: a possible new asthma-triggering mechanism. *J Allergy Clin Immunol* 1982; 69:418–428.
48. Borison HL, Ellis S, McCarthy LE. Central respiratory and circulatory effects of *Gymnodinium breve* toxin in anaesthetized cats. *Br J Pharmacol* 1980; 70:249–256.
49. Krzanowski J, Sakamoto Y, Duncan R, et al. The mechanism of *Ptychodiscus brevis* toxin induced rat vas deferens contraction. *Pharmacologist* 1984; 26:175.
50. Sakamoto Y, Krzanowski JJ, Lockey R, et al. The mechanism of *Ptychodiscus brevis* toxin induced contraction of rat vas deferens. *J Allergy Clin Immunol* 1985; 76:117–122.
51. Perl TM, Bedard L, Kosatsky T, et al. An outbreak of toxic encephalopathy caused by eating mussels contaminated with domoic acid. *N Engl J Med* 1990; 322:1775–1780.
52. Teitelbaum JS, Zatorre RJ, Carpenter S, et al. Neurologic sequelae of domoic acid intoxication due to the ingestio of contaminated mussels. *N Engl J Med* 1990; 322:1781–1787.
53. Glavin GB, Bose R, Pinsky C. (Letter). *Arch Intern Med* 1990; 150:2425.
54. Subba Rao DV, Quilliam MA, Pocklington R. Domoic acid—a neurotoxic amino acid produced by the marine diatom *Nitzschia pungens* in culture. *Can J Fish Aquat Sci* 1988; 45:2076–2079.

55. Quilliam MA, Wright JLC. The amnesic shellfish poisoning mystery. *Anal Chem* 1989; 61:1053–1059.
56. Fang G, Araujo V, Guerrant RL. Enteric infections associated with exposure to animals or animal products. *Infect Dis Clin N Am* 1991; 5(3): 681–701.
57. Wozniak DF, Stewart GR, Miller JP, et al. Age-related sensitivity to kainate neurotoxicity. *Exp Neutrol* 1991; 114:250-253.
58. Sims JK. Pufferfish poisoning: emergency diagnosis and management of mild human tetrodotoxin. *Ann Emerg Med* 1986; 15:1094–1098.
59. Fuhrman FA. Tetrodotoxin, tarichatoxin, and chiriquitoxins. Historical perspectives. *Ann N Y Acad Sci* 1986; 479:1–14.
60. Bower D, Hart R, Matthews P, et al. Nonprotein neurotoxins. *Clin Toxicol* 1981; 18:813–863.
61. Yokoo A. Chemical studies on tetrodotozin. Reprot III. isolation of shperoidine. *J Chem Soc Japan* 1950; 71:591–592.
62. Halstead BW. *Poisonous and Venomous Marine Animals of the World.* Washington, D.C., U.S. Government Printing Office, 1965.
63. Cook J. *A Voyage Towards the South Pole and Round the World.* London, Strahan and Cadell, 1777.
64. Hughes JM, Tauxe RV. Foodborne diseases. In: Mandell GL, Douglas RG Jr, Bennett JE (eds): *Principles and Practice of Infectious Diseases.* New York, Churchill Livingstone, 1990: pp. 893–905.
65. Lawrence DN, Enriquez MB, Lumish RM, et al. Ciguatera fish poisoning in Miami. *JAMA* 1980; 244:254–258.
66. Morris PD, Campbell DS, Freeman JI. Ciguatera fish poisoning: an outbreak associated with fish caught from North Carolina coastal waters. *South Med J* 1990; 83:379–382.
67. Morris JG. Ciguatera fish poisoning: barracuda's revenge. *South Med J* 1990; 83:371–372.
68. Bagnis R, Kuberski T, Laugier S. Clinical observations on 3,009 cases of ciguatera (fish poisoning) in the South Pacific. *Am J Trop Med Hyg* 1979; 28:1067–1073.
69. Withers NW. Ciguatera fish poisoning. *Ann Rev Med* 1982; 33:97–111.
70. Yasumoto T, Inoue A, Bagnis R. Ecological survey of a toxic dinoflagellate associate with ciguatera. In: Taylor, Seliger (eds): *Toxic Dinoflagellate Blooms.* New York, Elsevier/North Holland, 1979:221–224.
71. Hessel DW, Halstead BW, Peckham NH. Marine biotoxins. 1. Ciguatera poison: some biological and chemical aspects. *Ann N Y Acad Sci* 1960; 90:788–797.
72. Gillespie NC, Lewis RJ, Pearn JH, et al. Ciguatera in Australia: occurrence, clinical features, pathophysiology, and management. *Med J Aust* 1986; 145:584–590.
73. Kodama AM, Hokama Y, Yasumoto T, et al. Clinical and laboratory findings implicating palytoxin as cause of ciguatera poisoning due to *Decapterus macrosoma* (Mackerel). *Toxicon* 1989; 27:1051–1053.
74. Rainer MD. Mode of action of ciguatoxin. *Fed Proc* 1972; 31:1139–1145.
75. Kobayashi M, Kondo S, Yasumoto T, et al. Cardiotoxic effects of maitotoxin, a principal toxin of seafood poisoning, on guinea pig and rat cardiac muscle. *J Pharmacol Exp Ther* 1986; 238:1077–1083.

76. Morris JG Jr, Miller HG, Wilson R, et al. Illness caused by *Vibrio damsela* and *Vibrio hollisae*. *Lancet* 1982; i:1294–1297.
77. Van der Sar A. Ciguatera poisoning and T-wave changes. *JAMA* 1982; 247:1345.
78. Palafox N, Jain L, Pinano A, et al. Successful treatment of ciguatera fish poisoning with intravenous mannitol. *JAMA* 1988; 259:2740–2742.
79. Bowman P. Amitriptylline and ciguatera. *Med J Aust* 1984; 143:802.
80. Lewis N. Disease and development: ciguatera fish poisoning. *Soc Sci Med* 1986; 23:983–993.
81. Morrow JD, Margolies GR, Rowland J, et al. Evidence that histamine is the causative toxin of scombroid-fish poisoning. *N Engl J Med* 1991; 324:716–720.
82. Bagnis R, Berglund F, Elias PF, et al. Problems of toxicants in marine food products. 1. Marine biotoxins. *Bull WHO* 1970; 42:69–88.
83. Centers for Disease Control. Restaurant-associated scombroid fish poisoning Alabama, Tennessee. *MMWR* 1986; 35:264–265.
84. Taylor SL, Stratton JE, Nordlee JA. Histamine poisoning (scombroid fish poisoning): an allergy-like intoxication. *J Toxicol Clin Toxicol* 1989; 27: 225–240.
85. Etkind P, Wilson ME, Gallagher K, et al. Bluefish-associated scombroid poisoning. *JAMA* 1987; 258(23):3409–3410.
86. Murray C, Hobbs G. Scombrotoxin and scombrotoxin-like poisoning from canned fish. *J Hyg* 1982; 88:215–219.
87. Lerke PA, Werner SB, Taylor SL, et al. Scombroid poisoning: report of an outbreak. *West J Med* 1978; 12:381–386.
88. Blakesley M. Scombroid poisoning: prompt resolution of symptoms with cimetidine. *Ann Emerg Med* 1983; 12:104–106.
89. World Health Organization. Aquatic (marine and freshwater) biotoxins. In: *Environmental Health Criteria*. Geneva, Switzerland: World Health Organization, 1986:73–75.
90. Bolleta G, Bacchiocchi I, Durante G, et al. [Letter]. *Arch Intern Med* 1990; 150:2425.
91. Kat M. Diarrhetic mussel poisoning in the Netherlands related to the dino-flagellate *Dinophysis acuminata*. *Antonie van Leeuwenhoek* 1983; 49:417–427.
92. Bryan FL, Anderson HW, Cook OD, et al. *Procedures to Investigate Food-borne Illness*. Ames, Iowa, 1987 International Association of Milk, Food, and Environmental Sanitarians, 1987.
93. Tison DL, Kelly MT. *Vibrio* species of medical importance. *Diag Microbiol Infect Dis* 1984; 2:263–276.
94. Joseph SW, Colwell RR, Kaper JB. *Vibrio parahaemolyticus* and related halophilic *Vibrios*. *CRC Crit Rev Microbiol* 1983; 10:77–124.
95. Janda JM, Powers C, Bryant RG, et al. Current perspectives on the epidemiology and pathogenesis of clinically significant *Vibrio* spp. *Clin Microbiol Rev* 1988; 1:245–267.
96. Baumann L, Furniss AL, Lee JV. Genus I. *Vibrio* Pacini 1854,411. In: Kreig NR, Holt JG (eds): *Bergy's Manual of Systematic Bacteriology*. Baltimore, The Williams & Wilkins Co., 1984:518–538.
97. Hill MK, Sanders CV. Localized and systemic infection due to *Vibrio* species. *Infect Dis Clin N Am* 1987; 1:687–707.

98. Doyle MP. Food-borne pathogens of recent concern. *Ann Rev Nutr* 1985; 5:25–41.

99. Rhodes JB, Smith HL, Ogg JE. Isolation of non-01 *Vibrio cholerae serovars* from surface waters in Western Colorado. *Appl Environ Microbiol* 1986; 51:1216–1219.

100. Hickman FW, Farmer JJ, Hollis DG, et al. Identification of *Vivrio hollisae sp. nov* from patients with diarrhoea, *J Clin Microbiol* 1982; 15:395–401.

101. West PA, Lee JV. Ecology of *Vibrio* species, including *Vibrio cholerae*, in natural wares of Kent, England. *J Appl Bacteriol* 1982; 52:435–448.

102. Colwell RR, West PA, Maneval D, et al. Ecology of pathogenic *Vibrios* in the Chesapeake Bay. In: Colwell RR (ed): *Vibrios in the Environment*. New York, John Wiley & Sons, Inc., 1984:367–387.

103. Bockemuhl J, Roch K, Wohlers B, et al. Seasonal distribution of facultatively enteropathogenic vibrios (*Vibrio cholerae, Vibrio mimicus, Vibrio parahaemolyticus*) in the freshwater of the Elbe River at Hamburg. *J Appl Bacteriol* 1986; 60:435–442.

104. Singleton FL, Attwell R, Jangi S, et al. Effects of temperature and salinity on *Vibrio cholerae* growth. *Appl Environ Microbiol* 1982; 44:1047–1058.

105. Williams LA, La Rock PA. Temporal occurrence of *Vibrio* species and *Aeromonas* hydrophilia in estuarine sediments. *Appl Environ Microbiol* 1985; 50:1490–1495.

106. Seidler RJ, Evans TM. Computer-assisted analysis of *Vibrio* field data: four coastal areas. In: Colwell RR (ed): *Vibrios in the Environment*. New York, John Wiley & Sons, Inc., 1984:411–426.

107. Tison DL, Nishibuchi M, Seidler RJ, et al. Isolation of non-01 *Vibrio cholerae* serovars from Oregon coastal waters. *Appl Environ Microbiol* 1986; 51:444–445.

108. Miller CJ, Drasar BS, Feacham RG. Response of toxigenic *Vibrio cholerae* 01 to physico-chemical stresses in aquatic enviroments. *J Hyg* 1984; 93: 474–496.

109. Singleton FL, Attwell RW, Jangi S, et al. Influence of salinity and organic nutrient concentration on survival and growth of *Vibrio cholerae* in aquatic microcosms. *Appl Environ Microbiol* 1982; 43:1018–1085.

110. Sarkar BL, Nair GB, Banerjee AK, et al. Seasonal distribution of *Vibrio parahaemolyticus in freshwater environs and* in association with freshwater fishes in Calcutta. *Appl Environ Microbiol* 1985; 49:132–136.

111. Kaneko T, Colwell RR. Ecology of *Vibrio parahaemolyticus* in Chesapeake Bay. *J Bacteriol* 1973; 113:24–32.

112. Kaneko T, Colwell RR. The annual cycle of *Vibrio parahaemolyticus* in Chesapeake Bay. *Microb Ecol* 1978; 4:135–155.

113. Oliver JD, Warner RA, Cleland DR. Distribution of *Vibrio vulnificus* and other lactose-fermenting vibrios in the marine environment. *Appl Environ Microbiol* 1983; 45:985–998.

114. Huq A, Huq SA, Grimes DJ, et al. Colonization of the gut of the blue crab (*Callinectes sapidus*) by *Vibrio cholerae*. *Appl Environ Microbiol* 1986; 52:586–588.

115. Huq A, West PA, Small EB, et al. Influence of water temperature, salinity, and pH on survival and growth of toxigenic *Vibrio cholerae* serovar 01

associated with live copepods in laboratory microcosms. *Appl Environ Microbiol* 1984; 48:420–424.

116. Karunasagar I, Venugopal NM, Segar K. Role of chitin in the survival of *Vibrio parahaemolyticus* at different temperatures. *Can J Microbiol* 1987; 32:889–891.

117. Eyles MJ, Davey GR, Arnold G. Behavior and incidence of *Vibrio parahaemolyticus* in Sydney Rock Oysters (*Crassostrea commercialis*). *Int J Food Microbiol* 1985; 1:327–334.

118. Karunasagar I, Venugopal NM, Nagesha CN. Survival of *Vibrio parahaemolyticus* in estuarine and seawater and in association with clams. *Sys Appl Microbiol* 1987; 9:316–319.

119. Salmaso S, Greco D, Bonfiglio B, et al. Recurrence of pelecypod-associated cholera in Sardinia. *Lancet* 1980; ii:1124–1127.

120. De Paola A. *Vibrio cholerae* in marine foods and environmental waters: a literature review. *J Food Sci* 1981; 46:66–70.

121. Palasuntheram C, Selvarajah S. *Vibrio parahaemolyticus* in Colombo environment. *Indian J Med Res* 1981; 73:13–17.

122. Binta GM, Tjaberg TB, Nyaga PN, et al. Market fish hygiene in Kenya. *J Hyg* 1982; 89:47–52.

123. Auerbach PS, Yajko DM, Nassos PS, et al. Bacteriology of the marine environment: Implications for clinical therapy. *Ann Emerg Med* 1987; 16:643–649.

124. Buck JD, Spotte S, Gadbaw JJ Jr. Bacteriology of the teeth from a great white shark: potential medical implications for shark bite victims. *J Clin Microbiol* 1984; 20:849–851.

125. Desenclos JA, Klontz KC, Wolfe LE, et al. The risk of *Vibrio* illness in the Florida raw oyster eating population, 1981–1988. *Am J Epidemiol* 1991; 134:290–297.

126. Farmer JJ, Hickman-Brenner FW, Kelly MT. *Vibrio*. In: Lennette EH, Balows A, Hausler, Shadomy (eds): *Manual of Clinical Microbiology*. Washington, D.C., American Society for Microbiology, 1985:282–301.

127. Hoge CW, Watsky D, Peeler RN, et al. Epidemiology and spectrum of *Vibrio* infections in a Chesapeake Bay community. *J Infect Dis* 1989; 160: 985–993.

128. Bonner JR, Coker AS, Berryman CR, et al. Spectrum of *Vibrio* infections in a Gulf Coast community. *Ann Intern Med* 1983; 99:464–469.

129. Rosenberg CE. *The Cholera Years: The United States in 1832, 1849, and 1866*. Chicago, University of Chicago Press, 1962.

130. Blake PA, Allegra DT, Snyder JD, et al. Cholera—a possible endemic focus in the United States. *N Engl J Med* 1980; 302: 305–309.

131. World Health Organization. *Principles and Practice of Cholera Control*. 1970.

132. Weissman JB, DeWitt WE, Thompson J, et al. A case of cholera in Texas, 1973. *Am J Epi* 1975; 100:487–498.

133. Johnston JM, Martin DL, Perdue J, et al. Cholera on a Gulf Coast oil rig. *N Engl J Med* 1983; 309:523–526.

134. Swerdlow DL, Ries AA. Cholera in the Americas. Guidelines for the clinician. *JAMA* 1992; 267:1495–1499.

135. Lin FY, Morris Jr. JG, Kaper JB, et al. Persistence of cholera in the United States: isolation of *Vibrio cholerae* 01 from a patient with diarrhea in Maryland. *J Clin Microbiol* 1986; 23:624–626.

136. Colwell RR, Seidler RJ, Kaper J, et al. Occurrence of *Vibrio cholerae* serogroup 01 in Maryland and Louisiana estuaries. *Appl Environ Microbiol* 1981; 41:555–558.

137. Kaper JB, Lockman H, Colwell RR, et al. Ecology, serology and enterotoxin production of *Vibrio cholerae* in Chesapeake Bay. *Appl Environ Microbiol* 1979; 37:91–103.

138. Bryant RG. Food microbiology update. Emerging foodborne pathogens. *Appl Biochem Biotechnol* 1983; 8:437–454.

139. Hood MA, Ness GE, Rodrick GE. Isolation of *Vibrio cholerae* serotype 01 from the Eastem oyster, *Crassotrea virginica*. *Appl Environ Microbiol* 1981; 41:559–560.

140. Rodrick GE, Hood MA, Blake NJ. Human *Vibrio* gastroenteritis. *Med Clin N Am* 1982; 66;665–673.

141. Twedt RM, Madden JM, Hunt JM, et al. Characterization of *Vibrio cholerae* isolated form oysters. *Appl Environ Microbiol* 1981; 41:1475–1478.

142. World Health Organization. Cholera and other *Vibrio*-associated diarrhoeas. *Bull WHO* 1980; 58:353–374.

143. Centers for Disease Control. Update: cholera outbreak—Peru, Ecuador, and Colombia. *MMWR* 1991; 40:108–110.

144. Centers for Disease Control. Cholera—Peru, 1991. *MMWR* 1991; 40:108–110.

145. Wachsmuth IK, Boxx CA, Fields PI, et al. Differences between toxigenic *Vibrio cholerae* 01 from South American and Gulf Coast. *Lancet* 1991; 337:1097–1098.

146. West PA. The human pathogenic *Vibrios*—a public health update with environmental perspectives. *Epidem Inf* 1989; 103:1–34.

147. Oberhofer TR, Podgore JK. Urea-hydrolyzing *Vibrio parahaemolyticus* associated with acute gastroenteritis. *J Clin Microbiol* 1982; 16:581–583.

148. Morris Jr. JG, Wilson R, Davis BR, et al. Non-0 group 1 *Vibrio cholerae* gastroenteritis in the United States: clinical, epidemiologic, and laboratory characteristics of sporadic cases. *Ann Intern Med* 1981; 94:656–658.

149. Yamamoto K, Takeda Y, Miwatani T, et al. Evidence that a non-01 *Vibrio cholerae* produces enterotoxin that is similar but not identical to cholera enterotoxin. *Infect Immun* 1983; 41:896–901.

150. Tison DL, Kelly MT. *Vibrio vulnificus* endometritis. *J Clin Microbiol* 1984; 20:185–186.

151. Bart KJ, Huq Z, Khan M, et al. Seroepidemiologic studies during a simultaneous epidemic of infection with El Tor, Ogawa and classical Inaba *Vibrio cholerae*. *J Infect Dis* 1970; 12(Suppl):17–24.

152. Samadi AR, Huq MI, Shahid NS. Classical *Vibrio cholerae* biotype displaces El Tor in Bangladesh. *Lancet* 1983; 1:805–807.

153. Greenough W.B. III *Vibrio cholerae*. In: Mandell GL, Douglas RGJr, Bennett JE (eds): *Principles and Practice of Infectious Diseases*. New York, Churchill Livingstone, 1990:1636–1646.

154. Holmberg S. *Vibrios* and *Aeromonas*. *Infect Dis Clin N Am* 1988; 2:655–676.

155. Herrington DA, Hall RH, Losonsky G, et al. Toxin, toxin-coregulated pili, and the toxR regulon are essential for *Vibrio cholerae* pathogenesis in humans. *J Exp Med* 1988; 168:1487–1492.
156. Holmgren J, Svennerholm A. Mechanisms of disease and immunity in cholerae. A review. *J Infect Dis* 1977; 136(Suppl):105–112.
157. Levine MM, Black RE, Clements ML, et al. Volunteer studies in development of vaccines against cholera and enterotoxigenic *E. coli*: a review. In: Holme, Holmgren, Merson, Mollby (eds): *Acute Enteric Infections in Children: New Prospects for Treatment and Prevention*. Amsterdam, Elsevier/North Holland, 1981:443–459.
158. Schiraldi O, Benvestito V, DiBari C, et al. Gastric abnormalities in cholera: epidemiologic and clinical considerations. *Bull WHO* 1974; 51:349–352.
159. Sircar BK, Dutta P, De SP, et al. ABO blood group distributions in diarrhoea cases including cholera in Calcutta. *Ann Human Biol* 1981; 8:289–291.
160. Field M. Modes of action of enterotoxins of *Vibrio cholerae* and *Escherichia coli*. *Rev Infect Dis* 1979; 1:918–921.
161. Bobak DA, Guerrant RL. New developments in enteric bacterial toxins. *Adv Pharmacol* 1992; 23:85–108.
162. Hirschhorn N, Kinzie JL, Sachar DB, et al. Decrease in net stool output in cholera during intestinal perfusion with glucose-containing solutions. *N Engl J Med* 1968; 279:176–181.
163. Morris JG, Picardi JL, Lieb S, et al. Isolation of non-toxigenic *Vibrio* 0 group 1 from a patient with severe gastrointestinal disease. *J Clin Microbiol* 1984; 19:296–297.
164. Morris Jr. JG, Black RE. Cholera and other vibrioses in the United States. *N Engl J Med* 1985; 312:343–350.
165. Honda T, Finkelstein a. Purification and characterization of a hemolysin produced by *Vibrio cholerae* biotype El Tor: another toxic substance produced by cholera *Vibrios*. *Infect Immun* 1979; 26:1020–1027.
166. Magnusson B, Gulasekharam J. A lecithin-hydrolyzing enzyme which correlates with hemolytic activity in El Tor *Vibrio* isolates. *Nature* 1965; 206:728.
167. Chatterjee GC, Das SK. Purification and some properties of *Vibrio* El Tor phospholipase B. *Enzyme* 1965; 28:346–354.
168. Peterson JW, Ochoa G. Role of prostaglandins and cAMP in the secretory effects of cholera toxin. *Reports* 1989;245:857–859.
169. Wickboldt IG, Sanders CV. *Vibrio vulnificus* infection; case report and update since 1970. *J Am Acad Dermatol* 1983; 9:243–251.
170. Wallace CK, Pierce NF, Anderson PN, et al. Probable gallbladder infection in convalescent cholera patients. *Lancet* 1967; 1:865–868.
171. Gorbach SL, Banwell JG, Pierce NF, et al. Intestinal microflora in a chronic carrier of *Vibrio cholerae.J Infect Dis* 1970; 121:383–390.
172. Johnston JM, McFarland LM, Bradford HC, et al. Isolation of nontoxigenic *Vibrio cholerae* 01 from a human wound infection. *J Clin Microbiol* 1983; 17:918–920.
173. Morris Jr. JG, Tenney JH, Drusano GL. In vitro susceptibility of pathogenic *Vibrio* species to norfloxacin and six other antimicrobial agents. *Antimicrob Agents Chemother* 1985; 28:442–445.
174. Bhattacharya SK, Bhattacharya MK, Dutta P, et al. Double-blind, randomized, controlled clinical trials of norfloxacin for cholera. *Antimicrob Agents Chemother* 1990; 34:939–940.

175. Centers for Disease Control. ACIP: cholera vaccine. *MMWR* 1988; 37: 617–624.
176. Rhodes JB, Schweitzer D, Ogg JE. Isolation of non-01 *Vibrio cholerae* associated with enteric disease of herbivores in Western Colorado. *J Clin Microbiol* 1985; 22:572–575.
177. Safrin S, Morris JG Jr, Adams M, et al. Non-0:1 *Vibrio cholerae* bacteremia: case report and review. *Rev Infect Dis* 1988; 10:1012–1017.
178. Cover TL, Dunn BE, Ellison RT, et al. *Vibrio cholerae* wound infection acquired in Colorado. *J Infect Dis* 1989; 160:1083.
179. Mulder GD, Ries TM, Beaver TR. Nontoxigenic *Vibrio cholerae* wound infection after exposure to contaminated lake water. *J Infect Dis* 1989; 159:809–810.
180. DeGerome JH, Smith MT. Noncholera *Vibrio* enteritis contracted in the United States by an American. *J Infect Dis* 1974; 2:587–589.
181. Dakin WPH, Howell DJ, Sutton GA, et al. Gastroenteritis due to non-agglutinable (non-cholera) *Vibrios*. *Med J Aust* 1974; 2:487–490.
182. World Health Organization. Outbreak of gastroenteritis by non-agglutinable (NAG) *Vibrios*. *WHO Weekly Epidemiol Record* 1969; 44:10.
183. Aldova E, Laznickova K, Stepankova E, et al. lsolation of nonagglutinable *Vibrios* from an enteritis outbreak in Czechoslovakia. *J Infect Dis* 1968; 118:25–31.
184. Wilson R, Lieb S, Roberts A, et al. Non-O group 1 *Vibrio cholerae* gastroenteritis associated with eating raw oysters. *Am J Epidemiol* 1981; 114(2): 293–298.
185. Hughes JM, Hollis DG, Gangarosa EJ, et al. Non-cholera *Vibrio* infections in the United States: clinical epidemiologic, and laboratory features. *Ann Intern Med* 1978; 88:602–606.
186. Yamamoto K, Ichinose Y, Nakasone N, et al. ldentity of hemolysins produced by *Vibrio* cholerae non-O-1 and V. cholerae 01, biotype EI Tor. *Infect Immun* 1986; 51;927–931.
187. Datta-Roy K, Banerjee K, De SP, et al. Comparative study of expression of hemagglutinins, hemolysins, and enterotoxins by clinical and environmental isolates of non-01 *Vibrio cholerae* in relation to their enteropathogenicity. *Appl Environ Microbiol* 1986; 52:875–879.
188. Arita M, Takeda T, Honda T, et al. Purification and characterization of *Vibrio cholerae* non-01 heat-stable enterotoxin. *Infect Immun* 1986; 52:45–49.
189. Nishibuchi M, Seidler RJ, Rollins DM, et al. *Vibrio* factors cause rapid fluid accumulation in suckling mice. *Infect Immun* 1983; 51:927–931.
190. Nishibuchi M, Seidler RJ. Medium-dependent production of extracellular enterotoxins by non-o-1 *Vibrio cholerae*, *Vibrio mimicus* and *Vibrio fluvialis*. *Appl Environ Microbiol* 1983; 45:228–231.
191. Honda T, Arita M, Takeda T, et al. Non-01 *Vibrio cholerae* produces two newly identified toxins related to *Vibrio parahaemolyticus* haemolysin and *Escherichia coli* heat-stable enterotoxin. *Lancet* 1985; July 20:163–164.
192. O'Brien AD, Chen ME, Holmes RK, et al. Environmental and human isolates of *Vibrio cholerae* and *Vibrio parahaemolyticus* produce a *Shigella dysenteriae* 1 (Shiga)-like cytotoxin. *Lancet* 1984; i:77–78.

193. Dhar R, Ghafoor MA, Nasralah AY. Unusual non-serogroup 01 *Vibrio cholerae* bacteremia associated with liver disease. *J Clin Microbiol* 1989; 27:2853–2855.

194. Klontz KC, Desenclos J-CA. Clinical and epidemiological features of sporadic infections with *Vibrion fluvialis* in Florida, USA. *J Diarrhoeal Dis Res* 1990; 8:24–26.

195. Thibaut K, Van de Heying P, Pattyn SR. Isolation of non-01 *Vibrio cholerae* from ear tracts. *Eur J Epidemiol* 1986; 2:316–317.

196. Florescu DP, Nacescu N. *Vibrio cholerae* non group 0:1 associated with middle ear infection. *Arch Roum Path Exp Microbiol* 1981; 40:369–372.

197. Peterson EM, Jemison-Smith P, de la Maza L, et al. Cholecystitis: its occurrence with cholelithiasis associated with a non-01 *Vibrio cholerae*. *Arch Pathol Lab Med* 1982;106:300–301.

198. Klontz KC. Fatalities associated with *Vibrio parahaemolytics* and *Vibrio cholerae* non-01 infections in Florida (1981 to 1988). *South Med J* 1990; 83:500–502.

199. Morgan DR, Ball BD, Moore DG, et al. Severe *Vibrio cholerae* sepsis and meningitis in a young infant. *Texas Med* 1985; 81:37–38.

200. Fearrington EL, Rand CH, Mewborn A, et al. Non-cholera *Vibrio* septicemia and meningoencephalitis (letter). *Ann Intern Med* 1974; 81:401.

201. Rubin LG, Altman J, Epple LK, et al. *Vibrio cholerae* meningitis in a neonate. *J Pediatr* 1981; 98:940–942.

202. Fanca SMC, Gibbs DL, Samuels P, et al. *Vibrio parahaemolyticus* in Brazilian .11coastal waters. *JAMA* 1980; 244:587–588.

203. Lam S, Yeo M. Urease-positive *Vibrio parahaemolyticus* strain. *J Clin Microbiol* 1980; 12:57–59.

204. Abbott SL, Powers C, Kaysner CA, et al. Emergence of a restricted bioserovar of *Vibrio parahaemolyticus* as the predominant cause of vibrio-associated gastroenteritis on the West Coast of the United States and Mexico. *J Clin Microbiol* 1989; 27:2891–2893.

205. Kelly MT, Stroh EMD. Urease-positive, Kanagawa-negative *Vibrio parahaemolyticus* from patients and the environment in the Pacific Northwest. *J Clin Microbiol* 1989; 27:2820–2822.

206. Molenda JR, Johnson WG, Fishbein M, et al. *Vibrio parahaemolyticus* gastroenteritis in Maryland: laboratory aspects. *Appl Microbiol* 1972; 24:444–448.

207. Blake PA, Weaver RE, Hollis DG. Diseases of humans (other than cholera) caused by *Vibrios*. *Ann Rev Microbiol* 1980; 34:341–367.

208. Lowry PW, McFarland LM, Peltier BH, et al. *Vibrio* gastroenteritis in Louisiana: a prospective study among attendees of a scientific congress in New Orleans. *J Infect Dis* 1989; 160:978–984.

209. Barker WH. *Vibrio parahaemolyticus* outbreaks in the United States. *Lancet* 1974; i, March:551–554.

210. Mazumder DNG, Ghosh AK, De SP, et al. *Vibrio parahaemolyticus* infection in man. *Indian J Med Res* 1977; 66:180–188.

211. Mhalu FS, Yusufali AM, Mbwana J, et al. Cholera-like diseases due to *Vibrio parahaemolyticus*. *J Trop Med Hyg* 1982; 85:169–171.

212. Gilman RH, Spira WM. Invasive *E. coli* and *V. parahaemolyticus* a rare cause of dysentery in Dacca. *Trans R Soc Trop Med Hyg* 1980.

213. Bolen J, Zamiska SA, Greenough WB. Clinical features in enteritis due to *Vibrio parahaemolyticus. Am J Med* 1974; 57:638–641.
214. Honda T, Taga S, Takeda T, et al. Identification of lethal toxin with the thermostable direct hemolysin produced by *Vibrio parahaemolyticus* and some physicochemical properties of purified toxin. *Infect Immun* 1975; 13:133–139.
215. Miyamoto Y, Obara Y, Nikkawa T, et al. Simplified purification and bio-physicochemical characteristics of Kanagawa phenomenon-associated hemolysin of *Vibrio parahaemolyticus. Infect Immun* 1980; 28:567–576.
216. Obara Y, Yamai S, Nikkawa T, et al. Histochemical changes in the small intestine of suckling mice challenged orally with purified hemolysin from Vibrio parahemolyticus In: Fujino, Sakaguchi, Sakazaki, Takeda (eds): *International symposium on Vibrio parahaemolyticus.* Tokyo, Saikon Publ. Co., 1974: 253–257.
217. Zen-yoji H, Kudoh Y, Igarashi H, et al. Purification identification of enteropathogenic toxins "a" and "a'" produced by *Vibrio parahaemolyticus* and their biological and pathological activities. In: Fujino, Sakaguchi, Sakazaki, Takeda (eds): *International symposium on Vibrio parahaemolyticus.* Tokyo, Saikon Publ. Co., 1974: 237–243.
218. Hoashi D, Ogata K, Taniguchi H, et al. Pathogenesis of *Vibrio parahaemolyticus*: intraperitoneal and orogastric challenge experiments in mice. *Microbiol Immunol* 1990; 34:355–366.
219. Shirai H, Ito H, Hirayama T, et al. Molecular epidemiologic evidence for association of thermostable direct hemolysin (TDH) and TDH-related hemolysin of *Vibrio parahaemolyticus* with gastroenteritis. *Infcet Immun* 1990; 58:3568–3573.
220. Hackney CR, Kleeman EG, Ray B, et al. Adherence as a method for differentiating virulent and avirulent strains of *Vibrio parahaemolyticus. Appl Environ Microbiol* 1980; 40:652–658.
221. Limpert GH, Peacock JE. Soft tissue infections due to noncholera *Vibrios. Am Fam Physician* 1988; 37:193–198.
222. Lam S, Monteiro E. Isolation of mucoid *Vibrio parahaemolytic* strains. *J Clin Microbiol* 1984; 19:87–88.
223. Plotkin BJ, Kilgore SG, McFarland L. Polyvibrio infections: *Vibrio parahaemolyticus* dual wound and multiple site infections. *J Infect Dis* 1990; 161:364–365.
224. Steinkuller PG, Kelly MT, Sands SJ, et al. *Vibrio parahaemolyticus* endophthalmitis. *J Pediatr Opthalmol Strabismus* 1980; 17:150–153.
225. Tacket CO, Barrett TJ, Sanders GE, et al. Panophthalmitis caused by *Vibrio parahaemolyticus. J Clin Microbiol* 1982; 16:195–196.
226. Yu SL, Uy-Yu O. *Vibrio parahaemolyticus* pneumonia (letter). *Ann Interm Med* 1984; 100:320.
227. Roland F, Bertini R, Jhang J. *Vibrio parahaemolyticus* osteomyelitis of 12 years duration. *Rhode Island Med J* 1985; 68:553–555.
228. Reichelt JL, Baumann P, Baumann L. Study of genetic relationships among marine species of the genus *Beneckea* and *Photobhacterium* by means of in vitro DNA/DNA hybridization. *Arch Microbiol* 1976; 110:101–120.
229. Hollis DG, Weaver RE, Baker CN, et al. Halophilic *Vibrio* species isolated from blood cultures. *J Clin Microbiol* 1976; 3:425–431.

230. Farmer JJ III. *Vibrio* ("Beneckea") *vulnificus*, the bacterium associated with sepsis, septicemia and the sea. *Lancet* 1979; ii:903.
231. Tamplin M, Rodrick GE, Blake NJ, et al. Isolation and characterization of *Vibrio vulnificus* from two Florida estuaries. *Appl Environ Microbiol* 1982; 44:1466–1470.
232. Davis JW, Sizemore RK. Incidence of *Vibrio* species associated with blue crabs (*Callinectes sapidus*) collected from Galveston Bay, Texas. *Appl Environ Microbiol* 1982; 43:1092–1097.
233. Ali MB, Raff MJ. Primary *Vibrio vulnificus* sepsis in Kentucky. *South Med J* 1990; 83:356–357.
234. Blake PA. *Vibrios* on the half shell: what the walrus and the carpenter didn't know. *Ann Intern Med* 1983; 99(4):558–559.
235. Case records of the Massachusetts General Hospital. Weekly clinicopathological exercises. Case 41-1989. A 65-year-old man with fever, bullae, erythema, and edema of the leg after wading in brackish water. *N Engl J Med* 1989; 321:1029–1038.
236. Nip-Sakamoto CJ, Pien FD. *Vibrio vulnificus* infection in Hawaii. *Int J Dermatol* 1989; 28:311–316.
237. Oliver JD. Lethal cold stress of *Vibrio vulnificus* in oysters. *Appl Environ Microbiol* 1981; 41:710–717.
238. Johnston JM, Andes WA, Glasser G. *Vibrio vulnificus* a gastronomic hazard. *JAMA* 1983; 249(13):1756–1757.
239. Johnston JM, Becker SF, McFarland LM. *Vibrio vulnificus* man and the sea. *JAMA* 1985; 253(19):2850–2853.
240. Tacket CO, Brenner F, Blake PA. Clinical features and an epidemiological study of *Vibrio vulnificus* infections. *J Infect Dis* 1984; 149 (4):558–561.
241. Kaye JJ. *Vibrio vulnificus* infections in the hand. *J Bone Joint Surg* 1990; 72-A:283–285.
242. Johnston JM, Becker SF, McFarland LM. Gastroenteritis in patients with stool isolates of *Vibrio vulnificus*. *Am J Med* 1986; 80:336–338.
243. Klontz KC, Lieb S, Schreiber M, et al. Syndromes of *Vibrio vulnificus* infections. Clinical and epidemiologic features in Florida cases, 1981–1987. *Ann Intern Med* 1988; 109(4):318–323.
244. Kelly MT, Avery DM. Lactose-positive *Vibrio* in seawater: a cause of pneumonia and septicemia in a drowning victim. *J Clin Microbiol* 1980; 11:278–280.
245. Cunningham LW, Promisloff RA, Cichelli AV. Pulmonary infiltrates associated with *Vibrio vulnificus* septicemia. *J Am Osteopath Assoc* 1991; 91:84–86.
246. Truwit JD, Badesch DB, Savage AM, et al. *Vibrio vulnificus* bacteremia with endocarditis. *South Med J* 1987; 80: 1457–1459.
247. Vartian CV, Septimus EJ. Osteomyelitis caused by *Vibrio vulnificus*. *J Infect Dis* 1990; 161:363.
248. DiGaetano M, Ball SF, Straus JG. *Vibrio vulnificus* corneal ulcer. *Arch Ophthalmol* 1989; 107:323–324.
249. Wright AC, Simpson LM, Oliver JD, et al. Phenotypic evaluation of acapsular transposon mutants of *Vibrio vulnificus*. *Infcet Immun* 1990; 58:1769–1773.
250. Yoshida S, Ogawa M, Mizuguchi Y. Relation of capsular materials and colony opacity to virulence of *Vibrio vulnificus*. *Infect Immun* 1985; 47: 446–451.

251. Morris JG Jr. *Vibrio vulnificus*—a new monster of the deep. *Ann Intern Med* 1988; 109:261–263.
252. Kreger A, DeChatelet L, Shirley P. Interaction of *Vibrio vulnificus* with human polymorphonuclear leukocytes: association of virulence with resistance to phagocytosis. *J Infect Dis* 1981; 144:244–248.
253. Simpson LM, Oliver JD. Siderophore production by *Vibrio vulnificus*. *Infect Immun* 1983; 41:644–649.
254. Kaysner CA, Wekell MM, Abeyta C Jr. Enhancement of virulence of two environmental strains of *Vibrio vulnificus* after passage through mice. *Diag Microbiol Infect Dis* 1990; 13:285–288.
255. Gray LD, Kreger AS. Purification and characterization of an extracellular cytolysin produced by *Vibrio vulnificus*. *Infect Immun* 1985; 48:62–72.
256. smith GC, Merkel JR. Collagenolytic activity of *vibrio vulnificus*: potential contribution to its invasiveness. *Infect Immun* 1982; 35:1155–1156.
257. Gray LD, Kreger AS. Detection of *anti-Vibrio vulnificus* cytolysin antibodies in sera from mice and a human surviving *V. vulnificus* disease. *Infect Immun* 1986; 51:964–965.
258. Wright AC, Simpson LM, Oliver JD. Role of iron in the pathogenesis of *Vibrio vulnificus* infections. *Infect Immun* 1981; 34:503–507.
259. Brennt CE, Wright AC, Dugga SK, et al. Growth of *Vibrio vulnificus* in serum from alcoholics: association with high transferrin iron saturation. *J Infect Dis* 1991; 164:1030–1032.
260. Sacks-Berg A, Strampfer J, Cunha BA. *Vibrio vulnificus* bacteremia report of a case and review of the literature. *Heart Lung* 1987; 16:706–709.
261. Park SD, Sohn HS, Koh JW. Effect of hydrogen ions on the growth of *Vibrio vulnificus*. *Kor J Dermatol* 1986; 24:354–357.
262. Eng RHK, Chmel H, Smith SM, et al. Early diagnosis of overwhelming *Vibrio vulnificus* infections. *South Med J* 1988; 81:410–411.
263. Pool MD, Oliver JD. Experimental pathogenicity and mortality in ligated ileal loop studies of the newly reported halophilic lactose-positive *Vibrio* sp. *Infect Immun* 1978; 20:126–129.
264. Park SD, Shon HS, Joh NJ. *Vibrio vulnificus* septemia in Korea: clinical and epidemiologic findings in seventy patients. *J Am Acad Dermatol* 1991; 24:397–403.
265. Blake PA, Merson MH, Weaver RE, et al. Disease caused by a marine *Vibrio*: clinical characteristics and epidemiology. *N Engl J Med* 1979; 300(1): 1–5.
266. Hoffman TJ, Nelson B, Darouiche R, et al. *Vibrio vulnificus* septicemia. *Arch Intern Med* 1988; 148:1825–1927.
267. Tefany FJ, Lee S, Shumack S. Oysters, iron overload and *Vibrio vulnificus* septicaemia. *Australia J Dermatol* 1990; 31:27–31.
268. Fonde EC, Britton J, Pollock H. Marine *Vibrio* sepsis manifesting as necrotizing fasciitis. *South Med J* 1984; 77:933–934.
269. Howard RJ, Lieb S. Soft-tissue infections caused by halophilic marine *Vibrios*. *Arch Surg* 1988; 123:245.
270. Bowdre JH, Hull JH, Cochetto DM. Antibiotic efficacy against *Vibrio vulnificus* in the mouse: superiority of tetracycline. *J Pharmacol Exp Ther* 1983; 225:595–598.
271. Meadors MC, Pankey GA. *Vibrio vulnificus* wound infection treated successfully with oral ciprofloxacin (letter). *J Infect* 1990; 20:88–89.

272. ANONYMOUS. Shuck your oysters with care. *Lancet* 1990; 336:215–216.
273. Auerbach PS. Marine envenomations. *N Engl J Med* 1991; 325:486–493.
274. Morris JG Jr, Tenney J. Antibiotic therapy for *Vibrio vulnificus* infection (letter). *JAMA* 1985; 253:1121–1122.
275. Davis BR, Fanning GR, Madden JM, et al. Characterization of biochemically atypical *Vibrio cholerae* strains, and designation of a new pathogenic species, *Vibrio mimicus*. *J Clin Microbiol* 1981; 14:631–639.
276. Chowdhury MAR, Yamanaka H, Miyoshi S, et al. Ecology of *Vibrio mimicus* in aquatic environments. *Appl Environ Microbiol* 1989; 55:2073–2078.
277. Chowdhury MAR, Aziz KMS, Rahim Z, et al. Toxigenicity and drug sensitivity of *Vibrio mimicus* isolated form fresh water prawns (*Macrobrachium malcolmsonii*) in Bangladesh. *J Diarrhoeal Dis Res* 1986; 4:37–40.
278. Shandera WX, Johnston JM, Davis BR, et al. Disease from infection with *Vibrio mimicus*, a newly recognized *Vibrio* species: clinical characteristics and epidemiology. *Ann Intern Med* 1983; 99:169–171.
279. Kodama H, Gyobu Y, Tokuman N, et al. Ecology of non-01 *Vibrio cholerae* in Toyama prefacture. *Microbiol Immunol* 1984; 28:311–325.
280. Watsky D. *Vibrio fluvialis* and *Vibrio mimicus* associated with terminal ileitis. *Clin Microbiol Newsletter* 1983; 5:111.
281. Furniss AL, Lee JV, Donovan TJ. Group F, a new *Vibrio*? *Lancet* 1977; (8037):565–566.
282. Huq MI, Alam AKMJ, Brenner DJ, et al. Isolation of *Vibrio*-like group, EF-6, from patients with diarrhea. *J Clin Microbiol* 1980; 11:621–624.
283. Lee JV, Shread P, Furniss AL, et al. Taxonomy and description of *Vibrio fluvialis sp. nov.* (synonym group F vibrios, group EF-6). *J Appl Bacteriol* 1981; 50:73–94.
284. Tacket CO, Hickman F, Pierce GV, et al. Diarrhea associated with *Vibrio fluvialis* in the United States. *J Clin Microbiol* 1982; 991:992.
285. Thekdi RJ, Lakhani AG, Rale VB, et al. An outbreak of food poisoning suspected to be caused by *Vibrio fluvialis*. *J Diarrhoeal Dis Res* 1990; 8:163–165.
286. Yoshii Y, Nishino H, Satake K, et al. Isolation of *Vibrio fluvialis*, an unusual pathogen in acute suppurative cholangitis. *Am J Gastroenterol* 1987; 82:903–905.
287. Khan MV, Shahidullah M. Epidemiologic pattern of diarrhoea caused by non-agglutinating Vibrio (NAG) and EF-6 organisms in Dacca. *Trop Geo Med* 1982; 34:19–27.
288. Lockwood DE, Kreger AS, Richardson SH. Detection of toxins produced by *Vibrio fluvialis*. *Infect Immun* 1982; 352:702–708.
289. Morris JG, Lewin P, Hargrett NT, et al. Clinical features of ciguatera fish poisoning: a study of the disease in the U.S. Virgini Islands. *Arch Intern Med* 1982; 142:1090–1092.
290. Nishibuchi M, Doke S, Toizumis S, et al. Isolation from a coastal fish of *Vibrio hollisae* capable of producing a hemolysin similar to the thermostable direct hemolysin of *Vibrio parahaemolyticus*. *Appl Environ Microbiol* 1988; 54:2144–2146.
291. Dilmore LA, Hood MA. *Vibrios* of some deep-water invertebrates. *FEMS Microbiol Letters* 1986; 35:221–224.

292. Lowry PW, McFarland LM, Threefoot HK. *Vibrio hollisae* septicemia after consumption of catfish. *J Infect Dis* 1986; 154:730–731.
293. Rank EL, Smith IB, Langer M. Bacteremia caused by *Vibrio hollisae*. *J Clin Microbiol* 1988; 26:375–376.
294. Yoh M, Honda T, Miwatani T. Purification and partial characterization of a *Vibrio hollisae* hemolysin that reates to the thermostable direct hemolysin of *Vibrio parahaemolyticus*. *Can J Microbiol* 1986; 32:632–636.
295. Kothary MH, Richardson SH. Fluid accumulation in infant mice caused by *Vibrio hollisae* and its extracellular enterotoxin. *Infect Immun* 1987; 55:626–630.
296. Nishibuchi M, Ishibashi M, Takeda Y, et al. Detection of the thermostable direct hemolysin gene and related DNA sequences in *Vibrio parahaemolyticus* and other *Vibrio* species by the DAN colony hybridization test. *Infect Immun* 1985; 49:481–486.
297. Loev M, Teebken-Fisher D, Hose JE, et al. *Vibrio damsela*, a marine bacterium, causes skin ulcers on the damselfish *Chromis punctipinnis*. *Science* 1981; 214:1139.
298. Coffey JA, Harris RL, Rutledge ML, et al. *Vibrio damsela*: another potentially virulent marine *Vibrio*. *J Infect Dis* 1986; 153:800–802.
299. Schandevyl P, Van Dyck E, Piot P. Halophilic *Vibrio* species from seafish in Senegal. *Appl Environ Microbiol* 1984; 48:236–238.
300. Dryden MM, Legarde M, Gottlieb T, et al. *Vibrio damsela* wound infections in Australia (letter). *Med J Aust* 1989; 151:540–541.
301. Kreger AS. Cytolytic activity and virulence of *Vibrio damsela*. *Infect Immun* 1984; 44:326–331.
302. Sakazaki R. Proposal of *Vibrio alginolyticus* for the biotype 1 of *Vibrio parahaemolyticus*. *JP J Med Sci Biol* 1968; 21:359–362.
303. Prociv P. *Vibrio alginolyticus* in Western Australia. *Med J Aust* 1978; 2:296.
304. Pien FD, Ang KS, Nakashima NT, et al. Bacterial flora of marine penetrating injuries. *Diag Microbiol Infect Dis* 1983; 1:229–232.
305. Schmidt V, Chmel H, Cobbs C. *Vibrio alginolyticus* infections in humans. *J Clin Microbiol* 1979; 10:666–668.
306. Janda JM, Brenden R, DeBenedetti JA, et al. *Vibrio alginolyticus* bacteremia in an immunocompromised patient. *Diag Microbiol Infect Dis* 1986; (5):337–340.
307. English VL, Lindberg RB. Isolation of *Vibrio alginolyticus* from wounds and blood of a bum patient. *Am J Med Technol* 1977; 43:989–993.
308. Hare P, Scott-Burden T, Woods DR. Characterization of extracellular alkaline proteases and collagenase induction in *Vibrio alginolyticus*. *J Gen Microbiol* 1983; 129:1141–1147.
309. Larsen JL, Faid JF. In vitro antibiotic sensitivity testing of *Vibrio alginolyticus*. *Acta Pathol Microbiol Scand* 1980; 88:307–310.
310. Lam S, Monteiro E. Unusual *Vibrio* species found in diarrhoeal stools. *Singapore Med J* 1981; 22:259–261.
311. Nacescu N, Ciufecu C, Florescu D. *Vibrio alginolyticus* enteritis. *Ann Slavo* 1980; 22:169–172.
312. Opal SM, Saxon JR. Intracranial infection by *Vibrio alginolyticus* following injury in saltwater. *J Clin Microbiol* 1986; 23:373–374.

313. Lessner AM, Webb RM, Rabin B. P *Vibrio alginolyticus* conjunctivitis. *Arch Ophthalmol* 1985; 103:229–230.

314. Taylor R, McDonald M, Russ G, et al. *Vibrio alginolyticus* peritonitis associated with ambulatory peritoneal dialysis. *Br Med J* 1981; 283:275.

315. Brenner DJ, Hickman-Brenner FW, Lee JV, et al. *Vibrio furnissii* (formerly aerogenic biogroup of *Vibrio fluvialis*) a new species isolated form human feces and the environment. *J Clin Microbiol* 1983; 18:816–824.

316. Centers for Disease Control. An outbreak of acute gastroenteritis during a tour of the Orient—Alaska. *MMWR* 1969; 18:150.

317. Centers for Disease Control. Follow-up outbreak of gastroenteritis during a tour of the Orient—Alaska. *MMWR* 1969; 18:168.

318. Hickman-Brenner FW, Brenner DJ, Steigerwalt AG, et al. *Vibrio fluvialis* and *Vibrio furnissi* isolated from a stool sample of one patient. *J Clin Microbiol* 1984; 20:125–127.

319. Lam SYS, Goi LT. Isolations of "Group F *Vibrios*" from human stools. *Singapore Med J* 1985; 26:300–302.

320. Lee JV, Donovan TJ, Furniss AL. Characterization, taxonomy, and amended description of *Vibrio metschnikovii*. *Int J Syst Bacteriol* 1978; 28:99–111.

321. Jean-Jacques W, Rajashekaraiah KR, Farmer JJ III, et al. *Vibrio metschnikovii* bacteremia in a patient with cholecystitis. *J Clin Microbiol* 1981; 14:711–712.

322. Miyake M, Honda T, Miwatani T. Purification and characterization of *Vibrio metschnikovii* cytolysin. *Infect Immun* 1988; 56:954–960.

323. Miyake M, Honda T, Miwatani T. Effects of divalent cations and saccharides on *Vibrio metschnikovii* cytolysin-induces hemolysis of rabbit erythrocytes. *Infect Immun* 1989; 57:158–163.

324. Bode RB, Brayton PR, Colwell RR, et al. A new *Vibrio* species, *Vibrio cincinnatiensis*, causing meningitis: successful treatment in an adult. *Ann Intern Med* 1986; 104:55–56.

325. Brayton PR, Bode RB, Colwell RR, et al. *Vibrio cincinnationsis sp. nov.*, a new human pathogen. *J Clin Microbiol* 1986; 23:104–108.

326. Grimes DJ, Stemmler J, Hada H, et al. *Vibrio* species associated with mortality of sharks held in captivity. *Microbiol Ecol* 1984; 10:271–282.

327. Pavia AT, Bryan JA, Maher KL, et al. *Vibrio carchariae* infection after a shark bite. *Ann Intern Med* 1989; 111:85–86.

328. Aronson JD. Spontaneous tuberculosis in saltwater fish. *J Infect Dis* 1926; 39:315–320.

329. Baker JA, Hagan WA. Tuberculosis of Mexican platyfish (*Platypoecilus maculatus*). *J Infect Dis* 1942; 70:248–252.

330. Linell F, Norden A. *Mycobacterium balnei*: a new acid-fast bacillus occurring in swimming pools and capable of producing skin lesions in humans. *Acta Tuberc Scand* (Suppl) 1954; 33:1–84.

331. Collins CH, Grange JM, Noble WC, et al. *Mycobacterium marinum* infections in man. *J Hyg Camb* 1985; 94:135–149.

332. Swift S, Cohen H. Granuiomas of the skin due to *Mycobacterium balnei* after abrasions from a fish tank. *N Engl J Med* 1962; 267:1244–1246.

333. Feldman RA, Long MW, David HL. *Mycobacterium marinum*: a leisure time pathogen. *J Infect Dis* 1974; 129:618–621.

334. Heineman HS, Spitzer S, Pianphongsant T. Fish tank granuloma. A hobby hazard. *Arch Intern Med* 1972; 130:121–123.

335. Clark RB, Spector H, et al. Osteomyelitis and synovitis produced by *Mycobacterium marinum* in a fisherman. *J Clin Microbiol* 1990; 28:2570–2572.

336. Lacy JN, Viegas SF, Calhoun J, et al. *Mycobacterium marinum* flexor tenosynovitis. *Clin Orthop Rel Res* 1989; 238:288–293.

337. *Mycobacteria.* In: Koneman EW, Allen SD, Dowell VR, Janda WM, Sommers HM, Winn WC (eds): *Color Atlas and Textbook of Diagnostic Microbiology.* Philadelphia, J.B. Lippincott Co., 1988:535–572.

338. Nilsen A, Boe O. Fish tank granuloma. *Acta Dermatovener* (Stockholm) 1980; 60:451–452.

339. Vincenzi G, Bardazzi F, Tosti A, et al. Fish tank granuloma: report of a case. *Cutis* 1992; 49:275–276.

340. Jolly HW, Seabury JH. Infections with *Mycobacterium marinum. Arch Dematol* 1972; 106:32–36.

341. Wagner Jr RW, Tawil AB, Colletta AJ, et al. *Mycobacterium marinum* teosynovitis in a Long Island fisherman. *NYSJ of Med* 1981; 81:1091–1094.

342. Burnett JW. Some natural jellyfish toxins. In: Hall, Sun T (eds): *Marine Toxins. Origin, Structure, and Molecular Pharmacology.* Washington, D.C., American Chemical Society, 1990: 333–335.

343. Enzenauer RJ, McKoy J, Vincent D. Disseminated cutaneous and synovial *Mycobacyerium marinum* infection in a patients with systemic lupus erythematosus. *South Med J* 1990; 83:471–474.

344. Gombert ME, Goldstein LC, Corrado ML, et al. Disseminated *Mycobacterium marinum* infection after renal transplantation. *Ann Intern Med* 1981; 94:486–487.

345. King AJ, Fairley JA, Rasmussen JE. Disseminated cutaneous *Mycobacterium marinum* infection. *Arch Dermatol* 1983; 119:268–270.

346. Jones MW, Wahid IA, Matthews JP. Septic arthritis of the hand due to *Mycobacterium marinum. J Hand Surg* 1988; 13B:333–334.

347. Schonherr U, Naumann GOH, Lang GK, et al. Sclerokeratitis caused by *Mycobacterium marinum. Am J Ophthalmol* 1989; 108:607–608.

348. Van Dyke JJ, Lake KB. Chemotherapy for aquarium granuloma. *JAMA* 1975; 233:1380–1381.

349. Hurst LC, Amadio PC, Badalamente MA, et al. *Mycobactyerium marinum* infections of the hand. *J Hand Surg* 1987; 12A:428–435.

350. Mollohan CS, Romer MS. Public health significance of swimming pool granuloma. *Am J Pub Health* 1961; 51:883–891.

351. Huminer D, Pitlik SD, Block C, et al. Aquarium-borne *Mycobacterium marinum* skin infection: report of a case and review of the literature. *Arch Dermatol* 1986; 122:698–703.

352. Hoyt RE, Bryant JE, Glessner SF, et al. *M. marinum* infections in a Chesapeake Bay community. *Virginia Med* 1989; 16:467–470.

353. Bruckner-Tuderman L, Blank AA. Unusual cutaneous dissemination of a tropical fish tank granuloma. *Cutis* 1985; 405:408.

354. Prevost E, Walker Jr. EM, Kreutner AJ, et al. *Mycobacterium marinum* infections: diagnosis and treatment. *South Med J* 1982; 75:1349–1352.

355. Ries KM, White Jr. GL, Murdock RT. Atypical mycobacterial infection caused by *Mycobacterium marinum. N Engl J Med* 1990; 322:633.

356. Chow SP, Ip FK, Lau HK, et al. *Mycobacterium marinum* infection of the hand and wrist. *J Bone and Joint Surg* 1987; 69A:1161–1168.

357. Williams CS, Riordan DC. *Mycobacterium marinum* (atypical acid-fast bacillus) infections of the hand: a report of six cases. *J Bone and Joint Surg* 1973; 55A:1042–1050.

358. Loria PR. Minocycline hydrochloride treatment for atypical acid-fast infection. *Arch Dermatol* 1976; 112:517–519.

359. Izumi AK, Hanke CW, Higaki M. *Mycobacterium marinum* infections treated with tetracycline. *Arch Dermatol* 1977; 113:1067–1068.

360. Brown JW III, Sanders CV. *Mycobacterium marinum* infections: a problem of recognition, not therapy? *Arch Intern Med* 1987; 147:817–818.

361. Donta ST, Smith PW, Levitz RE, et al. Therapy of *Mycobacterium marinum* infections: use of tetracyclines vs. rifampin. *Arch Intern Med* 1986; 146:902–904.

362. Ljungbert B, Christensson B, Grubb R. Failure of doxycycline treatment in aquarium-associated *Mycobacterium marinum* infections. *Scan J Infect Dis* 1987; 19:539–543.

363. Collins CH, Uttley HC. In vitro activity of seventeen antimicrobial compounds against seven species of mycobacteria. *J Antimicrob Chemother* 1988; 22:857–861.

364. Brown CK, Shepher SM. Marine trauma, envenomations, and intoxications, *Emerg Med Clin North Am* 1992; 10:385–408.

365. Auerbach PS. Hazardous marine animals. *Emerg Med Clin North Am* 1984; 2:531–544.

366. Baldridge HD, Williams J. Shark attack: feeding or fighting? *Milit Med* 1969; 134:130–133.

367. McCabe MJ, Hammon WM, Halstead BW, et al. A fatal brain injury caused by a needlefish. *Neuroradiology* 1978; 15:137–139.

368. Haddad LM, Lee RF, McConnell O, et al. Toxic marine life. In: Haddad LM, Winchester (eds): *Clinical Management of Poisoning and Drug Overdose*. Philadelphia, W.B. Saunders, 1983:303–317.

369. Sodeman WA Jr. Venomous marine animals. In: Strickland (ed): *Hunter's Tropical Medicine*. Philadelphia; W.B. Saunders Co., 1991:869–875.

370. Russell FE. Injuries by venomous animals in the U.S. *JAMA* 1961; 177:85.

371. Trestrail JH III, al-Mahasneh QM. Lionfish sting experiences of an inland poison center: a retrospective study of 23 cases. *Vet Hum Toxicol* 1989; 31:173–175.

372. Auerbach PS, Halstead B. Marine hazards: attacks and envenomations. *J Emerg Nurs* 1982; 8:115–122.

373. Tu AT. Neurotoxins from sea snake and other vertebrate venoms. In: Hall, Strichartz (eds): *Marine Toxins. Origin, Structure, and Molecular Pharmacology*. Washington, D.C., American Chemical Society, 1990:336–346.

374. Soppe GG. Marine envenomation and aquatic dermatology. *Am Fam Physician* 1989; 40:97–106.

375. Auerbach PS, Halstead BW. Hazardous aquatic life. In: Auerbach PS, Geehr EC (eds): *Management of Wilderness and Environmental Emergencies*. St. Louis, C.V. Mosby, 1989:933–1028.

376. Tu AT. Biotoxicology of sea snake venoms. *Ann Emerg Med* 1987; 16:-1023–1028.

377. Murphey DK, Septimus EJ, Waagner DC. Catfish-related injury and infection: report of two cases and review of the literature. *Clin Infect Dis* 1992; 14:689–693.
378. Halstead BW. Coelenterate (Cnidarian) stings and wounds. *Clin Dermatol* 1987; 5:8–13.
379. Burnett JW, Calton GJ. Jellyfish envenomation syndromes updated. *Ann Emerg Med* 1987; 16:1000–1005.
380. Togias AG, Burnett JW, Kagey-Sobotka A, et al. Anaphylaxis after contact with a jellyfish. *J Allergy Clin Immunol* 1985; 75:673–675.
381. Lumley J, Williamson JA, Fenner PJ, et al. Fatal envenomation by *Chironex fleckert*, the north Australian box jellyfish: the continuing search for lethal mechanisms. *Med J Aust* 1988; 148:527–534.
382. Fenner PJ, Williamson JA, Burnett JW, et al. The "Irukundji Syndrome" and acute pulmonary edema. *Med J Aust* 1988; 149:150–156.
383. Centers for Disease Control. Cercarial dermatitis outbreak in a state park—Delaware, 1991. *MMWR* 1992; 41:225–228.
384. Neafie RC, Meyers WM. Cutaneous larva migrans. In: Strickland (ed): *Hunter's Tropical Medicine*. Philadelphia, W.B. Saunders Co., 1991:773–775.
385. Sarnaik AP, Vohra MP, Sturman SW, et al. Medical problems of the swimmer. *Clin Sports Med* 1986; 5:47–64.
386. Ryan AJ. Nontraumatic medical problems. In: Ryan AJ, Allman FL (eds): *Sports Medicine*. San Diego, Academic Press, 1989.
387. Stewart JP. Chronic exudative otitis externa. *J Laryngol Otol* 1951;65: 24.
388. Becker GD, Parell GJ. Otolaryngologic aspects of scuba diving. *Otolaryngol Head Neck Surg* 1979; 87:569–572.
389. Cassissi N, Cohn A, Davidson T, et al. Diffuse otitis externa: clinical and microbiologic findings in the course of a multicenter study on a new otic solution. *Ann Otol Rhinol Laryngol* 1972; 86(Suppl):39.
390. Schuller DE, Bruce RA. Ear, nose, throat, and eye. In: Strauss RH (ed): *Sports Medicine*. Philadelphia, W.B. Saunders Co., 1991.
391. Robinson AC. Evaluation for waterproof ear protectors in swimmers. *J Larngol Otol* 1989; 103:1154–1157.
392. Meyerhoff WL, Morizono T, Wright CG, et al. Tympanostomy tubes and otic drops. *Laryngoscope* 1983; 93:1022–1027.
393. Lounsbury BF. Swimming unprotected with long-shafted middle ear ventilation tubes. *Laryngoscope* 1985; 95:340–343.
394. Jaffe BF. Are water and tympanostomy tubes compatible? *Laryngoscope* 1981; 91:563–564.
395. Wright DN, Alexander JM. Effect of water on the bacterial flora of swimmer's ears. *Arch Otolaryngol* 1974; 99:15–18.
396. Bergh O, Borsheim KY, Bratbak G, et al. High abundance of viruses found in aquatic environments. *Nature* 1989; 340:467–468.
397. Craun GF. Introduction. In: Craun GF (ed): *Waterborne Diseases in the United States*. Boca Raton, CRC Press, 1984.
398. Gerba CP, Goyal CM, LaBelle RI, et al. Failure of indicator bacteria to reflect the occurrence of enteroviruses in marine waters. *Am J Public Health* 1979; 69:1116–1119.

399. Melnick JL, Gerba CP. The ecology of enteroviruses in natural waters. *CRC Crit Rev Environ Cont* 1980; 10:65–93.
400. Goyal SM. Viral pollution of the marine environment. *CRC Crit Rev Environ Cont* 1984; 14:32.
401. Gerba CP, Goyal SM. Development of a qualitative pathogen risk assessment methodology for ocean disposal of municipal sludge. U. S. Environmental Protection Agency, ALAO-CIN-493. Cincinnati, 1986.
402. Cabelli VJ, DuFour AP, McCabe LJ, et al. Swimming associated gastroenteritis and water quality. *Am J Epidemiol* 1982; 115:606–616.
403. Saliba LJ, Helmer R. Health risks associated with pollution of coastal bathing waters. *Wld Hlth Statist Quart* 1990; 43:177–187.
404. D'Alessio DJ, Minor TE, Allen CI, et al. A study of the proportions of swimmers among well controls and children with enterovirus-like illness shedding or not shedding an enterovirus. *Am J Epidemiol* 1981; 113:533–541.
405. Mosely JW. Epidemiologic aspects of microbial standards for bathing beaches. Discharge of sewage from sea outfalls. *Proceedings of an international symposium* 1974; 80–93.
406. Centers for Disease Control. Gastroenteritis associated with lake swimming. *MMWR* 1979; 28(35):413.
407. Brown JM, Campbell EA, Rickards AD, et al. Sewage pollution of bathing water. *Lancet* 1987; ii:1208–1209.
408. Yamashita T, Sakae K, Ishihara Y, et al. A 2-year survey of the prevalence of enteric viral infections in children compared with contamination in locally-harvested oysters. *Epidemiol Infect* 1992; 108:155–163.
409. Mahoney FJ, Farley TA, Kelso KY, et al. An outbreak of hepatitis A associated with swimming in a public pool. *J Infect* Dis 1992; 165:613–618.
410. Wanke CA, Guerrant RL. Viral hepatitis and gastroenteritis transmitted by shellfish and water. *Infect Dis Clin North Am* 1987; 1:649–664.
411. Hu M, Li T, Hu X, et al. Isolation of HAV from experimentally infected shellfish (abstract). *Abstracts of the IXth International Congress of Infectious and Parasitic Diseases* (Munich). Munich, Infectious Disease Association, 1986.
412. Halliday ML, Kang L, Zhou T, et al. An epidemic of hepatitis A attributable to the ingestion of raw clams in shanghai, China. *J Infect Dis* 1991; 164:852–859.
413. West PA. Hazard analysis critical control point (HAACP) concept: application to bivalve shellfish purification systems. *J Roy Soc Hlth* 1986; 105:133–139.
414. DuPont HL. Consumption of raw shellfish—is the risk now unacceptable? *N Engl J Med* 1986; 314:707–708.
415. Heller D, Gill ON, Raynham D, et al. Epidemiology: an outbreak of gastrointestinal illness associated with consumption of raw depurated oysters. *Br Med J* 1986; 292:1726–1727.
416. Koff RS, Sear HS. Internal temperature of steamed clams. *N Engl J Med* 1967; 276:737–739.
417. McCollum RW, Zuckerman AJ. Viral hepatitis: report on a WHO informal consultation. *J Med Virol* 1981; 8:1–29.

418. Scheid R, Deinhardt F, Frosner G, et al. Inactivation of hepatitis A and B virus and risk of iatrogenic transmission. In: Szmuness W, Alter HJ, Maynard HE (eds): *Viral hepatitis*. Philadelphia, Franklin, Institute Press, 1982.

419. Mishu B, Hadler SC, Boaz VA. Foodborne hepatitis A: evidence that microwaving reduces risk. *J Infect Dis* 1990; 162:655–658.

420. Roos B. Hepatitis epidemic transmitted by oysters. *Svenska lak-tidning* 1956; 53:989–1003.

421. Portnoy BL, Mackowiak PA, Caraway CT, et al. Oyster-associated hepatitis: failure of shellfish certification programs to prevent outbreaks. *JAMA* 1975; 233:1065–1068.

422. Harris JR, Cohen ML, Lippy EC. Water-related disease outbreaks in the United States, 1981. *J Infect Dis* 1981; 148:759–762.

423. Ramia S. Transmission of viral infections by the water route: implications for developing countries. *Rev Infect Dis* 1985; 7:180–188.

424. Centers for Disease Control. Hepatitis surveillance report no. 51. 1987 US Department of Health and Human Services. Atlanta.

425. Centers for Disease Control. Table III, Cases of specified notifiable diseases, United States. *MMWR* 1989; 37:803.

426. Centers for Disease Control. Summary of notifiable diseases, United States. *MMWR* 1987; 36:54.

427. Centers for Disease Control. Hepatitis surveillance report no. 52. 1989 US Department of Health and Human Services. Atlanta.

428. Centers for Disease Control. Foodborne hepatitis A—Alaska, Florida, North Carolina, Washington. *MMWR* 1990; 39:228–232.

429. Desenclos J-CA, Klontz KC, Wilder MH. A multistate outbreak of hepatitis A caused by the consumption of raw oysters. *Am J Public Health* 1991; 81:1268–1272.

430. Tang YW, Wang JX, Xu ZY, et al. A serologically confirmed, case-control study, of a large outbreak of hepatitis A in China, associated with consumption of clams. *Epidemiol Infect* 1991; 107:651–657.

431. Appleton H. Foodborne viruses. *Lancet* 1990; 336:1362–1364.

432. Rosenblum LS, Mirkin IR, Allen DT, et al. A multifocal outbreak of hepatitis A traced to commercially distributed lettuce. *AJPH* 1990; 80:1075–1079.

433. Reid TMS, Robinson HG. Frozen raspberries and hepatitis A. *Epidemiol Infect* 1987; 98:109–112.

434. Fang G, Araujo V, Guerrant RL. Enteric infections associated with exposure to animals or animal products. *Infect Dis Clin North Am* 1991; 5:681–701.

435. Dolin R, Treanor JJ, Madore HP. Novel agents of viral enteritis in humans. *J Infect Dis* 1987; 155:365–375.

436. Gunn RA, Janowski HT, Lieb S, et al. Norwalk virus gastroenteritis following raw oyster consumption. *Am J Epidemiol* 1982; 115:348–351.

437. Kaplan JE, Goodman RA, Baron RC, et al. Epidemiology of Norwalk gastroenteritis and the role of Norwalk virus in outbreaks of acute nonbacterial gastroenteritis. *Ann Intern Med* 1982; 96:756–761.

438. Craun GF. "Recent statistics of waterborne outbreaks (1981–1983). In: Craun GF (ed): *Waterborne diseases in the United States*. Boca Raton, CRC Press, 1986.
439. Murphy M, Grohmann GS, Christopher PJ, et al. An Australia-wide outbreak of gastroenteritis from oysters caused by Norwalk virus. *Med J Australia* 1979; 2:329–333.
440. Morse DL, Guzewich JJ, Hanrahan JP, et al. Widespread outbreaks of clam- and oyster-associated gastroenteritis: role of Norwalk virus. *N Engl J Med* 1986, 314:678–681.
441. Goldsmith R, Yarbough PO, Reyes GR, et al. Enzyme-linked immunosorbent assay for diagnosis of acute sporadic hepatitis E in Egyptian children. *Lancet* 1992; 339:328–331.
442. Viswanathan R. Infectious hepatitis in Delhi (1955–56): a critical study; epidemiology. *Ind J Med Res* 1957; 45(Suppl):1–30.
443. Sreenivasan MA, Banerjee K, Pandya PG, et al. Epidemiologic investigations of an outbreak of infectious hepatitis in Ahmedabad City during 1975–76. *Ind J Med Res* 1978; 67:197–206.
444. Wong DC, Purcell RH, Sreenivasan MA, et al. Epidemic and endemic hepatitis in India: evidence for a non-A, non-B hepatitis etiology. *Lancet* 1980; ii:876–879.
445. Bradley DW. Enterically-transmitted non-A, non-B hepatitis. *Br Med Bull* 1990; 46:442–461.
446. Tsega E, Krawczynski K, Hansson BG, et al. Outbreak of hepatitis E virus infection among military personnel in Northern Ethiopia. *J Med Virol* 1991; 34:232–236.
447. Bader TF, Krawczynski K, Favorov MO. Hepatitis E in a U.S. traveler to Mexico [letter]. *N Engl J Med* 1991; 325:1659.
448. Bradley D, Andjaparidze A, Cook EH, et al. Aetiological agent of enterically transmitted non-A, non-B hepatitis. *J Gen Virol* 1988; 69:731–738.
449. Ticehurst J, Rhodes LLJ, Krawczynski K, et al. Infection of owl monkeys (Aotus trivirgatus) and cynomolgus monkeys (Macaca fascicularis) with hepatitis E virus from Mexico. *J Infect Dis* 1992; 69:835–845.
450. World Health Organization. Rotavirus and other viral diarrhoeas. *Bull WHO* 1980; 58:183–198.
451. Meurman OH, Laine MJ. Rotavirus epidemics in adults. *N Engl J Med* 1977; 296:1298–1299.
452. Bonsdorff CH, Hovi T, Makela P, et al. Rotavirus infections in adults in association with acute gastroenteritis. *J Med Virol* 1978; 2:21–28.
453. Gill ON, Cubitt WD, McSwiggan DA, et al. Epidemic of gastroenteritis cased by oysters contaminated with small round structured viruses. *Br Med J* 1983; 287:1532–1534.
454. Appleton H, Pereira MS. A Possible virus etiology in outbreaks of food-poisoning from cockles. *Lancet* 1977; i:780.

4
On Fresh Water

DAVID L. DWORZACK

Introduction

In this chapter, I will discuss infections acquired in nonmarine environments. Both natural fresh waters (lakes, ponds, rivers, streams) and man-made aquatic environments (swimming pools, hot-tubs, whirlpools, spas) may serve as the origin for numerous pathogenic microorganisms. I will limit consideration to infections associated more with immersion in aquatic environments than with ingesting them. Even with this limitation, however, the reader will appreciate the wide variety of potential pathogens which occasionally cause problems for patients taking their leisure in fresh water (Table 4.1).

Water-borne pathogens may enter the body through inhalation, aspiration, direct application to the intact or injured skin, or invasion of respiratory or gastrointestinal mucosa. Pathogens may be native to aquatic environments or they may proliferate there because of the influence of man or his waste products. These microorganisms can produce infections that are often merely nuisances, as well as those that threaten life or have long-term severe sequelae.

Skin and Soft Tissue Infections

Skin, soft tissue, and wound infections acquired in aquatic, nonmarine environments run the gamut from relatively benign conditions which resolve without specific therapy to life threatening processes requiring intensive medical and surgical care. Infections caused by pyogenic bacteria, mycobacteria, parasites, and algae have all been reported.

Pseudomonas Dermatitis/Folliculitis

This superficial infection, which usually is recognized in clusters or localized outbreaks, was first reported in 1975 by McCausland and Cox (1).

TABLE 4.1. Infections associated with exposure to fresh water.

Skin and soft tissue infections
    Pseudomonas aeruginosa dermatitis/folliculitis
    Acute diffuse otitis externa (swimmer's ear)
    Schistosome dermatitis (swimmer's itch, clam-digger's itch)
    Nontuberculous mycobacterial infections (*M marinum, M fortuitum, M chelonae*)
    Gram-negative bacillary infections (*Aeromonas* spp., *Edwardsiella tarda*)
    Prototheca infection
Ocular infections
    Pharyngoconjunctival fever (swimming pool conjunctivitis)
    Amoebic keratitis (*Acanthamoeba* spp.)
Pulmonary infections
    Legionella infections (pneumonia, Pontiac fever)
    Pseudomonas aeruginosa pneumonia
    Pneumonia following near drowning (*Pseudomonas aeruginosa, Aeromonas* spp.,
        Pseudallescheria boydii, Aspergillus spp.)
Disseminated infections
    Leptospirosis
    Chromobacterium violaceum
Central nervous system infections
    Primary amoebic meningoencephalitis (*Naegleria fowleri*)
    Pseudallescheria boydii brain abscess
    Coxsackievirus infection

This original outbreak, like most others reported since, was associated with exposure to heated water in a hotel whirlpool (1–5). Similar occurrences have followed the use of home spas as well as swimming pools (6). One large outbreak involved exposure at a water slide (7).

In most outbreaks, faulty maintenance of water in these man-made pools has been associated with overgrowth of *Pseudomonas aeruginosa*. Recommendations for treatment of pool water include maintaining pH between 7.2 and 7.8 and free chlorine levels >0.5 mg/L (8). In one outbreak, however, the pH and chlorine content of contaminated water was found to be within these guidelines, suggesting some strains of *P aeruginosa* may be more resistant to recommended chlorine concentrations (4).

There have been more outbreaks associated with whirlpools or spas than with swimming pools, indicating that the environment of the former is more conducive to the development of folliculitis. In part, this appears related to the difficulty in maintaining a stable free chlorine level in whirlpools as compared to swimming pools because of the higher temperature of the water, mechanical agitation and aeration by pressurized jets, and a higher concentration of organic material because of the large number of bathers per volume of water (9). For this reason, some have recommended higher concentrations of free chlorine (1 to 3 mg/L) in whirlpool or spa water (4,10). In addition to the predisposing environmental factors mentioned above, dilatation of skin pores because of the higher water temperature may facilitate entry of the *P aeruginosa* contained in the water (2).

Most outbreaks have been associated with serogroup O-11 *P aeruginosa*, although serogroups O-1 and O-9 have been implicated occasionally (4–6).

Clinically, *P aeruginosa* dermatitis/folliculitis presents after an incubation period which averages 48 hours with a range of 8 to 120 hours (6). Younger patients (<20 years) appear predisposed, as do those who are exposed to the contaminated water longer or more frequently (11). Showering after exposure to *P aeruginosa*-laden water does not appear to prevent development of the infection, suggesting that the organism rapidly gains access to the deeper regions of the skin pores during water exposure (4). Initially, the infection is manifested as pruritic follicular papules of 2 to 10 mm in diameter, generally located on the buttocks, thighs, arms, and axillae. These are areas in which apocrine sweat glands are located, which frequently open into hair follicles. Other skin areas can be involved as well. Women not infrequently develop a low-grade mastitis through infection of the glands of Montgomery (6). Several authors have reported a greater intensity of rash in areas covered by tight bathing suits (2,11). Application to the skin of felt pads wetted with water containing pseudomonads and covered with an occlusive dressing have been shown to induce a maculopustular rash on the superhydrated skin, similar to the eruptions described in these patients (12). The face and scalp are generally not affected, as these parts of the body are typically not immersed when the patient is using a whirlpool or spa. With time, pinpoint pustules develop in the center of the papules, and the rash generally heals in 2 to 5 days without scarring. Hyperpigmentation may persist at the site of the papules for some time, however (11). Fever, if present at all, is usually low grade. Occasional patients have complained of malaise or headache. Secondary infection to friends or family members has not been documented (6).

Systemic or topical antibiotic therapy is not required, and topical corticosteroid therapy may delay resolution of the folliculitis.

Acute diffuse otitis externa (swimmer's ear) also is usually caused by *P aeruginosa* and may be similar in its pathogenesis to *Pseudomonas* folliculitis. Swimmer's ear has been seen more frequently in swimming pool users than in whirlpool/spa users who usually keep their heads out of the water (6). However, an outbreak has been reported related to the use of redwood hot-tubs (13). Clinical manifestations of swimmer's ear include discharge from a pruritic or painful external auditory canal that, on examination, is erythematous, edematous, and filled with debris. Usually, systemic antibiotic therapy is unnecessary; the infection responds to 2% acetic acid otic solution which impairs the growth of *P aeruginosa*. Topical steroid and antibiotic-containing ear drops are also employed. Infection is often recurrent in swimmers.

Only rarely in normal hosts does *P aeruginosa* penetrate deeper structures surrounding the external auditory canal. However, in diabetics, acute diffuse otitis externa may give rise to life-threatening malignant otitis externa which is rapidly spreading and highly destructive of tissue. Most malignant otitis externa, although caused by *P aeruginosa*, does not appear to be related to swimmer's ear, however.

Schistosome Dermatitis (Swimmer's Itch, Clam Digger's Itch)

Schistosome dermatitis is caused when the cercariae of a number of nonhuman schistosomes penetrate the skin of man, are unable to proceed further, and are destroyed, causing a pruritic skin rash. The disease was first noted in the United States by Cort in 1928 among patients who had been wading in Douglas Lake, in Michigan (14). Since then, more than twenty species of cercariae from fresh water snails and at least four species from marine snails have been found to produce the illness (15). Snails are intermediate hosts for the schistosomes whose natural hosts are usually waterfowl or nonprimate mammals. The illness has been described in North, Central, and South America, as well as Oceania, India, and Africa. In the United States, illness following swimming or wading in lakes in the North Central states have been most frequent. Marine outbreaks in Florida, southern California, and Hawaii have also been reported.

Clinical manifestations include an initial "prickling" sensation, typically felt when the film of water evaporates on the skin. This is followed by urticaria which spontaneously subsides, usually within an hour, with the persistence of pruritic macules. With time, these macules may evolve into papules or pustules which reach their peak intensity in 48 to 72 hours. The severity of the reaction varies markedly from person to person and appears to increase with repeated exposures, as the patient becomes sensitized. In most patients, symptoms subside in 4 to 7 days, but severely allergic individuals may be symptomatic for more than a week.

Histopathologically, the cercariae are unable to penetrate human skin, become walled off, and evoke an acute inflammatory response with infiltration of lymphocytes, neutrophils, and eosinophils.

There is no specific antihelminthic therapy. The illness is treated with topical and systemic medications to control the pruritus. Prevention is largely keyed to control of the intermediate host by application of molluscacides, such as copper sulfate and copper carbonate, to water.

Skin and Soft Tissue Infections Caused by Nontuberculous Mycobacteria

Mycobacterium marinum is the most frequently identified mycobacterial species causing skin and subcutaneous tissue infections associated with immersion. The organism is a photochromagen which grows best at 32°C and poorly at 37°C or more (16). It inhabits both fresh- and saltwater environments as a free-living organism. It was first recognized as a pathogen in aquarium fish in 1927 by Aronson (17).

Human infection was described definitively in 1954. An outbreak of 80 cases of skin infection acquired in a swimming pool was reported. The responsible organism was initially identified as *M balnei*, later shown to be synonymous with *M marinum* (18).

Human infection is usually associated with trauma, such as abrasions, injuries from fish spines, or pricks from crustacean or shellfish shells, although the injury itself is often trivial. Usually, the infection is confined to cooler areas of the body such as the extremities. The incubation period appears to be several weeks, with initial lesions appearing as groups of small papules. Typically, there is progression to shallow ulcerations (16). However, there is considerable pleomorphism in the appearance of the infections with "sporotrichoid" variants in which nodules appear in the afferent lymphatics, simulating sporotrichosis (16).

Involvement of deeper structures in the hand, such as the synovium, tendons, and bones, has been demonstrated (19). Dissemination has been reported in both immunosuppressed and immunocompetent patients (20,21).

Diagnosis is made most readily from tissue biopsy. The specimen should be submitted for mycobacterial culture as well as histology, since the organism frequently cannot be identified in the biopsy microscopically. Growth of the organism in the laboratory is facilitated by incubation at 30 to 32°C (22). A range of histopathological findings is possible, with some lesions showing suppuration, and others, granulomas of varying organization.

Many *M marinum* lesions spontaneously resolve (16). This quality makes it difficult to judge the broad clinical applicability of anecdotal reports describing successful interventional drug or surgical therapy. Many smaller lesions are adequately resected at the time of biopsy and require no further therapy. Surgical debridement is sometimes required for infections involving the hand, where closed spaces may be involved. In vitro, *M marinum* is usually susceptible to rifampin, ethambutol, trimethoprim/sulfamethoxazole, tetracyclines, and amikacin. It is usually resistant to isoniazid and streptomycin (23). Because antimicrobial therapy is felt to shorten the duration of this frequently painful illness, patients are usually given such therapy, especially if the lesion is on the hand. Successes as well as failures have been reported with tetracyclines and trimethoprim/

sulfamethoxazole (24). Rifampin, with or without ethambutol, has generally been reported to produce favorable results, even in tetracycline failures (25). The proper duration of therapy is uncertain, with most authors recommending 6 to 12 weeks (16,25). Relapses have been reported frequently. They usually respond to the same antimicrobial agents, given for a longer period.

It is unusual to encounter community-acquired skin and soft tissue infections caused by mycobacteria other than *M marinum* in which immersion in fresh water is an epidemiological factor. Occasional rapidly growing mycobacterial infections (*M fortuitum*, *M chelonae*) have occurred following injuries in water, but far more common is a history of injury caused by objects contaminated with soil (26). These organisms are resistant to most antituberculous agents, but are often susceptible to amikacin, ciprofloxacin, cefoxitin, doxycycline, and rifampin (27). Extensive debridement, coupled with combination antimicrobial agent therapy appears to offer the best chance of cure.

Soft Tissue Infections Caused by Gram-Negative Bacilli

Aeromonas species are gram-negative straight or curved bacilli. They have been implicated as a cause of gastroenteritis, traumatic and surgical wound infections, myonecrosis, gangrene, osteomyelitis, and, rarely, lower respiratory tract and ocular infections (28).

Traumatic wound infections in which the organism appears to have been acquired from contaminated fresh or salt water have been reported frequently. These infections tend to occur on the lower extremities or hands and are often sustained while wading or swimming (29). The spectrum of severity is broad, ranging from mild cellulitis to rapidly-progressive, life-threatening myonecrosis with gangrene. Presumably, the virulence of the infecting strain as well as the severity of the injury and the immune status of the patient are all factors determining this severity. Janda has provided an excellent recent review of *Aeromonas* virulence factors and pathogenicity (30).

Cases of cellulitis have been described related not only to injuries that occur while immersed in environmental water, but also to an abrasion associated with a fish tank (31), to a boating accident (32), and following swimming in river water in which no injuries were sustained (33). Cellulitis "one-step removed" from fresh water has recently been reported as a complication of the use of the medicinal fresh water leech *Hirudo medicinalis* for treatment of vascular congestion after surgical procedures. *A hydrophila* is part of the normal gut flora of this annelid (34). No definite aeromonad infections have been reported in naturally-acquired leech bites.

More severe aeromonad tissue infections, including myonecrosis with or without gas gangrene, have been reported. In a number of these cases, the original injury occurred in association with fresh water (28,35). Some patients had underlying conditions associated with immune deficits, such as diabetes or corticosteroid use (36,37), while others appeared to be immunocompetent. The latter group includes the case of a 19-year-old man whose leg was lacerated by a motor boat propeller and that of an 88-year-old woman who cut her hand on a fish bone (35,38). Bacteremia may complicate these severe soft tissue infections and appears to significantly worsen the prognosis. Heckerling et al in their case report and literature review found no survivors among patients with *Aeromonas* myonecrosis complicated by bacteremia (38). In their article on human infections caused by *Aeromonas* species, Janda and Duffey reviewed studies of patients with bacteremia previously reported in the literature; mortality ranged from 29% to 73% in these studies (28). Most of these patients did not have severe soft tissue infections which caused their bacteremia. In fact, the precipitating event was not apparent in many patients, although some had a history of contact with water. *Aeromonas* bacteremia may give rise to ecthyma gangrenosum, which has the identical clinical appearance to that seen in *P aeruginosa* septicemia (28). In addition to traumatic injuries, hematologic malignancies, solid tumors, and hepatobiliary disorders all appear to predispose to *Aeromonas* bacteremia (29).

Aeromonas soft tissue infections which complicate trauma in fresh water can lead to contiguous osteomyelitis. Karam et al reported two such cases occurring in immunologically normal patients (39).

In vitro, *A hydrophila* is generally susceptible to "third-generation" cephalosporins, chloramphenicol, trimethoprim/sulfamethoxazole, fluoroquinolones, aztreonam, and aminoglycosides. *A sobria* tends to be more susceptible to cephalothin, but more variable in susceptibility to chloramphenicol and amikacin (40). Broad-based β-lactam resistance may develop in *Aeromonas* species through stable derepression of inducible chromosomal β-lactamases (41). Clinical reports have generally described therapy with combinations of antibiotics, often "third-generation" cephalosporins combined with aminoglycosides.

Edwardsiella tarda is a gram-negative bacterium that has been isolated from reptiles, fish, mammals, birds, and environmental water sources (42). Soft tissue infections caused by *E tarda* have been associated with injuries sustained in fresh water. Clinically, these infections appear to be similar to *Aeromonas* cellulitis (42,43). The organism is susceptible in vitro to ampicillin, chloramphenicol, aminoglycosides, cephalosporins, tetracyclines, fluroquinolones, and trimethoprim/sulfamethoxazole (44).

Prototheca Skin and Soft Tissue Infections

Prototheca are unicellular achloric algae. They are found in aquariums, fresh or stagnant water, and other moist environments (45). Human infections of two types have been described. Papulonodular or ulcerative skin lesions have generally followed minor trauma or surgical incisions, particularly on the extremities or face. Often, patients with these wound infections report exposure to environments known to harbor the organism. The other type of infection is olecranon bursitis, usually following minor (even nonpenetrating) trauma. In the United States, most *Prototheca* infections have been reported from southern or central states (46).

Diagnosis is best established by biopsy and culture. Microabscesses and granulomata are seen histologically. Fungal stains such as Gomori methenamine silver will usually identify the organism in the biopsied tissue. Prototheca grows on Sabouraud agar, producing whitish colonies (45).

Antimicrobial and/or surgical therapy is usually necessary; few lesions have resolved spontaneously. Amphotericin B or ketoconazole have been used in larger lesions; smaller ones can often be resected successfully (46).

Ocular Infections

Pharyngoconjunctival Fever (Swimming Pool Conjunctivitis)

This pediatric and occasionally adult syndrome has been associated with a number of adenoviruses, most commonly serotypes 3 and 7 in this country and serotype 4 in Asia and Latin America (47). Pharyngoconjunctival fever often occurs in outbreaks or small epidemics and has been reported as a hazard at childrens' summer camps (48).

The illness is characterized by fever as high as 38°C, bulbar and palpebral conjunctivitis, pharyngitis, and enlargement of the adenoids. Usually, symptoms begin in one eye, but ultimately involve both. Occasionally, symptoms other than conjunctivitis are lacking. The illness usually lasts 3 to 5 days, is not complicated by bacterial superinfections, and can be treated symptomatically (47,49). Outbreaks can usually be terminated or prevented by adequate chlorination of pool water ($\geq 0.2\,\text{mg/L}$) (48).

Amoebic Keratitis

Free-living amoeba of the *Acanthamoeba* genus have been responsible for several hundred reported cases of keratitis since the original description in a Texas rancher in 1975 (50). The number of cases has been increasing dramatically in the past 2 years as physicians have become more aware of the problem and as diagnostic tools have been refined. This infection has proven difficult to treat, often resulting in severe visual impairment or loss.

Acanthamoeba species are found in a variety of environmental settings, including soil, water, and air (51). They have even been isolated from the respiratory tracts of healthy people (52). The species reported to cause keratitis in man include *A hatchetti*, *A castellani*, *A polyphaga*, *A culbertsoni*, and *A rhysodes* (53). *Acanthamoeba* species exist in nature only in the trophozoite or cyst stages. Identifying markers of trophozoites include a diameter of 14 to 40 µm, a single nucleus containing a centrally placed, prominent nucleolus, and spine-like plasma membrane projections (acanthapodia). Motility is sluggish. Cysts are 12 to 16 µm in diameter and have a wrinkled, double layered wall with pores (54).

Acanthamoeba are capable of producing a granulomatous encephalitis in debilitated or immunosuppressed patients. By contrast, the keratitis that they produce can occur in healthy people as well as those with underlying diseases. Most, but not all, of these patients have been soft contact lens wearers (55). The illness has been associated with minor corneal trauma and with exposure to contaminated water. A case-control study in soft contact lens wearers found that patients with *Acanthamoeba* keratitis were more likely than controls to use home-made saline for rinsing and as a wetting agent, and to wear their lenses while swimming (56). Other authors have remarked on the use of chemical rather than thermal disinfection of contact lenses as a risk factor (57).

Histologically, both trophozoites and cysts are found within the cornea in association with an acute inflammatory infiltrate. Giant cells may be present. Corneal neovascularization is variably present. Involvement of the posterior chamber of the eye in amoebic keratitis occurs only rarely (58).

Symptoms of amoebic keratitis generally begin with a sensation of a foreign body followed by pain, photophobia, tearing, blepharospasm, and altered visual acuity. Progression of symptoms is variable and may take place over several days to several months. Periods of remission are not unusual, and when these coincide with a change in therapy, an erroneous impression as to the etiology may occur. Findings on examination in one-half or more of patients include iritis, a corneal ring-shaped infiltrate, and recurrent epithelial breakdown or cataracts. Less commonly found are hypopyon, increased intraocular pressure, or anterior nodular scleritis (58). The ring corneal infiltrate has been described as a characteristic finding in amoebic keratitis and is probably caused by the presence of antigen-antibody complexes in the cornea and resultant chemoattraction of neutrophils (58,59). Although this ring infiltration has occasionally been reported in other conditions such as herpes simplex, fungal, or bacterial keratitis, its presence should signal the need for microbiological studies to determine if amoebae are present. Elevated corneal epithelial lines also appear to be a clinical indication of *Acanthamoeba* infection.

Histopathological examination of scrapings of these lines has revealed both trophozoites and cysts (60). Recently, dendriform epithelial involvement has been reported as an early finding in *Acanthamoeba* keratitis (61).

The definitive diagnosis of amoebic keratitis requires a demonstration of *Acanthamoeba* on corneal scrapings, biopsy, or culture. Motile trophozoites can sometimes be identified in wet mounts of scrapings. Cysts and trophozoites can be identified in fixed material with several different stains, including hematoxylin-eosin, Wright, Giemsa, and periodic acid-Schiff (58). Calcofluor white, a chemofluorescent dye, has been reported to facilitate the identification of trophozoites and cysts in tissue (62). Routine culture methods are frequently misleading in the diagnosis of *Acanthamoeba* keratitis. Because of bacterial colonization of the corneal scrapings or contamination, cultures may reveal potential pathogens. A nonnutrient agar with an *Escherichia coli* or *Aerobacter aerogenes* overlayment has been shown to successfully grow *Acanthamoeba* from the majority of biopsy-positive specimens (58). Cultures of contact lens or lens solutions may also be helpful diagnostically (57).

Effective treatment of *Acanthamoeba* keratitis requires both surgical and medical components. Diagnosis early in the course can sometimes lead to successful management employing debridement of the abnormal epithelium in combination with topical medication for 3 to 4 weeks (61,63). In many cases, however, penetrating keratoplasty is necessary for pain relief and to improve vision. Topical medications that have been reported to be beneficial include:

1. A combination of 1% miconazole nitrate, 0.1% propamidine isethionate, and neosporin (61).
2. A combination of 1% clotrimazole, 0.1% propamidine isethionate, and neosporin (64).
3. 0.1% propramidine isethionate and 0.15% dibromopropamidine (65).

Unfortunately, propramidine and dibromopropramidine, both analogs of stilbamidine, are not available commercially in the United States. Topical steroids are also frequently, but not universally, employed to inhibit neovascularization of the cornea. However, some experimental evidence suggests that when used in *Acanthamoeba* keratitis, steroids may not be effective in this regard (66). Development of animal models for *Acanthamoeba* keratitis will undoubtedly help clarify optimal therapy (66,67).

Prevention of *Acanthamoeba* keratitis in contact lens wearers is possible. Heat disinfection of lenses is preferable to chemical disinfection (68). Home-made saline solutions should be avoided for lens cleaning and storage, and contact lenses should not be worn while swimming in fresh water (56).

Pulmonary Infections

Legionella

Members of the genus *Legionella* are fastidious, nonspore forming, gram-negative bacilli. There are currently 29 named species, 3 subspecies, 21 serogroups, 5 tentatively named species, and 6 proposed unnamed species in this genus. Among these, *L pneumophila* is the major pathogen for man, and may cause infections in normal hosts as well as in those with underlying diseases. Fourteen other *Legionella* species have been isolated from humans, usually immunosuppressed patients (69).

Most *Legionellae* have been found naturally in a variety of fresh water habitats. *L pneumophila* and other species have been isolated from flowing streams and rivers as well as lakes, thermal ponds, and groundwater (70). They can gain access to man-made water supplies, such as air conditioning cooling towers, potable water systems, and whirlpools/spas. They tolerate water temperature in excess of 60°C. Aerosols from both natural and man-made water sources appear to be the usual source for human respiratory tract infections investigated since the first identified outbreak in 1976. It has been thought that *Legionellae* are possibly nonfree living microorganisms. There is some evidence that they live on the products of blue-green and thermophilic algae, as well as other bacteria such as *Pseudomonas* and *Flavobacterium* which commonly share the same environment. In addition, *Legionellae* are capable of intracellular survival and multiplication in free-living ameobae, such as *Naegleria* and *Acanthamoeba* (69,71). It has been hypothesized that aerosolized *Legionella*-carrying ameobae may constitute a system whereby the bacterium is presented to the human host in a protected form (69).

L pneumophila causes pneumonia, Pontiac fever (an influenza-like illness with less severe respiratory symptoms), and occasional soft tissue infections. Although most outbreaks of *Legionella* pneumonia or Pontiac fever have resulted from exposure to airborne bacteria from air conditioning systems, hospital potable water systems, or machine tool grinding coolants, infections related to immersion have also been reported. An outbreak of Pontiac fever related to the use of a whirlpool/spa was reported to have occurred in 1982 (72). Fourteen female members of a church group who used a health club whirlpool developed chills, fever, chest pain, cough, and nausea within 2 days. Most of these patients seroconverted to antigen from *L pneumophila* serogroup 6. This organism was recovered from the whirlpool water. It was hypothesized that *Legionellae* seeded the whirlpool from an air conditioner condensation pan with a blocked drain. The organism can reach high numbers in heated, agitated, underchlorinated whirlpool water. Whirlpool aerators produce droplets of 2 to 8 μm in size which are capable of reaching the alveolar air spaces when inhaled. Two similar outbreaks, one involving 34 cases of Pontiac fever and the other, 7 cases of pneumonia, were reported in 1982, associated with a whirlpool at a Vermont inn (73). More recently, six college students on a ski trip to Vermont developed Pontiac fever (five cases) or Legionnaires' disease (one case) after using a whirlpool spa (74).

A hospital-associated wound infection caused by *L pneumophila* serogroup 4 was related to immersion in a Hubbard tank (75). The pathogenic isolate as well as other *L pneumophila* serogroups were grown from the Hubbard tank as well as a small whirlpool tank near it. Povidone iodine, which was used to disinfect the tank and added to the water used to immerse the patient, was ineffective in killing *L pneumophila* at concentrations under 1,000 parts per million.

Two cases of *L bozemani* pulmonary infection following near drowning in dirty water have also been reported (76,77). Underlying immunosuppressive illness was an apparent predisposing factor in the etiology of this pneumonia.

Most patients with Pontiac fever have recovered from their illness without specific antibiotic therapy. This holds true for those reported in the above-mentioned whirlpool-associated outbreaks. Erythromycin, with the frequent addition of rifampin in severe cases, remains the therapy of choice for *L pneumophila* pneumonia as well as infections caused by other species of *Legionella*. Tetracycline, trimethoprim/sulfamethoxazole, and ciprofloxacin have been used with success in small numbers of patients (78,79).

Disinfection of hospital water systems colonized by *Legionella* has been accomplished through hyperchlorination, as well as thermally. *Legionellae* are relatively chlorine-tolerant and even more resistant to bromine, used occasionally for whirlpool disinfection (72). Levels of 2 to 6 parts per million residual chlorine are effective but, as discussed earlier, difficult to maintain in whirlpools, spas, and hot tubs.

Pseudomonas aeruginosa

While pneumonia associated with the aspiration of fresh water has been reported to be caused by *P aeruginosa*, in a number of cases it is unclear whether the organism was acquired at the time of near drowning or later, during hospitalization. The organism is a well-recognized agent of nosocomial pneumonia.

Pneumonia caused by *P aeruginosa* has been reported in a patient with a 50 pack-year history of smoking, but no other underlying medical problems, who sat in a whirlpool/spa for 90 minutes one day prior to the onset of respiratory symptoms (80). Both the sputum culture and cultures of the spa grew the identical serogroup of *P aeruginosa*. It was hypothesized that prolonged inhalation of *Pseudomonas*-laden aerosol from the spa was responsible for the development of pneumonia in this patient whose pulmonary clearance mechanisms were probably impaired from heavy smoking. In this regard, the pathogenesis is similar to the development of nosocomial *P aeruginosa* pneumonia after inhaling contaminated humidified air during mechanical ventilation (81).

Aspergillus

Invasive pulmonary aspergillosis has been reported following the near drowning of a 27-year-old man in a ditch after a motor vehicle accident (82). Pre-existing bronchiectasis was present in this patient. He was successfully treated with amphotericin B and flucytosine.

Pseudallescheria boydii

P boydii has been isolated from polluted water, sewage sludge (83), soil, and animal manure (84). This fungus has caused pulmonary infections in severely immunocompromised patients and, occasionally, in previously normal individuals who have aspirated contaminated water (85,86). The organism appears to have a propensity to spread from the initial site of infection in the lung, often producing widespread metastases, including brain abscesses (87). On one occasion, infected kidneys from a patient with a fatal disseminated case were transplanted into two recipients, both of whom developed *P boydii* infections (86). Therapy with antifungal drugs has been disappointing, overall. In vitro susceptibility tests usually indicate resistance to amphotericin B and flucytosine with susceptibility to miconazole and, to a lesser extent, ketoconazole. Both of the latter two agents have been used successfully to treat human pulmonary and bone infections (87,88).

Aeromonas

In addition to soft tissue infections associated with immersion, discussed earlier in this chapter, *Aeromonas* species can also cause pneumonia, complicated by septicemia in the setting of near drowning. Several such cases have been reported, but it is difficult to discern whether there has been actual pulmonary parenchymal infection in all cases (89,90). Sometimes the patient's pulmonary findings have been more compatible with noncardiogenic pulmonary edema and the *Aeromonas* has been recovered only from blood cultures (90). Although *A hydrophila* was identified as the species causing infection in the above cases, more recently differentiated *Aeromonas* species, such as *A sobria*, *A caviae*, or *A veronii*, may have been responsible (30).

Susceptibility of *Aeromonas* species and therapy of infections is discussed in the section on soft tissue infections.

Disseminated Infections

Leptospirosis

Leptospires are aerobic, motile, spiral, flexible microorganisms with hooked ends. They can be cultured in artificial media containing rabbit serum or bovine serum albumin and long-chain fatty acids, although the incubation time for optimal growth can range from a few days to a few weeks (91).

Two species are recognized: *L biflexa* is considered saprophytic and is found in surface and potable water. *L interrogans* is pathogenic and may be carried for prolonged periods in proximal renal tubular cells of many different mammalian species. Members of the two *Leptospira* species can be distinguished biochemically, but within each species members can be identified into serovars only on the basis of their agglutinogenic characteristics with rabbit antiserum. More than 200 serovars of *L interrogans* are known (91). From the site of infection in the kidney, leptospires are shed into the urine in variable numbers. With some serovars in some hosts, this excretion may be life-long. With other host-serovar combinations, however, urine shedding may persist for only a few months (92).

Human leptospirosis is an occupational risk for cattle, dairy, or swine farmers, as well as veterinarians and abattoir workers (93). Humans can also be infected by exposures such as swimming or wading in water contaminated with animal urine (94–96). The first reported water-borne outbreak of leptospirosis occurred in 1939 (97). Since then, similar outbreaks and small epidemics have occurred regularly. Crawford et al have reviewed twelve such outbreaks in the United States associated with swimming in natural fresh water pools, streams, and rivers. In several, contamination of the water with animal urine or offal was proven. They point out that sporadic cases of leptospirosis may occur as a result of various kinds of contact, but epidemics are usually associated with swimming or other types of water immersion (96).

Many human cases of leptospirosis are asymptomatic. Human illness varies in severity form a mild influenza-like syndrome to severe renal and hepatic failure accompanied by hemorrhage, shock, and confusion. The severe form of leptospirosis is called Weil's disease or Weil syndrome after the initial describer of the illness.

Leptospires may enter the body through intact mucosal membranes, the conjunctiva, or abraded skin. They are rapidly disseminated hematologically. The incubation period is usually 7 to 12 days. During the influenza-like septicemic phase of anicteric leptospirosis, the organism can be cultured from blood, cerebrospinal fluid, and other tissues. Despite its presence in spinal fluid, patients usually have no meningeal signs in this phase of the illness, although headache is usually present, as is fever, myalgia, and fatigue. After 4 to 7 days, the illness resolves for a day or two to be followed in many patients by an "immune" stage of the illness which can last up to a month. Circulating antibody can be detected, and patients may have meningismus, uveitis, and rash. Blood and cerebrospinal fluid cultures are usually negative during this second phase, but the organism can be found in the urine and aqueous humor of the eye. The meningitis seen in the "immune" stage, although sterile, is characterized by cerebrospinal fluid pleocytosis, a variably elevated protein, and a normal glucose. Eye findings of photophobia, ocular pain, and conjunctival hemorrhage are common (93,98).

In icteric leptospirosis, there is less distinction between septicemic and immune phases, although the renal and hepatic complications generally are not present before 3 to 7 days. The jaundice usually does not reflect hepatocellular necrosis, and no residual hepatic dysfunction has been found in survivors. Elevation of liver enzymes is relatively modest. Creatine kinase levels are quite high, however. Renal failure usually does not progress to the point where the patient requires dialysis, and this dysfunction also resolves completely (93,98). Thrombocytopenia occurs in about one-half of patients and is correlated with renal failure (99). Death is usually related to vascular collapse, thought to be caused by vasculitis and hemorrhagic myocarditis, which occurs in about 50% of fatal cases.

Diagnosis may be established by serologic means or by culturing the organism from clinical specimens (usually blood, cerebrospinal fluid, or urine). Tween 80-albumin agar is commercially available and is used in many clinical laboratories. Cultures are incubated for 5 to 6 weeks in the dark; growth is usually apparent by 2 weeks, however. Leptospires can also be identified in clinical specimens by dark field examination and by immunostaining. No commercial kits are yet available for the latter procedure, however. In tissue specimens, the organism can be detected by silver staining (91).

Most diagnoses are made serologically. The microscopic agglutination test is used most frequently, but is highly serovar-specific. In the United States, almost all human infections are caused by one of eight serovars (copenhageni, grippotyphosa, canicola, wolffi, pomona, djatzi, autumnalis, and patoc), and use of these serovars as antigens should detect the majority of human infections. Titers ≥1:100 are considered significant. Macroscopic agglutination tests using single or pooled Formalin-fixed antigens are also commercially available (91). Enzyme-linked immunosorbent assay tests have also been developed for use in the diagnosis of human infection and have the advantage of using a genus-specific antigen that detects a wide range of serovars (91).

Traditional antibiotic therapy for leptospirosis has been penicillin G or tetracycline. Recent evidence in humans indicates that therapy is effective even in severe disease treated after the initial septicemic period (100). Animal studies indicate that penicillins, tetracycline, and some cephalosporins are effective, while other cephalosporins are not (101).

Intravenous penicillin or ampicillin should be used for severe disease; oral ampicillin or doxycycline for mild symptoms. Therapy should be given for 5 to 7 days.

Chromobacterium violaceum

C violaceum is a gram-negative, facultatively anaerobic, fermentative bacillus which is a normal inhabitant of soil and water and has caused human infections primarily in tropical and subtropical areas (102). Most reports have not linked infection to freshwater exposure, but two cases have been reported in which immersion appears to play a role. One case occurred in a 44-year-old woman who sustained a wasp sting while bathing in a Paraguayan lagoon. One month later, she developed septicemia in association with inflammation of the sting site and purplish ulcerating nodular lesions on her thigh, abdomen, and back. Blood and skin lesions grew *C violaceum*. She responded to mezlocillin and gentamicin therapy despite shock and renal failure. However, the infection relapsed 2 weeks after the antibiotic course was completed, leading to her demise (103).

A second patient (a 53-year-old man) who nearly drowned in a Florida river, developed multiple liver abscesses, lung infiltrates, and a pustular skin rash 2 months after the accident. Blood and pustule cultures grew *C violaceum*, and the patient responded to chloramphenicol, ampicillin, and carbenicillin (104).

The interesting features of the disseminated infections in these two previously healthy patients were the long incubation periods and the skin lesions associated with the septicemia.

Central Nervous System Infections

Primary Amoebic Meningoencephalitis

Amoebic meningoencephalitis was first described in 1965 in Australia (105). Although originally thought to be caused by an *Acanthamoeba* species, it was ultimately recognized that acute infections of this type, termed primary amoebic meningoencephalitis (PAM), result from *Naegleria fowleri* infections. PAM was so named to distinguish it from metastatic amoebic abscesses involving the brain caused by *Entamoeba histolytica*. *Acanthamoeba*, instead, causes a subacute central nervous system infection in debilitated or immunosuppressed patients called granulomatous amoebic encephalitis, the pathogenesis of which does not appear to be related to immersion. Rather, the *Acanthamoeba* species reach the brain via the hematogenous route from a primary focus usually thought to be the lung or skin. It is hypothesized that these primary foci become infected by dusts, aerosols, or air containing the *Acanthamoeba* cysts (106).

N fowleri is a small amoeba measuring 10 to 35 μm. In unfavorable environments, it transforms to a pear-shaped biflagellate stage. The amoeba may also encyst. The cysts are spherical, smooth walled, have mucous-plugged pores, and measure 7 to 15 μm (51). *N fowleri* is a thermophilic organism and tolerates water as warm as 45°C. It has a world wide distribution in naturally warm as well as thermally polluted waters (107). The concentration of amoebae in warm water frequently exceeds one organism per 25 mL (108). With its wide distribution in water frequently used for recreation, it is apparent that millions of people have been exposed. Human cases, however, number in the 150 to 200 range, with 63 cases reported in the United States as of September 1, 1989. What factors provide immunity to *N fowleri* in the majority of exposed individuals are uncertain. Antibody to the amoeba can be demonstrated in human populations, but its protective role is unclear (107,109).

The organism is thought to enter the central nervous system via the nasal route. Amoebae from contaminated water are deposited on olfactory mucosal epithelium and penetrate the submucosal nervous plexus and cribiform plate. Olfactory neuroepithelium is capable of active phagocytosis, and the amoebae travel to the terminus of the olfactory nerve in the olfactory bulb which is in the subarachnoid space and surrounded by cerebrospinal fluid. Multiplication of the amoebae occurs in the meninges and in neural tissue and, eventually, a diffuse meningoencephalitis develops. Cortical gray matter is severely affected, with hemorrhage and edema, often leading to uncal or cerebellar herniation. Trophozoites can be identified in the necrotic olfactory bulbs as well as the adventitia and perivascular spaces of small to medium sized arteries and cerebrospinal fluid. No cysts are found (106,107). Tissue necrosis in response to *Naegleria* infections, seen in nasal mucosa as well as neural tissue, has been ascribed to the release of lysosomal enzymes or cytopathic toxins by the amoebae, or to enzymes on the surface of the organism (110–112).

Unfortunately, there is little in the clinical picture of PAM to distinguish it from acute bacterial meningitis. As a result, clinicians often do not consider PAM in their initial differential diagnosis when a patient presents with purulent meningitis. The period between exposure and the onset of symptoms may vary from 2 to 14 days, although most cases have occurred within 5 days. The majority of cases have involved children and young adults. Initially, the patient may notice some alteration of taste or smell. This is rapidly followed by fever, headache, anorexia, nausea, vomiting, and meningismus. The majority of patients also exhibit confusion at the time of presentation. This progresses to coma, and the infection is usually fatal within a week (106,113). Outside the central nervous system, focal myocarditis has been described in fatal cases of

PAM. The pathogenesis is unclear, however, since amoebae have not been demonstrated in myocardial tissue (114).

PAM should be considered in any case of acute pyogenic meningitis which occurs in a patient with a history of swimming in water potentially contaminated with amoebae. Cerebrospinal fluid pressure is often elevated, and the fluid generally has an increased number of red blood cells, sometimes sufficient to appear grossly hemorrhagic. White blood cell counts in the cerebrospinal fluid can vary widely, but there is a predominance of neutrophils. Glucose levels are usually low, with an elevated protein. It is of paramount diagnostic importance to do a wet mount microscopic examination of the spinal fluid to detect motile trophozoites. These are not usually recognized on the gram stain because of disruption of the amoebae by the fixation process (106,115). Computed tomographic x-ray studies have been reported in only two patients. One patient showed diffuse contrast enhancement of the gray matter and obliteration of the ambiens, interpeduncular, and quadrigeminal cysterns (115). The other patient's study was normal except for minimal edema (116).

Only a few survivors of PAM have been documented in the literature (116,117). Amphotericin B is the drug that has shown the greatest clinical activity and has been employed in the therapy of all the survivors. The drug is given in high dose both intravenously and intrathecally. Even when given within 24 hours of admission, its use has not been universally successful, however (118). Rifampin has also been given in combination with amphotericin B in several survivors.

Pseudallescheria boydii

As noted earlier in this chapter, *P boydii* can be found in polluted water as well as other sources. Most central nervous system infections have been preceded by aspiration of potentially contaminated material in near drownings, often associated with loss of consciousness from closed head trauma or asphyxiation (87). Usually, but not always (119), pneumonia in which *P boydii* is cultured from the sputum precedes the development of central nervous system infection. Both meningitis and brain abscess have been reported, although most cases of meningitis have been associated with abscess formation. Rarely, meningitis has occurred alone in association with trauma and contiguous infection, or spinal anesthesia (120,121). Both solitary and multiple brain abscesses may occur, although patients who develop central nervous system infection after aspiration and pneumonia usually have multiple abscesses. That these abscesses are caused by fungemia is evidenced by the frequency of documented abscesses elsewhere in these patients (thyroid, kidney, heart, lungs, skin) (122).

Surgical therapy appears to be effective in solitary or contiguous brain abscesses where adequate drainage can be performed. Indeed, one patient with a solitary abscess survived after drainage even though amphotericin

B (to which the isolate was resistant in vitro) was used therapeutically (123). In addition to the feasibility of surgical drainage, factors which may improve survival include prolonged high dose antifungal drug administration and avoidance of corticosteroid therapy (87).

Most isolates have been resistant to amphotericin B and flucytosine, and somewhat more susceptible to miconazole than to ketoconazole. Survival of two patients who developed multiple brain abscesses (as well as other foci of infection) was reported following prolonged, high dose intravenous miconazole therapy (up to 90 mg/kg/day). One of these patients also had probable meningitis and was treated intrathecally with miconazole as well. It was noted in both patients that frequent dosage increases were necessary in order to keep blood levels above the minimum inhibitory concentrations for the isolates (87). Miconazole is extensively metabolized by hepatic enzymes, and it is possible that with prolonged dosing, this metabolism is facilitated (124).

Coxsackieviruses

Coxsackieviruses are members of the genus *Enterovirus*, along with polioviruses, echoviruses, and enteroviruses 68 through 72. Coxsackieviruses are divided into groups A and B based on their infection pattern in mice and growth in primate cells. Twenty-four serotypes of Group A and six serotypes of group B have been recognized (125).

Most infections caused by Coxsackieviruses are either asymptomatic or take the form of undifferentiated febrile illnesses. Aseptic meningitis, encephalitis, paralysis, myopericarditis, pleurodynia, conjunctivitis, exanthems, enanthems, pharyngitis, and lower respiratory tract infections are additional infection patterns that can be caused by various Coxsackievirus serotypes.

Apparent water-borne infections caused by Coxsackie B_5 and A_{16} have been described. Hawley et al. reported a summer outbreak of illness caused by Coxsackie B_5 which included conjunctivitis, meningitis, and/or gastroenteritis that occurred at a boys' summer camp on Lake Champlain in Vermont. The virus was also recovered from a roped-off swimming area in the lake adjacent to the camp (126).

Denis et al. reported an illness which consisted of fever, vomiting, anorexia, diarrhea, and myalgia in five children who had swum in a lake in France. Coxsackie A_{16} was cultured from a patient and the lake water. Of two boys tested, both had an increased antibody titer to this virus (127).

Enteroviruses are thought to be transmitted between humans mostly by the fecal-oral route. Coxsackieviruses are postulated to be spread additionally by the respiratory-oral route, since they often can be recovered from the pharynx in convalescence (128). Urban sewage sampling, especially in summer months, commonly shows enteroviruses, and it may be that freshwater Coxsackievirus outbreaks are caused by contamination with sewage or the presence of swimmers who are spreading the virus (129).

References

1. McCausland WJ, Cox PJ. *Pseudomonas* infection traced to motel whirlpool. *J Environ Health* 1975; 37:455–459.
2. Washburn J, Jacobson JA, Marston E, Thorson B. *Pseudomonas aeruginosa* rash associated with a whirlpool. *JAMA* 1976; 235:2205–2207.
3. Sausker WF, Aeling JL, Fitzpatrick JE, Judson FN. *Pseudomonas* folliculitis acquired from a health spa whirlpool. *JAMA* 1978; 239:2362–2365.
4. Khabbaz RF, McKinley TW, Goodman RA, Hightower AW, Highsmith AK, Tait KA, Band JD. *Pseudomonas aeruginosa* 0:9: New cause of whirlpool-associated dermatitis. *Am J Med* 1983; 74:73–77.
5. Vogt R, LaRue D, Parry MF, Brokopp CD, Klauke D, Allen J. *Pseudomonas aeruginosa* skin infections in persons using a whirlpool in Vermont. *J Clin Microbiol* 1982; 15:571–574.
6. Gustafson TL, Band JD, Hutcheson RH, Schaffner W. *Pseudomonas* folliculitis: An outbreak and review. *Rev Infect Dis* 1983; 5:1–8.
7. Centers for Disease Control. An outbreak of *Pseudomonas* folliculitis associated with a waterslide—Utah. *MMWR* 1983; 32:425–427.
8. David BJ. Whirlpool operation and the prevention of infection. *Infect Control* 1985; 6:394–397.
9. Rinke CM. Hot tub hygiene. *JAMA* 1983; 250:2031.
10. Centers for Disease Control. Suggested health and safety guidelines for public spas and hot tubs. Atlanta, GA: 1981. (*HHS Publication* No. 99–960).
11. Gregory DW, Schaffner W. *Pseudomonas* infections associated with hot tubs and other environments. *Infect Dis Clin N Am* 1987; 1:635–648.
12. Hojyo-Tomoka MT, Marples RR, Klingman AM. *Pseudomonas* infection in superhydrated skin. *Arch Dermatol* 1973; 107:723–727.
13. Centers for Disease Control. Otitis due to *Pseudomonas aeruginosa* serotype 0:10 associated with mobile redwood hot tub system—North Carolina. *MMWR* 1982; 31:541–542.
14. Cort WW. Schistosome dermatitis in the United States (Michigan). *JAMA* 1928; 90:1027–1029.
15. Beck JW, Davies JE. *Medical Parasitology*, 3rd ed. St. Louis, CV Mosley Co., 1981: pp. 255–256.
16. Walinsky E. Nontuberculosis mycobacteria and associated diseases. *Am Rev Resp Dis* 1979; 119:107–159.
17. Aronson JD. Spontaneous tuberculosis in saltwater fish. *J Infect Dis* 1926; 39:315–319.
18. Linell F, Nordin A. *Mycobacterium balnei*: A new acid-fast bacillus occurring in swimming pools and capable of producing skin lesions in humans. *Acta Tuberc Scand* 1954; 33(Suppl):1–5.
19. Williams CS, Riordan DC. *Mycobacterium marinum* (atypical acid-fast bacillus) infections of the hand: A report of six cases. *J Bone Joint Surg (Am)* 1973; 55:1042–1047.

20. Gombert ME, Goldstein EJC, Corrado ML, Stein AJ, Butt KMH. Disseminated *Mycobacterium marinum* infection after renal transplantation. *Ann Intern Med* 1981; 94:486–487.
21. King AJ, Fairley JA, Rasmussen JE. Disseminated cutaneous *Mycobacterium marinum* infection. *Arch Dermatol* 1983; 119:268–270.
22. Roberts GD, Koneman EW, Kim YK. Mycobacterium. In: Balows A, Hausler WJ, Herrman KL, Isenberg HD, Shadomy HJ (eds): *Manual of Clinical Microbiology*, 5th ed. Washington D.C., American Society for Microbiology 1991; pp. 304–339.
23. Sanders WJ, Wolinsky E. In vitro susceptibility of *Mycobacterium marinum* to eight antimicrobial agents. *Antimicrob Agents Chemother* 1980; 18: 529–531.
24. Izumi AK, Hanke CW, Higaki M. *M. marinum* infections treated with tetracycline. *Arch Dermatol* 1977; 113:1607–1608.
25. Donta ST, Smith PW, Levitz RE, Quintiliani R. Therapy of *Mycobacterium marinum* infections: Use of tetracyclines vs rifampin. *Arch Intern Med* 1986; 902–904.
26. Wallace RJ, Swensen JM, Silcox VA, Good RC, Tschen JA, Stone MS. Spectrum of disease due to rapidly-growing mycobacteria. *Rev Infect Dis* 1983; 5:657–679.
27. Wallace RJ, Swensen JM, Silcox VA, Bullen MG. Treatment of nonpulmonary infections due to *Mycobacterium fortuitum* and *Mycobacterium chelonei* on the basis of in vitro susceptibilities. *J Infect Dis* 1985; 152: 500–514.
28. Janda JM, Duffey PS. Mesophilic aeromonads in human disease: Current taxonomy, laboratory identification, and infectious disease spectrum. *Rev Infect Dis* 1988; 10:980–997.
29. Khardori N, Fainstein V. *Aeromonas* and *Plesiomonas* as etiologic agents. *Ann Rev Microbiol* 1988; 42:395–419.
30. Janda JM. Recent advances in the study of the taxonomy, pathogenicity, and infectious syndromes associated with the genus *Aeromonas*. *Clin Microbiol Rev* 1991; 4:397–410.
31. Warrier RP, Ducos R, Azeemuddin S, Ruff A. *Aeromonas* infection in an infant with aplastic anemia. *Pediatr Infect Dis* 1984; 3:491.
32. Young DF, Barr RJ. *Aeromonas hydrophila* infection of the skin. *Arch Dermatol* 1981; 117:244.
33. Delbeke E, DeMarcq MJ, Roubin C, Baleux B. Contamination aquatique de plaies par *Aeromonas sobria* apres bain de riviere. *Presse Med* 1985; 14:1292.
34. Adams SL. The medicinal leech: A page from the annelids of internal medicine. *Ann Intern Med* 1988; 109:399–405.
35. Smith JA. *Aeromonas hydrophila*: Analysis of 11 cases. *Can Med Assoc J* 1980; 122:1270–1272.
36. Levin ML. Gas-forming *Aeromonas hydrophila* infection in a diabetic. *Postgrad Med* 1973; 54:127–129.
37. Shilkin KB, Annear DI, Rowett LR. Infection due to *Aeromonas hydrophila*. *Med J Aust* 1968; 1:351–353.
38. Heckerling PS, Stine TM, Pottage JC Jr, Levin S, Harris AA. *Aeromonas hydrophila* myonecrosis and gas gangrene in a nonimmunocompromised host. *Arch Intern Med* 1983; 143:2005–2007.

39. Karam GH, Ackley M, Dismukes WE. Posttraumatic *Aeromonas hydrophila* osteomyelitis. *Arch Intern Med* 1983; 143:2073–2074.
40. San Joaquin VH, Scribner RK, Picket DA, Welch DF. Antimicrobial susceptibility of *Aeromonas* species isolated from patients with diarrhea. *Antimicrob Agents Chemother* 1986; 30:794–795.
41. Bakken JS, Sanders CS, Clark RB, Hori M. β-lactam resistance in *Aeromonas* spp. caused by inducible β-lactamases active against penicillins, cephalosporins, and carbapenems. *Antimicrob Agents Chemother* 1988; 32: 1314–1319.
42. Clarridge JE, Musher DM, Fainstein V, Wallace RJ, Jr. Extraintestinal human infection caused by *Edwardsiella tarda*. *J Clin Microbiol* 1980; 11: 511–514.
43. Vartian CV, Septimus EJ. Soft tissue infection caused by *Edwardsiella tarda* and *Aeromonas hydrophila*. *J Infect Dis* 1990; 161:816.
44. Reinhardt JF, Fowlston S, Jones J. Comparative in vitro activities of selected antimicrobial agents against *Edwardsiella tarda*. *Antimicrob Agents Chemother* 1985; 27:966–967.
45. Sudman MS. Prototothecosis, a critical review. *Am J Clin Pathol* 1974; 61: 10–19.
46. Pegram PS, Jr, Kerns FT, Wasilauskas BL, Hampton KD, Scharyj M, Burke JG. Successful ketoconazole treatment of Prototothecosis with ketoconazole-associated hepatotoxicity. *Arch Intern Med* 1983; 143:1802–1805.
47. Wadell G. *Adenoviridae*: The adenoviruses. In: Lennette EH, Halonen P, Murphy FA (eds): *Laboratory Diagnosis of Infectious Diseases, Vol II; Viral, Rickettsial and Chlamydial Diseases*. New York, Springer Verlag, 1988: pp. 284–300.
48. D'Angelo LJ, Hierholzer JC, Keenlyside RA, Anderson LJ, Martone WJ. Pharyngoconjunctival fever caused by adenovirus type 4: Report of a swimming pool related outbreak with recovery of virus from pool water. *J Infect Dis* 1979; 140:42–47.
49. Caldwell GG, Lindsey NJ, Wulff H, Donnelly DD, Bohl FN. Epidemic of adenovirus type 7 acute conjunctivitis in swimmers. *Am J Epidemiol* 1974; 99:230–234.
50. Jones DB, Visvesvara GS, Robinson NM. *Acanthamoeba polyphaga* keratitis and *Acanthamoeba* uveitis associated with fatal meningoencephalitis. *Trans Ophthalmol Soc UK* 1975; 95:221–232.
51. Krogstad DJ, Visvesvara GS, Walls KW, Smith JW. Blood and tissue protozoa. In: Balows A, Hausler WJ Jr, Herrmann KL, Isenberg HD, Shadomy HJ (eds): *Manual of Clinical Microbiology*, 5th ed. Washington D.C., American Society for Microbiology, 1991: pp. 727–750.
52. Wang SS, Feldman HA. Isolation of *Hartmanella* species from human throats. *N Engl J Med* 1967; 277:1174–1179.
53. Centers for Disease Control. *Acanthamoeba* keratitis in soft contact lens wearers—United States. *MMWR* 1987; 36:397–398, 403–404.
54. Martinez AJ. Free-living amoebae: Pathogenic aspects. A review. *Protozool Abst* 1983; 7:293–305.
55. Sharma S, Srinivasan M, George C. *Acanthamoeba* keratitis in non-contact lens wearers. *Arch Ophthalmol* 1990; 108:676–678.

56. Stehr-Green JK, Bailey TM, Brandt FH, Carr JH, Bond WW, Visvesvara GS. *Acanthamoeba* keratitis in soft contact lens wearers: A case-control study. *JAMA* 1987; 258:52–60.

57. Cohen EJ, Parlato CJ, Arentsen JJ, Genvert GI, Eagle RC, Wieland MR, Laibson PR. Medical and surgical treatment of *Acanthamoeba* keratitis. *Am J Ophthalmol* 1987; 103:615–625.

58. Auran JD, Starr MB, Jakobiec FA. *Acanthamoeba* keratitis: A review of the literature. *Cornea* 1987; 6:2–26.

59. Theodore FH, Jakobiec FA, Juechter, Ma P, Troutman RC, Pang PM, Iwamoto T. The diagnostic value of a ring infiltrate in acanthamoebic keratitis. *Ophthalmology* 1985; 92:1471–1479.

60. Florakis GJ, Folberg R, Krachmer JH, Tse DT, Roussel TJ, Vrabec MP. Elevated corneal epithelial lines in *Acanthamoeba* keratitis. *Arch Ophthalmol* 1988; 106:1202–1206.

61. Lindquist TD, Sher NA, Doughman DJ. Clinical signs and medical therapy of early *Acanthamoeba* keratitis. *Arch Ophthalmol* 1988; 106:73–77.

62. Wilhelmus KR, Osato MS, Font RL, Robinson NM, Jones DB. Rapid diagnosis of *Acanthamoeba* keratitis using calcofluor white. *Arch Ophthalmol* 1986; 104:1309–1312.

63. Holland GN, Donzis PB. Rapid resolution of early *Acanthamoeba* keratitis after epithelial debridement. *Am J Ophthalmol* 1987; 104:87–89.

64. Driebe WT Jr, Stern GA, Epstein RJ, Visvesvara GS, Adi M, Komadina T. *Acanthamoeba* keratitis: Potential role for topical clotrimazole in combination chemotherapy. *Arch Ophthalmol* 1988; 106:1196–1201.

65. Wright P, Warhurst D, Jones BR. *Acanthamoeba* keratitis successfully treated medically. *Br J Ophthalmol* 1985; 69:778–782.

66. John T, Lin J, Sahm D, Rockey JH. Effects of corticosteroids in experimental *Acanthamoeba* keratitis. *Rev Infect Dis* 1991; 13(Suppl):S440–S442.

67. Badenoch PR, Johnson AM, Christy PE, Coster DJ. A model of *Acanthamoeba* keratitis in the rat. *Rev Infect Dis* 1991; 13(Suppl 5):S445.

68. Ludwig IH, Mecsler DM, Rutherford I, Bican FE, Langston RH, Visvesvara GS. Susceptibility of *Acanthamoeba* to soft contact lens disinfection systems. *Invest Ophthalmol Vis Sci* 1986; 27:626–269.

69. Rodgers FG, Pasculle AW. *Legionella*. In: Balows A, Hausler WJ Jr, Herrmann KL, Isenberg HD, Shadomy HJ (eds): *Manual of Clinical Microbiology*, 5th ed. Washington D.C., American Society for Microbiology, 1991; pp. 442–453.

70. Fliermans CB. Ecological niche of *Legionella pneumophila*. In: Katz SM (ed): *Legionellosis, Vol 2*. Boca Raton, Fl, CRC Press, 1985: pp. 75–116.

71. Edelstein PH. Environmental aspects of *Legionella*. *ASM News* 1985; 51:460–467.

72. Mangione EJ, Remis RS, Tait KA, McGee HB, Gorman GW, Wentworth BB, Baron PA, Hightower AW, Barbaree JM, Broome CV. An outbreak of Pontiac fever related to whirlpool use. *JAMA* 1985; 253:535–539.

73. Spitalny K, Vogt R, Witherell L, Ociari L, Orrison L, Etkind P, Novick L. Legionnaires' disease and Pontiac fever associated with a whirlpool. *22nd Interscience Conference on Antimicrobial Agents and Chemotherapy*. Miami Beach, Fl. 1982: Abstract 87.

74. Thomas DL, Mundy LM, Tucker PC. An outbreak of hot-tub Legionellosis. *31st Interscience Conference on Antimicrobial Agents and Chemotherapy.* Chicago, Il. 1991: Abstract 310.
75. Brabender W, Hinthorn DR, Asher M, Lindsey NJ, Liu C. *Legionella pneumophila* wound infection. *JAMA* 1983; 250:3091–3092.
76. Bozeman FM, Humphries JW, Campbell JM. A new group of Rickettsia-like agents recovered from guinea pigs. *Acta Virol* 1968; 12:87–93.
77. Thomason BM, Harris PP, Hicklin MD, Blackman JA, Moss CW, Matthews F. A legionella-like bacterium rleated to WIGA in a fatal case of pneumonia. *Am Intern Med* 1979; 91:673–676.
78. Ching WTW, Meyer RD. *Legionella* infections. *Inf Dis Clin N Am* 1987; 1:595–614.
79. Fang GD, Yu VL, Vickers RS. Disease due to the *Legionellaceae* (other than *Legionella pneumophila*). *Medicine* 1989; 68:116–132.
80. Rose HD, Franson TR, Sheth NK, Chusid MJ, Macher AM, Zierdt CH. *Pseudomonas* pneumonia associated with use of a home whirlpool spa. *JAMA* 1983; 250:2027–2028.
81. Goodison RR. *Pseudomonas* cross-infection due to contaminated humidified water. *Br Med J* 1980; 281:1288.
82. Vieira DF, VanSaene HKF, Miranda DR. Invasive pulmonary aspergillosis after near drowning. *Intensive Care Med* 1984; 10:203–205.
83. Cooke WB, Kabler P. Isolation of potentially pathogenic fungi from polluted water and sewage. *Public Health Rep* 1955; 70:689–694.
84. Bell RG. The development in beef cattle manure of *Petriellidium boydii* (Shear) Malloch, a potential pathogen for man and cattle. *Can J Microbiol* 1976; 22:552–556.
85. Meadow WL, Tipple MA, Rippon JW. Endophthalmitis caused by *Petriellidium boydii*. *Am J Dis Child* 1981; 135:378.
86. Van der Vliet JA, Tidow G, Kootstra G. Transplantation of contaminated organs. *Br J Surg* 1980; 67:596.
87. Dworzack DL, Clark RB, Borkowski WJ, Smith DL, Dykstra M, Pugsley MP, Horowitz EA, Connolly TL, McKinney DL, Hostetler MK, Fitzgibbons JF, Gallant M. *Pseudallescheria boydii* brain abscess: Association with near drowning and efficacy of high-dose prolonged miconazole therapy in patients with multiple abscesses. *Medicine* 1989; 68:218–224.
88. Galgiani JN, Stevens DA, Graybill JR, Stevens DL, Tillinghast AJ, Levine HB. *Pseudallescheria boydii* infections treated with ketoconazole. *Chest* 1984; 86:219–224.
89. Reines HD, Cook FV. Pneumonia and bacteremia due to *Aeromonas hydrophila*. *Chest* 1981; 80:264–266.
90. Genoni L, Domenighetti G. Beinahe-Ertrinken beim erwachsenen: Gunstiger verlauf nach 20 minutiger submersionszeit. *Schweiz Med Wochenschr* 1982; 112:867–868.
91. Alexander AA. Leptospira. In: Balows A, Hausler WJ Jr, Herrmann KL, Isenberg HD, Shadomy HJ (eds): *Manual of Clinical Microbiology*, 5th ed. Washington D.C., American Society for Microbiology, 1991: pp. 554–559.
92. Van der Heoden J. Epizooitiology of leptospirosis. *Adv Vet Sci* 1958; 4: 277–339.

93. Feigen RD, Anderson DC. Human leptospirosis. *CRC Crit Rev Clin Lab Sci* 1975; 5:413–424.

94. Alston JM, Broom JC. *Leptospirosis in Man and Animals*. Edinburgh, E and S Livingstone, 1958.

95. Kaufman AF. Epidemiological trends of leptospirosis in the United States 1965–1974. In: Johnson RC (ed): *The Biology of Parasitic Spirochetes*. New York, Academic Press, 1976: pp. 177–189.

96. Crawford RP, Heineman JM, McCulloch WF, Diesch SL. Human infections associated with waterborne leptospires and survival studies on serotype pomona. *J Am Vet Med Assoc* 1971; 159:1477–1484.

97. Havens WP, Bucher CJ, Reinmann HA. Leptospirosis: A public health hazard. Report of a small outbreak of Weil's disease in bathers. *JAMA* 1941; 116:289–291.

98. Edwards GA, Donn BM. Human Leptospirosis. *Medicine* 1960; 39:117–128.

99. Edwards CN, Nicholson GD, Hassell TA. Thrombocytopenia in leptospirosis: The absence of evidence for disseminated intravascular coagulation. *Am J Trop Med Hyg* 1986; 35:352–354.

100. Watt G, Tuazon ML, Santiago E, Padre LP, Calubaquib C, Ranoa LP, Laughlin LW. Placebo-controlled trial of intravenous penicillin for severe and late leptospirosis. *Lancet* 1988; 1:433–435.

101. Alexander AD, Rule PL. Penicillins, cephalosporins, and tetracyclines in treatment of hamsters with fatal leptospirosis. *Antimicrob Agents Chemother* 1986; 30:835–839.

102. Petrillo VF, Severo V, Sontos MM, Edelweiss EL. Recurrent infection with *Chromobacterium violaceum*: First case report from South America. *J Infect* 1984; 9:167–169.

103. Kaufman SC, Ceraso D, Shugurensky A. First case report of fatal septicemia caused by *Chromobacterium violaceum*. *J Clin Microbiol* 1986; 23: 956–958.

104. Starr AJ, Cribbett LS, Poklepovic J, Friedman H, Ruffolo EH. *Chromobacterium violaceum* presenting as a surgical emergency. *South Med J* 1981; 74:1137–1139.

105. Fowler M, Carter RF. Acute pyogenic meningitis probably due to *Acanthomoeba* sp.: A preliminary report. *Br Med J* 1965; 2:740–741.

106. Ma P, Visvesvara GS, Martinez AJ, Theodore FH, Daggett PM, Sawyer TK. *Naegleria* and *Acanthamoeba* infections: A review. *Rev Infect Dis* 1990; 12:490–513.

107. John DT. Primary amebic meningoencephalitis and the biology of *Naebleria fowleri*. *Ann Rev Microbiol* 1982; 36:101–123.

108. Wellings FM, Amuso PT, Chang SL. Isolation and identification of pathogenic *Naegleria* from Florida lakes. *Appl Environ Microbiol* 1977; 34: 661–667.

109. Cursons RTM, Brown TJ, Keys EA. Immunity to pathogenic free-living amoebae. *Lancet* 1977; 2:875–876.

110. Cursons RTM, Brown TJ, Keys EA. Virulence of pathogenic free-living amebas. *J Parasitol* 1978; 64:744–748.

111. Dunnebacke TH, Schuster FL. The nature of a cytopathogenic material present in amebae of the genus *Naegleria*. *Am J Trop Med Hyg* 1977; 26:412–414.

112. Feldman MR. *Naegleria fowleri*: Fine structural localization of acid phosphatase and heme proteins. *Exp Parasitol* 1977; 41:290–292.
113. Thong YH. Primary amoebic meningoencephalitis: Fifteen years later. *Med J Aust* 1980; 1:352–353.
114. Markowitz SM, Martinez AJ, Duma RJ, Schiel FOM. Myocarditis associated with primary amebic (*Naegleria*) meningoencephalitis. *Am J Clin Pathol* 1974; 62:619–628.
115. Martinez AJ. *Free Living Amebas: Natural History, Prevention, Diagnosis, Pathology and Treatment of Disease*. Boca Raton, Fl., CRC Press, 1985.
116. Brown RL. Successful treatment of primary amebic meningoencephalitis. *Arch Intern Med* 1991; 151:1201–1202.
117. Duma RJ. Disease caused by free-living amebae. *Inf Dis Newsletter* 1989; 8:25–32.
118. Stevens AR, Shulman ST, Lansen TA, Cichon MJ, Willaert E. Primary amebic meningoencephalitis: A report of two cases and antibiotic and immunologic studies. *J Infect Dis* 1981; 143:193–199.
119. Fisher JF, Shadomy S, Teabeut JR, Woodard J, Michaels GE, Newman MA, White E, Cook P, Seagraves A, Yaghman F, Rissing JP. Near-drowning complicated by brain abscess due to *Petriellidium boydii*. *Arch Neurol* 1982; 39:511–513.
120. Schiess RJ, Coscia MF, McClellan GA. *Petriellidum boydii* pachymeningitis treated with miconazole and ketoconazole. *Neurosurgery* 1984; 14:220–224.
121. Wolf A, Benham R, Mount L. Maduromycotic meningitis. *J Neuropath Exp Neurol* 1948; 7:112–113.
122. Berenguer J, Diaz-Mediavilla J, Urra D, Munoz P. Central nervous system infection caused by *Pseudallescheria boydii*: Case report and review. *Rev Infect Dis* 1989; 11:890–896.
123. Bell WE, Myers MG. *Allescheria (Petriellidium) boydii* brain abscess in a child with leukemia. *Arch Neurol* 1978; 35:386–388.
124. Brugmans JP, Van Cutsem J, Heykants J, Schuermans V, Thierpont D. Systemic antifungal potential, safety, biotransport and transformation of miconazole nitrate. *Eur J Clin Pharmacol* 1972; 5:93–102.
125. Menegus MA. Enteroviruses. In: Balows A, Hausler WJ Jr, Herrmann KL, Isenberg HD, Shadomy HJ (eds): *Manual of Clinical Microbiology*, 5th ed. Washington D.C., American Society for Microbiology, 1991: pp. 943–947.
126. Hawley HB, Morin DP, Geraghty ME, Tomkow J, Phillips JA. Coxsackie B epidemic at a boys' summer camp. Isolation of virus from swimming water. *JAMA* 1973; 226:33–36.
127. Denis FA, Blanchovin E, DeLignieres A, Flamen P. Coxsackie A_{16} infection from lake water. *JAMA* 1974; 228:1370–1371.
128. Kogon A, Spigland I, Frothingham TE. The virus watch program. A continuing surveillance of viral infections in metropolitan New York families. *Am J Epidemiol* 1969; 89:51–60.
129. Horstman DM, Emmons J, Gimpel L. Enterovirus surveillance following a community-wide oral poliovirus vaccination program: A seven-year study. *Am J Epidemiol* 1973; 97:173–178.

5
The Camper's Uninvited Guests

GORDON E. SCHUTZE and RICHARD F. JACOBS

Venturing into the wilderness can be exhilarating, and each year millions of people take time off to enjoy this pastime. During this relaxing endeavor the majority of adventurers will come into contact with different species of biting arthropods. Ticks, mosquitoes, lice, fleas, mites, bees, wasps, scorpions, and spiders, can make time spent in the outdoors unpleasant, and are potential carriers of disease. These biting arthropods may identify humans not only as an enemy, but also as a potential source of food. Biting, therefore, can be an act of feeding, probing, or defending. Contact with the host can be transient (mosquito) or prolonged (tick) and may result in the inoculation of salivary fluids or regurgitation of digestive tract contents. Organisms present in these fluids are able to cause many different diseases in their human hosts.

In the United States, the majority of illnesses attributed to biting arthropods are due to ticks and mosquitoes. Although potentially serious, the majority of bites from bees, wasps, scorpions, and spiders are simply painful. Physicians should consider arthropod transmitted diseases during all seasons, but suspicions should be heightened during the summer months when arthropods are most abundant. Children are especially prone to encounter ticks due to their frequent contact with animals and tick habitats. The spectrum of diseases caused by these arthropods is broad and can be confusing for the clinician. A history of rural travel, travel to areas endemic for arthropod-borne diseases, tick bites, or wilderness exposure may aid in obtaining a diagnosis.

Many an adventurer will attempt to avoid these uninvited guests by seeking refuge in lakes or streams. These bodies of water, especially those contaminated by wild animals such as beavers, are themselves not without risk of disease. Although the biting arthropods may be avoided, other uninvited guests, such as *Giardia lamblia*, have the potential to make a vacation equally unpleasant.

TABLE 5.1. Infectious diseases transmitted by ticks.

Disease	Agent
Lyme disease	*Borrelia burgdorferi*
Ehrlichiosis	*Ehrlichia chaffeensis*
Rocky Mountain spotted fever	*Rickettsia rickettsii*
Tularemia	*Francisella tularensis*
Relapsing fever	Borrelia species
Colorado tick fever	Arbovirus
Babesiosis	*Babesia* species
Fievre boutonneuse	*Rickettsia conorii*
Siberian tick typhus	*Rickettsia siberica*
Queensland tick typhus	*Rickettsia australis*
Powassan encephalitis	Flavivirus

Ticks

Infections diseases transmitted by ticks are listed in Table 5.1. In the United States, the major infections transmitted to humans by ticks are Lyme disease, ehrlichiosis, Rocky Mountain spotted fever, and tularemia. Each of these disorders has a causative agent that is passed from a specific tick to the host. The two types of ticks usually encountered are the soft (argasid) tick and the hard (ixodid) tick. The hard ticks are of greater concern since they are more frequently encountered, are difficult to remove, and are more likely to transmit disease to humans.

Lyme disease is the leading vector-borne disease reported in the United States (1). This multisystem inflammatory disease is caused by the spirochetal organism *Borrelia burgdorferi*. This spirochete was identified in the stomach of the main tick vector (*Ixodes dammini*) and subsequently recognized as the causative agent for this disease (2). Other ticks implicated in transmission of this disease include *Ixodes pacificus*, *Ixodes cookei*, and *Amblyomma americanum* (Lone Star tick) (3,4). Even when engorged these ticks are quite small, therefore histories of tick bites are infrequently obtained. Lyme disease has been reported in most states, but cases remain concentrated in well-established areas in the Northeast, North Central, and Pacific Coast states. Approximately 80% of reported cases come from seven states in these regions (5).

The clinical presentation of Lyme disease is divided into three stages. These stages are defined by the chronological relationship to the original tick bite (Table 5.2). The major manifestation of the first stage of this disease is the localized skin rash termed erythema migrans which is present in up to 80% of patients (Fig. 5.1) (6). This rash usually begins anywhere from 4 to 21 days after the tick bite and consists of an erythematous papule which gradually enlarges to form a large plaque-like annular lesion. The average duration of the untreated lesion is approximately 3 weeks. If appropriate medications are given, the rash may resolve in several days. Patients in this first stage of disease may also have fever, regional adenopathy, or other minor constitutional symptoms (7).

The second stage of Lyme disease is the result of dissemination by the spirochete into the circulation. Although the potential clinical manifestations of this dissemination are extensive, the major characteristics are seen in the skin and the nervous and musculoskeletal systems. Patients in this stage may appear quite ill with debilitating malaise and fatigue as major symptoms. A secondary annular skin lesion may occur in approximately one-half of the patients. The musculoskeletal discomfort is generally migratory in joints, bursae, tendons, muscle, and bone lasting only a few hours or days in one location (8). Disease of the nervous system is found in approximately 15% of the reported cases and usually begins approximately 4 weeks after the tick bite. The characteristic triad of findings include meningitis, cranial nerve palsies, and a peripheral radiculoneuropathy (9). The most common manifestation of meningitis is usually a headache and a stiff neck which is not generally associated with a Kernig's or Brudzinski's sign. Unilateral or bilateral facial nerve involvement (Bell's palsy) is the most common nerve palsy and may represent the only neurological abnormality (10). Other cranial nerves may also be involved. Cardiac involvement is limited to fewer than 10% of patients, with problems ranging from atrioventricular block to myopericarditis and left ventricular dysfunction (11). The length of cardiac involvement can be as brief as 3 days.

The third stage is highlighted by chronic complaints of arthritis. Although present very early in children, episodes of arthritis in adults become

TABLE 5.2. Major clinical manifestations of Lyme disease.

Stage 1 (early infection)	Stage 3 (late disease)
Erythema migrans	Acrodermatitis chronica atrophicans
Headache	Prolonged arthritis
Arthralgias	Chronic neurological syndromes
Regional lymphadenopathy	Keratitis
Stage 2 (disseminated disease)	
Recurrent erythema migrans	
Migratory bone and joint pain	
Meningitis	
Bell's palsy	
Peripheral radiculoneuropathy	
Atrioventricular block	
Myocarditis	
Pancarditis	
Conjunctivitis	
Mild hepatitis	
Hematuria, proteinuria	
Malaise and fatigue	

Adapted from references 8,9, with permission.

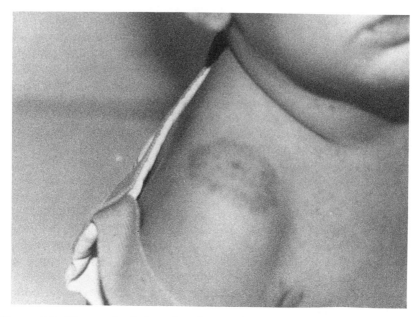

FIGURE 5.1. The annular lesion of erythema migrans on the shoulder of a child.

longer during the second and third years of illness, lasting months instead of weeks or days. Large joints, often those that were very close to the initial rash, are most commonly involved. The knee is the principal joint that is involved in the majority of patients (12). The involved joints tend to become swollen, warm, and painful, but rarely red. Other clinical manifestations of the third stage of disease include acrodermatitis chronica atrophicans, a progressive dermatological condition which develops with increasing erythema and pigmentation changes of the skin on the extensor surfaces. Chronic neurological complications, keratitis, and fatigue may also be seen.

Pregnant women may be at risk for transplacental passage of this spirochetal organism to their fetus. Preliminary data indicate that there is only a slight possibility for an adverse outcome. Although there has been no direct link to fetal abnormalities, there have been adverse outcomes for fetuses born to mothers with Lyme disease. All poor outcomes, however, have had different reasons for their demise and could not be conclusively linked to this disorder. The risk of an adverse outcome is quite low (13).

Lyme disease can be easily diagnosed if erythema migrans is present. Without this characteristic rash a broad range of diseases should be considered. The primary rash is sometimes confused with staphylococcal or streptococcal cellulitis, erythema multiforme, or erythema marginatum. Other forms of arthritis that can be confused with Lyme disease include pauciarticular juvenile rheumatoid arthritis; Reiter syndrome; psoriatic arthritis; gonococcal arthritis; reactive arthritis due to *Salmonella*, *Shigella*, or *Yersinia*; and postinfectious or septic arthritis.

The specific diagnosis is made with clinical and epidemiological data and can be established early if erythema migrans is present. Others will need serologic studies to establish the diagnosis. Antibodies may not rise until 2 to 3 weeks following the infection and may be aborted with antimicrobial therapy (14). These factors make the serologic diagnosis very difficult. Most untreated patients with long-standing disease will have a positive antibody titer. Both an indirect fluorescent antibody and an enzyme-linked immunosorbent assay (ELISA) test are available, but these tests are not yet standardized due to the lack of a common antigen. Therefore, test results will vary depending on the expertise of the laboratory. The use of the Western blot may aid to identify those patients with a false positive ELISA (15).

For patients with stage 1 disease (early infection), isolated Bell's palsy, arthritis, or mild carditis, oral antimicrobial therapy is currently recommended (14). For those patients over 9 years of age tetracycline, doxycycline, or amoxicillin are currently recommended. Children less than 9 years of age should receive amoxicillin or penicillin. Erythromycin can be substituted in those patients who are penicillin allergic, but it may be less effective. The oral regimens are given until the patients demonstrate a clinical response, which usually occurs after 10 to 30 days of therapy. For those patients with persistent arthritis, severe carditis, meningitis, or encephalitis, parenteral medications should be used. Penicillin G, ceftriaxone, or cefotaxime for 14 to 21 days are currently recommended as the medications of choice.

Ehrlichiosis is a tick-borne disease that is caused by *Ehrlichia chaffeensis*. This organism is an intraleukocytic rickettsia spread from a tick bite to the human host. Ehrlichiosis has been recognized as a disease in dogs since 1935, but human disease caused by this organism in the United States has only been recognized since 1986 (16,17). The tick vector for canine Ehrlichia has been identified as *Rhipicephalus sanguineus* but the principle vector for the spread to humans has not yet been identified. The canine vector is unlikely to transmit this disease to humans since this tick rarely feeds on humans (18).

Human ehrlichiosis has been described in 19 states, with a substantial male predominance (74%) (19). Although cases have been described in all ages, nearly half of the patients are over 50 years old. One-half of reported cases have occurred in May or June, and approximately 80% of individuals have a history of tick exposure (19). The incubation period required for human infection after a tick bite averages 10 to 14 days (range, 1 to 3 weeks) (20,21).

The most commonly encountered clinical manifestations of this disease are fever and headache (Table 5.3) (21,22). Fever (range, 38 to 41°C)

TABLE 5.3. Manifestations of Ehrlichia infections.

Clinical	%	Laboratory	%
Fever	100	Elevated LFT*	83
Headache	77	Leukopenia	74
Chills/rigors	65	Thrombocytopenia	72
Malaise	61	Elevated CSF WBC#	71
Nausea	54	Anemia	50
Myalgia	53		
Anorexia	50		
Vomiting	49		
Rash	47		

Adapted from reference 21, with permission.
* LFT—Liver function tests
# CSF WBC—Cerebrospinal fluid white blood cell count

is seen in almost 100% of patients during the first week of illness. Headaches encountered in this disorder are usually quite severe. Other commonly encountered symptoms include chills or rigors, myalgias, nausea, anorexia, and malaise (23). Rashes are found in up to 50% of patients but are more prominent in children. The classic rash is macular and is usually discovered upon presentation. The skin abnormalities usually start on the extremities, but do not progress as does the rash of Rocky Mountain spotted fever (21,22). Other physical abnormalities include cough, diarrhea, pharyngitis, arthralgia, weight loss, lymphadenopathy, dyspnea, abdominal pain, tick bite lesions, diaphoresis, splenomegaly, hepatomegaly, jaundice, meningismus, pulmonary edema, and pedal edema.

Hematological abnormalities are present in the majority of patients. Leukopenia, frequently associated with lymphopenia, is the most common abnormality (24). Lymphocyte counts are often below 1,500 per mm^3. Thrombocytopenia (<150,000 per mm^3) and anemia can be encountered as well as hyponatremia, elevated liver function tests, hypoalbuminemia, and cerebrospinal fluid pleocytosis (21,25). Infections with Ehrlichia cause clinical symptoms similar to Rocky Mountain spotted fever except for a decreased frequency of rash and a more profound pancytopenia. Differential diagnosis should also include the other tick-borne diseases including tularemia, Colorado tick fever, and Lyme disease.

The laboratory test for ehrlichiosis is an indirect fluorescent antibody (IFA) technique and a titer of greater than 1:80 provides a presumptive diagnosis of Ehrlichia; however, paired sera in the form of acute and convalescent sera should be submitted. (26) A fourfold rise or fall in the paired sera is considered diagnostic.

Treatment for patients over 9 years of age includes tetracycline or doxycycline given orally for 10 to 14 days. For those patients less than 9 years of age, chloramphenicol should be considered as an alternative antimicrobial agent.

Rocky Mountain spotted fever (RMSF) is the most important and severe disease in the spotted fever group. This disease is caused by *Rickettsia rickettsii* which is an organism transmitted by the bite of a tick. The wood tick (*Dermacentor andersoni*) in the West, the dog tick (*Dermacentor variabilis*) in the East, and the Lone Star tick (*Amblyomma americanum*) in the Southwest are all natural vectors of this disease. This disorder is most commonly seen in the spring and summer months with the majority of cases occurring between May and June. The peak incidence for RMSF is found in the 5 to 9-year age group (27).

The incubation period is short, with an average of 5 to 7 days after the tick bite (range, 3 to 12 days). Fever, headache, rash, toxicity, mental confusion, and myalgias are the major clinical symptoms of RMSF (Table 5.4) (28). The fever with RMSF tends to remain relatively high (40°C) and is associated with an intense headache that is not easily relieved with medications. The rash seen with RMSF can be pathopneumonic for this disorder. The skin lesions begin as small erythematous papules which blanch with pressure. They progress and rapidly become maculopapular, then petechial, and occasionally hemorrhagic. A regular occurrence with this rash is the involvement of the palms of the hands and the soles of the feet (Fig. 5.2A, 5.2B). When the rash becomes ecchymotic it may be mistaken for meningococcemia. Patients may appear to be irritable, restless, or apprehensive and may rapidly progress to mental confusion and delirium.

The diagnosis of RMSF is based upon clinical features (29). In the spring–summer season, an illness with fever and a rash may be enough to start empiric therapy against this rickettsial infection, especially if the patient is from an endemic area. Patients with this disorder can be thought to have meningococcemia or measles. An immunization and exposure history can aid in diagnosis.

Specific antibody can be demonstrated in patients from 5 to 10 days after the onset of illness. The serologic diagnosis is made by demonstrating a fourfold rise in specific antibody. Currently, enzyme-linked immunosorbent assay (ELISA) and microimmunofluorescence assays are

TABLE 5.4. Signs and symptoms of Rocky Mountain spotted fever.

Fever	94%
Rash	85%
Headache	80%
Myalgia	71%
Tick exposure	60%
Triad: fever/rash/headache	48%

Adapted from references 23,27–29, with permission.

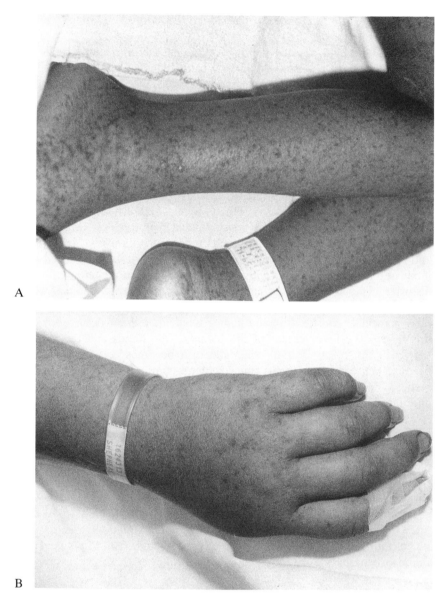

FIGURE 5.2. (A) The maculopapular rash of Rocky Mountain spotted fever on the leg and (B) hand.

available commercially for serologic diagnosis. In the past, the Weil–Felix agglutination reaction was presumptive evidence of infection. This test depended on the fact that the rickettsiae possessed common antigens with certain strains of *Proteus* bacteria. Strains *OX19* and *OX2* either singly or together would show rising titers during the course of the infection. Results of 1:20 to 1:80 were often found in uninfected patients and a titer of 1:160 or greater was required for the diagnosis. This test should no longer be used since specific antibody tests are now available. Other hematological abnormalities that may aid in the diagnosis are leukopenia, thrombocytopenia, and hyponatremia.

Tetracycline, doxycycline, and chloramphenicol are the antibiotics which have been proven to be effective against RMSF. Tetracycline and doxycycline are used when patients are over 9 years of age. When patients less than 9 years of age are to be treated, chloramphenicol is the drug of choice. A closer evaluation of tetracycline use has demonstrated that the tooth discoloration described in children may be due to multiple courses of tetracycline. Therefore, it is felt that children less than 9 years of age with a tetracycline-sensitive disease such as RMSF may be treated safely with one course of medications. The specific reasons and risks for the use of tetracycline should be outlined for the families prior to its use (30). Recently, the quinolones have been proven to be effective against rickettsial agents, but cannot be used in children (31). The total duration of therapy is usually between 7 to 10 days.

Tularemia is a bacterial infection caused by *Francisella tularensis*. This acute febrile illness is a zoonotic disease in which humans are a susceptible host. There are over 100 species in the animal kingdom that carry this bacteria (32). This organism is usually associated with lagomorphs (hares and rabbits), but is quite commonly found among rodents, racoons, opossums, and cats. The infection is transmitted to humans by ingestion of infected animal tissue; by direct contact with infected animals; through the bite of infected animals, ticks, or other arthropods; by inhalation of infected vapors; or by consumption of water that is contaminated.

Two types of *F tularensis* have been recognized. Biovar *tularensis*, also called Jellison type A, has been isolated in North America, whereas biovar *palaearctica* or Jellison type B, is found wherever tularemia is found. Biovar *tularensis* is highly virulent in man, whereas biovar *palaearctica* has always been considered to be less virulent. There has been, however, more human disease attributed to biovar *palaearctica* recently, and it may be that the extent of disease caused by this second type is not fully understood (33).

F tularensis is a highly infectious bacterium with as few as 10 organisms required to produce systemic disease in humans. This organism will gain access to the body through the skin, oropharynx, conjunctiva, respiratory tract, or gastrointestinal tract. After the organism gains entry into the body, further dissemination may occur via the blood or lymphatic system.

Ticks are the major vector for the transmission of this disease in the southern parts of the United States. *Amblyomma americanum* (Lone Star tick), *Dermacentor andersoni* (wood tick), and *Dermacentor variabilis* (dog tick) are the principle tick vectors known not only to transmit but also to serve as reservoirs for this disease. Other vectors such as fleas, mites, deer flies, and mosquitoes are also known to transmit the disease.

The incubation period for this disorder is usually 3 to 4 days (range, 1 to 21 days). The onset of symptoms is usually quite abrupt and consists of fever, chills, headache, myalgias, vomiting, and photophobia. Children are more likely to suffer from adenopathy and fever compared to adults. There are six forms of the disease which have been described. The most common is the ulceroglandular form but others include the glandular, oculoglandular, oropharyngeal, typhoidal, and pneumonic forms (Table 5.5) (34,35).

In the ulceroglandular form of the disease the organisms gain entry through the skin via an embedded tick. After approximately 2 days, patients will complain of tender, swollen lymph nodes most commonly found in the axillary or inguinal regions in adults and cervical nodes in children (33). At the site of entry there is often a painful, swollen papule. This papule will rupture, leaving a punched-out ulcer with raised borders. This ulcer may persist for months. The swollen lymph node may become inflamed and in many cases will suppurate and drain. The glandular form is very similar except the skin lesion is lacking.

The conjunctival space is thought to be the portal of entry causing the oculoglandular form of tularemia. The eye becomes involved due to contact with infected secretions, most often from rubbing the eyes. The eyelids become edematous and inflamed and extremely painful. Occasionally multiple small yellowish nodules or ulcers will appear on the palpebral conjunctiva or sclera (Fig. 5.3). Preauricular, submaxillary, and cervical adenopathy may also be evident.

In oropharyngeal tularemia the organisms are introduced to the oropharyngeal mucosa through contaminated food and water. The complaint of a sore throat is usually out of proportion to the pharyngitis seen on exam. Cervical adenopathy may also be present (36).

The typhoidal form often presents as an acute septicemia. The onset is usually quite abrupt with fever, myalgias, and vomiting. Patients may often have meningitis, delirium, and pulmonary involvement. In children, where typhoidal tularemia can be the result of the ingestion of the organism, necrotic lesions may be present throughout the bowel (37).

TABLE 5.5. Common forms of tularemia.

Ulceroglandular	50%
Glandular	9%
Oculoglandular	1%
Oropharyngeal	2%
Typhoidal	8%
Pneumonic	15%
Unclassified	15%

Adapted from references 34,35, with permission.

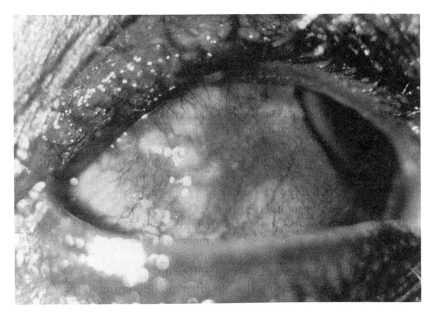

FIGURE 5.3. Note the small nodules on the palpebral conjunctiva and the sclera of a patient with oculoglandular tularemia.

The pneumonic form of tularemia is uncommon but when it presents it is quite severe. This disorder has been limited to laboratory workers in the past (38). Pneumonia, however, may occur in up to 15% of cases of ulceroglandular disease and 80% of typhoidal tularemia.

The overall mortality rate for tularemia is approximately 2% (39). Patients with a poor outcome are more likely to have electrolyte or renal abnormalities, pneumonia and pleural effusion, rhabdomyolisis with elevated serum creatine phosphokinase, and *F. tularensis* bacteremia (40).

The diagnosis of tularemia is established based upon history, physical exam, and serology. The agglutination test is the usual method employed for diagnosing tularemia. Antibody usually develops in the second week of illness. A titer of $\geq 1:160$ is a presumptive diagnostic test which suggests a current or past infection, while a fourfold rise of the convalescent sera with titers in the $1:1,280$ to $1:2,560$ range is an easy way to document a current infection. Cultures for *F tularensis* should not be attempted in the routine clinical laboratory due to the risk of infecting the workers.

The differential diagnosis of ulceroglandular and glandular tularemia include diseases caused by routine pathogens such as *Streptococcus* and *Staphylococcus*. Also included are diseases due to *Mycobacterium tuberculosis*, atypical *Mycobacterium*, cat scratch disease, sporotrichosis, and infectious mononucleosis. Typhoidal tularemia can be confused with acute bacterial sepsis. Tularemia pneumonia can resemble pneumonia that is caused by a number of organisms including *Mycoplasma, Legionella, Chlamydia, Coxiella, Mycobacterium*, and those of fungal and viral etiologies.

Streptomycin is currently the drug of choice for tularemia. Gentamicin, however, may become the principal medication due to side effects and manufacturing problems with streptomycin. Although tetracycline and chloramphenicol have been demonstrated to cause a prompt response in patients with tularemia, a relatively high rate of relapse makes these medications less desirable. After institution of appropriate medications, patients demonstrate improvement within 24 to 48 hours. Treatment duration is usually 7 to 10 days with at least 4 afebrile days prior to discontinuing the medications.

Prevention

A proper wardrobe is essential in preventing tick-transmitted diseases. Protective clothing that covers the arms, legs, and other exposed areas, ankle-high footwear, pants' legs that cinch at the ankles or are worn tucked into the socks can help protect the wilderness adventurer from unwanted travel companions. Permethrin can be sprayed upon clothing to prevent tick attachment, and insect repellents that employ N,N-diethyl-m-toluamide (DEET) can be applied to the skin for further protection. Caution should be employed when using repellents with DEET on small children due to the potential of central nervous system complications (seizures). Concentrations of more than 35% DEET should also be avoided since they are not proven to be more effective than the lower concentrations and have a greater risk for complications due to overdose (41).

Close and regular inspections of all body parts is essential for the adventurer. Adult ticks are usually on the body for 1 to 2 hours prior to attchment. The duration of tick feeding may be directly related to disease transmission (42). If ticks are discovered they should be removed. The recommended method for tick removal is to grasp the tick as close to the skin as possible with tweezers or protected fingers. The tick is then pulled straight out with steady even pressure. Care should be taken to avoid twisting or jerking the tick as this might cause mouthparts to break off and be left in the skin. Crushing or puncturing the body of the tick is also not suggested since the body fluids may contain infective agents. After the tick is removed the bite site should be disinfected (43). Traditional methods of tick removal such as fingernail polish or isopropyl alcohol application to the tick, or the use of a hot match may only induce the tick to salivate or regurgitate into the wound, thus spreading their infected secretions. The empiric use of antimicrobial agents after a tick bite to prevent the acquisition of tick-borne diseases has been demonstrated not to be useful (42).

Mosquitoes/Lice/Fleas/Mites

There are many diseases transmitted by mosquitoes across the world but very few are encountered in the United States (Table 5.6). For the most part, those diseases that are encountered are transmitted from a host, such as wild birds, to humans or other animals by the moquito. The type of encephalitis that is found in humans will vary according to geographic location. For example, western equine encephalitis is found in the western and midwestern states; eastern equine encephalitis is located in the eastern, Gulf Coast, and southern states; St. Louis encephalitis can be found in the western, central, and southern states; and California encephalitis (LaCrosse variant) is found in the central and eastern states.

The hallmark of these viral disorders is an acute onset of a febrile illness. The clinical findings reflect disease progression as the cells of the central nervous system become infected. These findings include headache, fever, altered mental states, disorientation, behavioral and speech disturbances, and other diffuse neurological signs. Outcome and permanent sequelae are dependent on the type of encephalitis.

The proper use of clothing can help prevent these diseases. Items that should be considered include long sleeved shirts, protective facial netting, and mosquito netting for sleeping. These garments should be used in areas with large mosquito populations. Insect repellents that employ DEET will also aid in the battle against these biting arthropods (41).

Lice are the main vector for epidemic typhus. This disease, which is rarely reported in North America, is caused by *Rickettsia prowazekii*. Louse-borne disease is especially prominent in areas of poverty, overcrowding, and poor sanitation. Disease in the United States has been attributed to contact with flying squirrels in Virginia, West Virginia, and North Carolina (44). This disease is characterized by an influenza-like illness with headache, fever, and malaise. A rash begins approximately 4

TABLE 5.6. Mosquito-borne infections.

Disease	Agent
Western equine encephalitis	Alphavirus
Eastern equine encephalitis	Alphavirus
St. Louis encephalitis	Flavivirus
California virus encephalitis	Bunyavirus
Dengue	Flavivirus
Venezuelan encephalitis	Alphavirus
Tularemia	*Francisella tularenisis*

to 7 days into the illness. This rash usually begins on the trunk and then spreads to involve the extremities. Illness usually varies from moderate to fatal and if left untreated will last approximately 2 weeks. The treatment for epidemic typhus is tetracycline or chloramphenicol.

The flea is instrumental in the transmission of an ancient infection, the plague. This disorder is generally characterized by fever and painful lymphadenitis (bubonic plague). The plague is caused by the organism *Yersinia pestis* and is mainly seen in the southwestern part of the United States. The flea usually lives on wild rodents such as rats or rabbits and can also be transmitted to domestic pets. This enables the flea to come into contact with the human host and transmit the disease. The plague can be severe and is treated with tetracycline or chloramphenicol.

A second zoonotic infection transmitted by the flea is murine (endemic) typhus. This disorder is caused by the organism *Rickettsia typhi* and is transmitted from the rat to the human by the rat flea. Fever, headache, malaise, and rash are the common clinical symptoms of this disease. Endemic typhus is located in the southwestern regions of the United States and is treated with tetracycline or chloramphenicol (45).

Infections due to mites have been recognized for many years. The larval form of the mite is commonly referred to as the chigger and is responsible for many of these diseases. Scabies, rickettsial pox, and scrub typhus are all transmitted by mites. In the wilderness, most humans have trouble only with the bite of the chigger. Within 24 to 48 hours these bites become intensely pruritic and may develop small hemorrhagic papules or nodules. The inflammation is proportional to the hosts hypersensitivity to the oral secretions of the mite. These bites may persist for 5 to 6 days and occur mostly on the lower legs or other exposed regions.

Other Arthropods

Some other arthropod envenomations may be particularly severe. Hymenoptera stings (bees, wasps, hornets, and ants) are the most common cause of envenomations, especially in children. They usually produce local pain, swelling, and erythema. If a stinger remains after the envenomation, it should be removed by carefully brushing it away. Grasping the stinger to remove it may squeeze the remaining venom into the wound (46). The application of ice or cool compresses often helps to reduce the pain and swelling. In older children, the use of oral antihistamines may provide relief. Early signs of generalized pruritus, urticaria, angioedema, or bronchospasm necessitates a medical evaluation emergency. If the patient cannot be evaluated, epinephrine is the drug of choice for systemic reactions and should be given in the field (41).

Although lethal scorpion bites are a serious problem throughout the world, in the United States the only dangerous species encountered is

Centruroides exilicauda. This scorpion is found mostly in the southwestern desert climate. Symptoms are usually limited to local pain, but children younger than 2 years of age may demonstrate multisystem organ failure (47). The brown recluse (*Loxosceles reclusa*) and the black widow (*Latrodectus mactans*) spiders may also cause painful bites. If signs of systemic envenomation develop, the victim requires medical evaluation. Antivenin is available for black widow and *C exilicauda* bites.

Giardia

In certain high-risk regions or populations, *Giardia lamblia* is an important cause of diarrhea. Travelers to the Rocky Mountains or consumers of contaminated water, are at high risk for this parasite (48). Infection may occur after ingestion of only 10 to 100 cysts contained in only a few micrograms of stool (49). These cysts are very hardy and may be viable for up to 3 months in moist environments. Person to person transmission is the most common route of infection.

After the organisms are ingested, patients will demonstrate a varied response. They may be asymptomatic or develop an acute infectious diarrhea that has a sudden onset. This diarrhea is associated with watery, foul smelling, explosive stools. Flatulence, abdominal distention, nausea, and anorexia are often present as well. Patients may also develop chronic diarrhea with persisitent gastrointestinal symptoms that last for months.

The diagnosis of *Giardia* can be made by examination of a fresh stool. Duodenal biopsy is believed to be the most sensitive method of detection, but is expensive and not readily available. Certain medications such as antibiotics, antacids, and antidiarrheal compounds may all interfere with the morphology of the organism and prevent identification (50). Patients should not receive these compounds for 48 to 72 hours prior to stool examination. Recently, detection of *Giardia* by an enzyme immunoassay has become available (51). These tests can be used on stool specimens or rectal swabs. Exams such as these will alleviate problems due to intermittent shedding or low numbers of parasites which make the diagnosis difficult.

Treatment of patients with acute diarrhea due to *Giardia* is recommended. Currently, acceptable medications include furazolidone, quinacrine, and metronidazole. The optimal period of treatment is from 5 to 7 days. Other household contacts with symptoms should also be evaluated and treated.

References

1. Dennis DT. Lyme disease: Tracking an epidemic. *JAMA* 1991; 266:1269–1270.
2. Steere AC, Grodzicki RL, Kornblatt AN, et al. The spirochetal etiology of Lyme disease. *N Engl J Med* 1983; 308:733–740.

3. Magnarelli LA, Swihart RK. Spotted fever group *Rickettsiae* or *Borrelia burgdoferi* in *Ixodes cookei* (*Ixodidae*) in Connecticut. *J Clin Microbiol* 1991; 29:1520–1522.
4. Schulze TL, Bowen GS, Bosler EM, et al. *Amblyomma americanum*: A potential vector of Lyme disease in New Jersey. *Science* 1984; 244:601–603.
5. Centers for Disease Control. Lyme disease surveillance—United States, 1989–1990. *MMWR* 1991; 40:417–421.
6. Steere AC, Bartenhagen NH, Craft JE, et al. The early clinical manifestations of Lyme disease. *Ann Intern Med* 1983; 99:76–82.
7. Steere AC, Taylor E, Wilson ML, et al. Longitudinal assessment of the clinical and epidemiological features of Lyme disease in a defined population. *J Infect Dis* 1986; 154:295–300.
8. Steere AC. Lyme disease. *N Engl J Med* 1989; 321:586–596.
9. Stechenberg BW. Lyme disease: The latest great imitator. *Pediatr Infect Dis* 1988; 7:402–409.
10. Clark JR, Carlson RD, Sasaki CT, et al. Facial paralysis in Lyme disease. *Laryngoscope* 1985; 95:1341–1345.
11. Olson LJ, Okafor EC, Clements IP. Cardiac involvement in Lyme disease: Manifestations and management. *Mayo Clin Proc* 1986; 61:745–749.
12. Doughty RA. Lyme disease. *Pediatr Rev* 1984; 6:20–25.
13. Markowitz LE, Steere AC, Benach JL, et al. Lyme disease during pregnancy. *JAMA* 1986; 255:3394–3396.
14. Plotkin SA, Peter G, Easton JG, et al. Treatment of Lyme borreliosis. *Pediatrics* 1991; 88:176–179.
15. Rose CD, Fawcett PT, Singsen BH, et al. Use of Western blot and enzyme-linked immunosorbent assay to assist in the diagnosis of Lyme disease. *Pediatrics* 1991; 88:465–470.
16. Donatien A, Lestoquard F. Existence en algerie d'une *Rickettsia* du chien. *Bull Soc Pathol Exot* 1935; 28:418–419.
17. Maeda K, Markowitz N, Hawley RC, et al. Human infection with *Ehrlichia canis*, a leukocytic *Rickettsia*. *N Engl J Med* 1987; 316:853–856.
18. Nelson VA. Human parasitism by the brown dog tick. *J Econ Entomol* 1969; 62:710–712.
19. Walker DH, Fishbein DB. Epidemiology of rickettsial diseases. *Eur J Epidemiol* 1991; 7:237–245.
20. Taylor JP, Betz TG, Fishbein DB, et al. Serological evidence of possible human infection with *Ehrlichia* in Texas. *J Infect Dis* 1988; 158:217–220.
21. Eng TR, Harkess JR, Fishbein DB, et al. Epidemiologic, clinical, and laboratory findings of human ehrlichiosis in the United States, 1988. *JAMA* 1990; 264:2251–2258.
22. Harkess JR, Ewing SA, Brumit T, et al. Ehrlichiosis in children. *Pediatrics* 1991; 87:199–203.
23. Centers for Disease Control. Rocky Mountain spotted fever and human ehrlichiosis—United States, 1989. *MMWR* 1990; 39:281–284.
24. Fishbein DB, Sawyer LA, Holland CJ, et al. Unexplained febrile illness after exposure to ticks: Infection with an *Ehrlichia*? *JAMA* 1987; 257:3100–3104.
25. Fishbein DB, Kemp A, Dawson JE, et al. Human ehrlichiosis: Prospective active surveillance in febrile hospitalized patients. *J Infect Dis* 1989; 160:803–809.

26. Dawson JE, Fishbein DB, Eng TR, et al. Diagnosis of human ehrlichiosis with the indirect flourescent antibody test: Kinetics and specificity. *J Infect Dis* 1990; 162:91–95.
27. Centers for Disease Control. Rocky Mountain spotted fever—United States, 1990. *MMWR* 1991; 40:451–454.
28. Helmick CG, Bernard KW, D'Angelo LJ. Rocky Mountain spotted fever: Clinical, laboratory, and epidemiological features of 262 cases. *J Infect Dis* 1984; 150:480–488.
29. Linnemann CC, Janson PJ. The clinical presentations of Rocky Mountain spotted fever: Comments on recognition and management based on a study of 63 patients. *Clin Pediatr* 1978; 17:673–679.
30. Abramson JS, Givner LB. Should tetracycline be contraindicated for presumed of presumed Rocky Mountain spotted fever in children less than 9 years of age? *Pediatrics* 1990; 86:123–124.
31. Guchiol F, Pallares R, Carratala J, et al. Randomized double-blind evaluation of ciproflaxacin and doxycycline for Mediterranean spotted fever. *Antimicrob Agents Chemother* 1989; 33:987–988.
32. Hopla CE. The ecology of tularemia. *Adv Vet Sci Comp Med* 1974; 18:25–53.
33. Uhari M, Syrjala H, Salminen A. Tularemia in children caused by *Francisella tularensis* biovar *palaearctica*. *Pediatr Infect Dis* 1990; 9:80–83.
34. Jacobs RF, Condrey YM, Yamauchi T. Tularemia in adults and children: A changing presentation. *Pediatrics* 1985; 76:818–822.
35. Jacobs RF, Narain JP. Tularemia in children. *Pediatr Infect Dis* 1983; 2: 487–491.
36. Hughes WT, Etteldof JN. Oropharyngeal tularemia. *J Pediatr* 1957; 51: 363–372.
37. Dienst FT. Tularemia: A perusal of three hundred thirty-nine cases. *J La State Med Soc* 1963; 115:114–127.
38. Overhold EL, Tigert WD, Kadull PJ, et al. An analysis of forty-two cases of laboratory-acquired tualremia. *Am J Med* 1961; 30:785–806.
39. Taylor JP, Istre GR, McChesney TC, et al. Epidemiologic characteristics of human tularemia in the Southwest-Central States, 1981–1987. *Am J Epidemiol* 1991; 133:1032–1038.
40. Penn RL, Kinasewitz GT. Factors associated with a poor outcome in tularemia. *Arch Intern Med* 1987; 147:265–268.
41. Gentile DA, Kennedy BC. Wilderness medicine for children. *Pediatrics* 1991; 88:967–981.
42. Costello CM, Steere AC, Pinkerton RE, et al. A prospective study of tick bites in an endemic area for Lyme disease. *J Infect Dis* 1989; 159:136–139.
43. Needham GR. Evaluation of five popular methods for tick removal. *Pediatrics* 1985; 75:997–1002.
44. Duma RJ, Sonenshine DE, Bozeman FM, et al. Epidemic typhus in the United States associated with flying squirrels. *JAMA* 1981; 245:2318–2323.
45. Dumler JS, Taylor JP, Walker DH. Clinical and laboratory features of murine typhus in South Texas 1980 through 1987. *JAMA* 1991; 266:1365–1370.
46. Maguire JF, Geha RS. Bee, wasp, and hornet stings. *Pediatr Rev* 1986; 8:5–11.
47. Berg RA, Tarantino MD. Envenomation by the scorpion *Centuroides exilicauda* (*C sculpturatus*): Severe and unusual manifestations. *Pediatrics* 1991; 87:930–933.

48. Craft JC. Giardia and giardiasis in childhood. *Ped Infect Dis* 1982; 1:196–211.
49. Rendtorff RC. The experimental transmission of human intestinal protozoan parasites: II. *Giardia lamblia* cysts given in capsules. *Amer J Hyg* 1954; 59:209–220.
50. Wolfe MS. Giardiasis. *N Engl J Med* 1978; 298:319–321.
51. Rosoff JD, Sanders CA, Sonnad SS, et al. Stool diagnosis of giardiasis using a commercially available enzyme immunoassay to detect Giardia-specific antigen 65 (GSA-65). *J Clin Microbiol* 1989; 27:1997–2002.

6
With Man's Best Friend

ROBERT S. JONES and BENNETT LORBER

The relationship between man and dog is an ancient one. The dog has been man's workmate, protector, guide, and companion. No one would question the merit of the long history of valuable service the dog has provided to man; it is the stuff of legend and literature. We even have evidence that a dog companion is good for our physical health (1). Occasionally, however, pathogens may be transmitted from dog to human beings resulting in problems ranging from a trivial rash to a life-threatening bacteremia. These infections are reviewed in this chapter.

Considering that there are an estimated 55 million pet dogs in the United States (2) physicians need to be familiar with the potential illnesses that can result from canine exposure. An inquiry into animal contact is an important part of the medical history. Some clinical conditions along with etiologies to be considered in persons with a canine exposure are listed in Table 6.1.

Infections Following Dog Bites

Epidemiology

Animal bites are a major public health problem and account for about 1% of emergency room visits; dogs are responsible for 75% to 90% of reported bites (2,3). In most instances the dog belongs to the bite victim, a friend, or neighbor (4). One-half to two-thirds of bites occur in children, with a peak incidence in those 5 to 9 years of age; in adult life, letter carriers, veterinarians, and animal control officers have a high incidence.

The risk of infection following a dog bite is considerably lower than with cats, and is generally reported in the 5% range (3). Suturing does not seem to increase the risk of subsequent infection (5).

TABLE 6.1. Etiologies to consider in patients with canine exposure.

Clinical Picture	Pathogen
Skin and soft tissue	
Local infection after a bite:	
less than 24 hours	*Pasteurella multocida*
more than 24 hours	*Streptococcus* spp., *P multocida*
	Staphylococcus spp., anaerobes
chronic	*Blastomyces dermatitidis*
Dermatitis (tinea, ringworm)	*Microsporum canis*
Creeping eruption	*Ancylostoma* species
Erythema migrans	*Borrelia burgdorferi**
Lymph nodes	
Regional lymphadenopathy	Cat Scratch agent (*Rochalimaea henselae*)
	Francisella tularensis
	Yersinia pestis
Respiratory	
Pharyngitis	*Streptococcus pyogenes**
Pneumonitis	*Toxocara canis*
Pulmonary embolism	*Dirofilaria immitis*
Solitary pulmonary nodule	*Dirofilaria immitis*
Gastrointestinal	
Diarrhea	*Campylobacter jejuni*
	Salmonella enteritidis
	Cryptosporidium species
	Isospora belli
	*Giardia lamblia**
	Dipylidium caninum
Pruritis ani	*Dipylidium caninum*
Hepatitis	*Leptospira interrogans*
Hepatomegaly	*Toxocara canis*
Articular	
Arthritis	*Borrelia burgdorferi**
Neurological	
Aseptic meningitis	*Leptospira interrogans*
	*Borrelia burgdorferi**
Pyogenic meningitis	*Capnocytophaga canimorsus*
	Pasteurella multocida
Visual disturbances	*Toxocara canis*
Systemic	
Septicemia (shock, D.I.C.)	*Capnocytophaga canimorsus*
	Pasteurella multocida
Endocarditis	*Capnocytophaga canimorsus*
	Pasteurella multocida
Fever and rash	*Rickettsia rickettsii*
Fever without localizing symptoms	*Salmonella enteritidis*
	Brucella canis
	Ehrlichia species*
	Leptospira interrogans
Other	
Visceral mass	*Echinococcus granulosus*
Eosinophilia	*Toxocara canis*

* = transmission from dogs is controversial or unproven

Microbiology

The oral flora of the dog is complex, plentiful, and made up of many aerobic and anaerobic species. Uninfected bite wounds should not be cultured since they will typically grow multiple species, and initial cultures show little correlation with later cultures from bites that become infected (2,3).

Most infections following a dog bite are polymicrobial, typically yielding 2.5 to 4 species on wound culture. Common organisms are *Streptococcal* species, *Staphylococcal* species, anaerobes, and *Pasteurella multocida* (less common in dog bite infections than in those due to cat bites or scratches) (6). Rarely, chronic cutaneous infection with the fungus, *Blastomyces dermatididis*, has been reported after a dog bite injury from an infected dog (7).

Initial Bite Management

Wounds should be irrigated with large amounts of sterile saline using a large syringe and 18-gauge needle to create a high pressure jet (3). Standard recommendations for rabies and tetanus prophylaxis should be adhered to. Suturing may be used when needed; deep puncture wounds should probably not be sutured.

Antibiotic Prophylaxis

Controlled studies have not shown a beneficial effect of antibiotics in preventing infection (8), but these studies were small and may be subject to statistical error since infection rates following canine bites are low to begin with. Many authorities recommend prophylactic antibiotics for wounds of the hands and face, deep puncture wounds that cannot be irrigated adequately, and for immunocompromised persons, particularly those postsplenectomy (5). There is no consensus regarding drug choice. Amoxicillin-clavulanate 250 mg po t.i.d. is a reasonable choice, with tetracycline 500 mg po q.i.d. as an alternative for penicillin allergic individuals.

Treatment of Infection

There are really no good large-scale trials evaluating antibiotic treatment of infected dog bite wounds. Most infections are polymicrobial and treatment should be adequate for staphylococci, streptococci, *P multocida*, and anaerobes. Those persons whose infection began more than 24 hours following the bite should have therapy guided by gram stain and culture when possible (2). Amoxicillin-clavulanate, ciprofloxacin or ofloxacin plus clindamycin, or trimethoprim-sulfamethoxasole plus clindamycin are reasonable therapeutic choices. Infections which manifest (pain, erythema) within a few hours to 24 hours of the bite are usually due to *Pasteurella multocida*; penicillin is the drug of choice, with tetracycline, or trimethoprim-sulfamethoxasole as alternatives in penicillin allergic persons.

Capnocytophaga canimorsus *(Dog Bite Septicemia)*

Capnocytophaga canimorsus, formerly DF-2 (dysgonic fermenter 2) is a fastidious gram-negative rod which can cause serious systemic illness following a dog bite. Since first reported less than 20 years ago, more than 50 human cases have been described (9). The bacterium has been isolated from the normal gingival flora of 16% of dogs (3).

Eighty percent of patients have had a predisposing condition, most commonly splenectomy. More than 50% have reported antecedent dog bites or scratches, and another 20% have had exposure to dogs without knowledge of a bite or scratch.

The clinical illness is typically one of a severe septicemia; shock and disseminated intravascular coagulation are common. Patients may evidence an infected wound with an eschar or cellulitis; petechiae are often present. Endocarditis and meningitis may occur. The mortality rate has been about 25% (9).

Capnocytophaga canimorsus infection must be considered in a febrile, severely ill patient with a history of a dog bite or dog exposure (cats may also transmit this infection). Diagnosis depends on isolation of the organism from blood, other fluids, or tissues. Organisms may be seen in buffy coat smears, particularly in splenectomized patients.

Penicillin is thought to be the drug of choice. The bacterium is also susceptible to third generation cephalosporins, tetracyclines, and quinolones, but is relatively resistant to aminoglycosides and trimethoprim-sulfamethoxasole.

Patients who have had splenectomies should be warned about this rare but devastating infection and advised to take prophylactic antibiotics following a dog bite or contamination of an open wound with dog saliva.

Rabies

The important problem of rabies and its ancient association with dog bites is considered elsewhere in this volume.

Prevention of Dog Bites

Large breeds of dogs (e.g., shepherds) and guard dogs account for a disproportionate percentage of bites. Children should not be left unattended with large dogs, should be educated never to startle feeding or sleeping dogs of any size, and encouraged to avoid unfamiliar animals entirely.

Bacterial Infection

Bacterial zoonoses transmissible from dogs to human beings include campylobacteriosis, salmonellosis, leptospirosis, and brucellosis.

Campylobacteriosis

Campylobacteriosis is found throughout the world and is an important cause of human bacterial diarrhea, being as common or more common than salmonellosis and shigellosis. The vast reservoir of *Campylobacter* in animals is probably the ultimate source for most human enteric infections; a number of outbreaks have followed ingestion of raw milk. *Campylobacter jejuni* is a cause of canine diarrhea, but is often found in the stools of apparently healthy animals. Isolation rates are higher in puppies than in mature dogs and higher in kennel populations than among household dogs (10).

Several case studies have shown an association with patients who had *Campylobacter* enteritis and close contact with sick puppies (11,12). Epidemiological investigation of these cases revealed the only common factor was common exposure to sick dogs. Young children have particularly close exposure to puppies and are, therefore, more susceptible to fecal-oral transmission.

The clinical picture of *Campylobacter* enteritis is usually one of abrupt onset with fever, abdominal pain, and diarrhea, sometimes with malaise, headache, myalgia, arthralgia, nausea, and vomiting. A history of grossly bloody stools is common, and many patients have at least one day of illness with eight or more bowel movements (13). Most patients recover within a week.

Confirmation of the diagnosis of *C jejuni* is based upon positive stool cultures which must be placed on special selective media. Serologic testing can be done but a low titer may reflect previous infection (19).

Fluid and electrolyte replacement are important therapies in any diarrheal illness. *Campylobacter* enteritis is largely self-limited and only in cases with severe prolonged symptoms are antibiotics warranted. *C jejuni* is sensitive to a wide variety of antibiotics including erythromycin, tetracyclines, and quinolones. Erythromycin has been replaced by quinolones as the drug of choice.

Salmonellosis

Nontyphoidal *Salmonella* species are relatively common inhabitants of the canine intestinal tract. In one study 27.6% of rectal swabs from dogs were positive for *Salmonella* (15). Younger dogs may have higher prevalence than older dogs. Despite this high prevalence and evidence that dogs may act as a reservoir for human infection with transmission through the fecal-oral route (16,17), transmission to humans is rare.

The clinical features of canine infection vary with the virulence of the strain, inoculum size, and host factors. Most dogs shedding *Salmonella* in their stools are asymptomatic. The common clinical presentation of canine salmonellosis consists of fever, vomiting, and diarrhea (varying from watery to mucoid to bloody.) Abortion and stillbirth may occur and have epidemiological importance as the meconium, membranes, and discharge contain the organism.

Humans who have acquired salmonellosis have similar clinical findings with fever, nausea, vomiting, colicky abdominal pain, and diarrhea (with or without mucous and blood).

Diagnosis is confirmed by isolation of the organism from stool or blood.

Clinical management should be based upon severity of disease. Human *Salmonella* gastroenteritis is self-limited and requires treatment only in special cases (the very young, the very old, the immunocompromised). Trimethoprim-sulfamethoxasole, fluoroquinolones and third generation cephalosoporins can be used as initial therapy in high-risk patients or those suspected to be bacteremic. The intracellular nature of *Salmonellae* may occasionally create discrepancies between in vitro sensitivity and clinical response.

With regard to public health risk, infected dogs typically shed *Salmonella* for 20 to 40 days, but sometimes for up to 100 days. If one or more family members have confirmed salmonellosis without a known focus of exposure, the family pet should be cultured regardless of symptoms. A thorough investigation should attempt to identify a common source for both human and pet.

Leptospirosis

Leptospires are finely coiled, motile spirochetes that are unique from other pathogenic spirochetes in that they can be cultivated readily on artificial media. Pathogenic leptospires belong to the species *Leptospira interrogans* which has over 200 serovars.

Leptospirosis is a common zoonosis of livestock, pet animals, and wildlife in the United States and other parts of the world. Man is an accidental host, becoming infected through close contact with these animals or their urine. Dogs are important vectors of human illness. Infected canines may be asymptomatic or have fever, jaundice, conjunctivitis, and hemoglobinuria (18).

Infection of man can occur: 1) directly from the urine or tissue of affected animals, 2) indirectly through contact with water or soil that has been contaminated. Most human infection occurs through exposed mucous membranes or abrasions of the skin (19). Leptospirosis can occur at all ages and in all seasons, but it is primarily a disease of young adults, of hot weather, and of males. Optimal factors that determine length of survival of leptospires in the environment are acid urine, neutral or slightly alkaline environment, temperature 22° C or higher, and an aqueous or wet soil. Given these conditions the leptospire may survive for several weeks.

Canine shedder or carrier states develop after infection; leptospires can survive in the distal convoluted tubules of the host kidney after they have disappeared from the host tissues. In the carrier state the host may have leptospiruria for months or for the remainder of its life. Man does not develop a carrier state.

Most humans will have a subclinical infection or anicteric febrile disease which may initially be misdiagnosed as a viral syndrome or aseptic meningitis. Leptospirosis may follow a biphasic illness after an incubation of 7 to 12 days, initially characterized by clinical manifestations of an acute systemic infection (septicemic phase) with fever, headache, myalgia, conjunctival suffusion, leptospiremia, and proteinuria. This terminates after 4 to 7 days. During this first phase leptospires can be isolated from blood, cerebrospinal fluid (CSF), and most tissues. The second phase is immunologically mediated and manifested by meningitis, recurrent fever, uveitis, myositis, and leptospiruria. A detailed description of individual organ manifestations can be found in the review by Edwards and Domm (19). The severe form of leptospirosis is known as Weil's disease and is characterized by hepatic and renal dysfunction, hemorrhage, and circulatory collapse (20).

There are several vaccines available to prevent leptospirosis in dogs and they appear to be effective in preventing clinical illness. However, there have been isolated case reports of dogs that have had leptospires isolated from their urine despite vaccination within the previous year (18).

Definitive diagnosis requires isolation of leptospires from a clinical specimen or demonstration of seroconversion. Leptospires can be isolated from the blood, CSF, or tissue in the first 10 days of infection and identified by dark phase microscopy or culture. Growth may be very slow and culture should be incubated for 6 weeks at 30° C, in the dark (20). The laboratory diagnosis is usually made on the basis of serologic tests. Macroscopic and microscopic slide agglutination tests are available as well as more recently developed enzyme-linked immunosorbent assays (ELISA). Agglutinins appear between the sixth to twelfth day of illness. Identification of the serotype may supply important epidemiological information (*L canicola*—dogs; *L icterohemorrhagiae*—rats).

Treatment of leptospirosis remains controversial, as it is usually a nonfatal, self-limited disease. Some studies suggest that penicillin G or doxycycline may shorten the duration of fever and reduce complications, but only if started before the fourth day of illness (21). In moderate to severe cases most authorities would recommend penicillin G or ampicillin, even if the patient has been ill for several days (20). The Jarisch-Herxheimer reaction is frequently observed during treatment (22).

Recent controlled studies of U.S. troops training in a high-risk environment in Panama demonstrated a significant decrease in the attack rate of leptospirosis in a doxycycline prophylaxis group (200 mg weekly) compared to placebo (23).

Brucellosis

Dogs infected with *Brucella canis*, which is transmitted during mating, may have disease manifested by spontaneous abortion, orchitis, epididymitis, fever, and lymphadenopathy. Infected dogs characteristically have prolonged bacteremia (24).

Human infection due to *Brucella canis* is rare but, like other forms of brucellosis, it may be protean in its manifestations (25). Patients may have a nonspecific febrile illness with headache and myalgias or may demonstrate findings consistent with focal infection.

Blood cultures may be negative and, since antibodies to *Brucella canis* do not react with the standard antigens used when testing for *B abortus*, *B suis*, and *B melitensis*, specific serology for *B canis* must be performed when this diagnosis is suspected (25).

Tetracycline is the standard therapy for brucellosis; streptomycin is added in severe cases (26). It may be difficult to eradicate canine infection, and some authorities have recommended euthanasia for infected dogs.

Ehrlichiosis

Ehrlichia canis is an intraleukocytic rickettsial organism which is a cause of tick-borne canine infection worldwide. Affected dogs have pancytopenia.

Recently, human infection with an *Ehrlichia* species resembling *Ehrlichia canis* has been reported. Human ehrlichiosis is manifested by acute onset of fever, malaise, and headache; rash is absent. Laboratory features include leukopenia, thrombocytopenia, and liver function abnormalities (27). Most patients have a history of tick bite, and diagnosis has been established serologically. Tetracycline has been reported to be effective therapy.

Recent studies (28,29) indicate that human ehrlichiosis is caused by a species distinct from *Ehrlichia canis*. Dog to human transmission appears very unlikely.

Cat Scratch Disease

Cat scratch disease, reviewed elsewhere in this text, rarely has been reported following dog bites or scratches.

Streptococcosis

Group A beta-hemolytic streptococcus (*Streptococcus pyogenes*) is a common cause of pharyngitis in children and adults. There are reports of dogs acting as reservoirs for this organism.

In one report, a family of four had recurrent Group A streptococcal pharyngitis which was not eradicated until the family dog was treated (30).

Canine reservoirs for human streptococcal pharyngitis are probably exceedingly rare; that they occur at all is a controversial issue. Nevertheless, it is probably prudent to consider a canine source in families with recurrent hemolytic streptococcal infection and a pet dog.

Parasitic Infections

Many dogs harbor intestinal parasites; autopsy data have shown that more than 50% are infested with one or more such parasites (31). Some of these canine parasites may be transmitted to human beings in whom they may produce symptomatic illness.

Cryptosporidiosis and Isosporiasis

Cryptosporidium is a ubiquitous coccidian protozoan parasite of the gastrointestinal tract, related to *Isospora* and *Toxoplasma*, which has been identified in a large variety of animals. It has six major developmental stages that all occur within a single host.

Transmission of the oocyst is by a fecal-oral route. Dogs can act as reservoirs for this organism (32–35). The disease seems to be limited to puppies, but one study showed antibodies to cryptosporidia in 80% of all dogs tested (36).

Human cryptosporidiosis is characterized by watery diarrhea and cramping abdominal pain; fever is not prominent. The importance of this organism as a cause of human disease was recognized in AIDS patients in whom it causes protracted wasting diarrheal illness; in immunocompetent hosts it produces a self-limited illness of 1 to 2 weeks.

To date there are no documented cases of transmission from dogs or puppies to man. However, considering the prevalence of this organism and the similarity in the mode of transmission to other pathogens, it seems likely that it will be noted in time. Outbreaks involving veterinary students suggest that human *Cryptosporidium* infection may be acquired from dogs and/or cats (37).

Diagnosis is made by microscopic identification of the organism in a fresh stool sample; leukocytes and blood are absent. After diagnosis, treatment of immunocompetent individuals may not be necessary. For immunocompromised patients who are unable to clear the infection on their own, treatment has been frustrating and unsuccessful in most cases (33). Supportive therapy may be the only treatment available.

The related protozoan, *Isospora belli*, causes clinical illness similar to *Cryptosporidium* and is diagnosed by identification of oocysts in fecal specimens. The size and shape (large and ovoid) of *Isospora* distinguishes it from *Cryptosporidium* which is round and smaller; both are acid fast.

Isospora infection is common in dogs; one study (38) showed 9% of puppies from Atlanta pet stores to harbor the parasite. Transmission to humans has not been proven. Treatment of humans with a week of oral trimethoprim-sulfamethoxasole is curative; AIDS patients have a high frequency of recurrence but respond to retreatment.

Giardiasis

The flagellated enteric protozoan, *Giardia lamblia*, is an important world-wide cause of water-borne diarrhea in humans. Fecal-oral spread may also occur, particularly in day care settings, custodial institutions, and among sexually active male homosexuals.

Human infection is manifested by watery diarrhea without fever. Cramps, bloating, flatulence, and sulfuric belching are common.

Giardia may cause diarrhea in dogs, but its role in transmission of giardiasis to human beings has not been defined (2). *Giardia* species were identified in 34% of puppies in Atlanta pet stores (38).

Giardiasis should be considered in all patients with prolonged diarrhea or malabsorptive symptoms. Diagnosis is achieved by seeing cysts or trophozoites in stool specimens or by sampling duodenal contents. Treatment is with metronidazole or quinacrine; furazolidone is used in children.

Dirofilariasis

The dog heartworm, *Dirofilaria immitis* (Latin: dirus = evil; filum = thread) is found worldwide in warm climates. In the United States, canine and human dirofilariasis is most prevalent along the East Coast, Gulf Coast, Great Lakes, and Mississippi River Valley (39).

Mosquito vectors transmit the microfilarial form of the parasite from dog to dog and from dog to human being. In the canine host the adult worm lives in the right ventricle and pulmonary artery. Infected dogs are often asymptomatic but may have hemoptysis or evidence of heart failure secondary to right ventricular outflow obstruction.

In humans, larvae cannot develop into adults; most die before reaching the heart. Occasionally, a larva may reach the right ventricle, die, and embolize to the lung. Symptoms are rare, but, when present, may mimic thromboembolic pulmonary embolism (pleuritic pain, fever, hemoptysis) (40,41). The granulomatous lung reaction to the embolized larva produces the roentgenographic finding of a solitary pulmonary nodule (42,43). Human infection is confirmed only when larvae are identified histologically following resection of solitary pulmonary nodule. Eosinophilia is rarely noted, and serologic studies have not proved useful (39).

Canine infection is diagnosed by demonstrating microfilariae in smears of peripheral blood; treatment in dogs and prophylaxis in endemic areas should be under veterinary supervision. Human infection should be considered in the differential diagnosis of solitary lung nodule; diagnosis is established following resection, and further treatment is unnecessary.

Toxocariasis

Toxocara canis is a roundworm that infects most puppies and many adult dogs in the United States, and is the primary cause of visceral larva migrans (VLM) in humans.

Adult worms live an average of 4 months in the proximal small intestine of dogs. By the time a dog has aged 6 months, the majority of worms have been expelled. During that time, however, an adult female roundworm can produce 200,000 eggs per day. Eggs are then passed in the feces but are unembryonated and, therefore, uninfective. Embryonation occurs in the expelled feces over approximately a 2-week period; depending on temperature and moisture of the environment, eggs can remain viable for months.

Infection in adult dogs follows ingestion of embryonated eggs, ingestion of larvae in other infected hosts, or larvae or immature adults from the vomitus or feces of infected pups. After hatching in the stomach the larvae penetrate the intestinal mucosa, enter lymph and blood vessels, reach the liver within 24 hours, and pass to the heart and lungs. From the lungs some of the larvae pass through the bronchioles to the trachea and pharynx where they are swallowed and can complete their life cycle and develop into adults in the intestine (44). There the larvae, as in human infections, rarely complete their life cycle. This results in the somatic migration of larvae which become encysted in various tissues. Hormonal changes in a pregnant bitch stimulate the larvae, resulting in transplacental migration of the larvae to the litter or passage of larvae in bitch's milk (45).

Transmission to humans may occur by ingestion of eggs from the soil or on contaminated hands and fomites. Children 1 to 6 years of age are most prone to infection, particularly those with a history of pica and exposure to puppies. Up to 20% to 30% of soil samples recovered from backyards of residences, public parks, and childrens' sandboxes are contaminated with *T canis* eggs (46). Despite uniformly high levels of toxocariasis in dogs throughout the United States, the diagnosis of visceral larva migrans in children is made most frequently in the south central and southeastern regions.

Human infection begins following ingestion of the infective egg; hatching occurs in the small intestine, releasing the larvae (47). The larvae penetrate the mucosa, migrate to the liver via the portal system, follow vascular channels to the lungs, and enter the systemic circulation. Larvae are stopped when the diameter of the blood vessel becomes too small to allow passage. They then bore through the vessel wall and migrate aimlessly. In man, larvae migrate most frequently to the liver, but virtually any tissue can be invaded, where larvae become dormant and may remain viable for many years. At a later time, they may reactivate and resume their migration.

Light infections are generally asymptomatic and probably occur most frequently; eosinophilia may be the only indicator of infection. In three human subjects who received 100 to 200 larvae as a single dose, moderate eosinophilia lasted for more than a year but there were no other signs or symptoms of disease (45).

Common signs and symptoms include cough, wheeze, pallor, malaise, irritability, and weight loss. Pruritic eruptions may occur, especially over the trunk and lower extremities. Pulmonary involvement is common, with approximately half of the patients developing transient infiltrates on chest radiograph. Patients may present with bronchitis, asthma, pneumonitis, or any combination of these signs.

Leukocyte counts ranging from 30,000 to 100,000 per cubic millimeter, with 30% or more eosinophils are not unusual. Eosinophilia may persist for months or years, even after other manifestations of the disease have abated.

In a study by Huntley et al (48) of 51 patients with VLM, the most common symptoms were cough (80%) and wheezing (63%); fever (80%), hepatomegaly (65%), rales, and malnutrition were the most common physical findings.

A question has been raised as to whether *Toxocara* is responsible for neurological disease in children. Skin testing for *Toxocara* in healthy individuals and those with epilepsy showed positive tests in 2.1% and 7.5%, respectively. Twenty-eight percent of the patients in the Huntley study had a history of seizures. Testing by Glickman in 1979 (44) showed significantly higher *Toxocara* titers in epileptic children compared to nonepileptic controls. Children with toxocara are more likely to have lead poisoning than noninfected children; both share the same risk factors—pica and lower socioeconomic status. Further studies are necessary to define the significance of *T canis* in children with respect to neurological function and to distinguish the effects from those of lead (46).

Ocular larva migrans (OLM) is caused by the larva of *Toxocara* entering the eye; it is typically a unilateral disease, but occasionally occurs bilaterally.

Presenting complaints are varied, and there is no pathognomonic pattern. Patients may complain of failing vision, strabismus, leukocoria, eye pain, fixed pupil, or red eye. Fundoscopic exam may vary from a solitary posterior pole lesion or peripheral granuloma in an asymptomatic eye to severe exudative endophthalmitis with retinal detachment.

Generally, ocular cases differ from VLM in several important aspects. Ocular cases are more frequently reported in adults and are usually seen in the absence of visceral symptoms; unlike VLM, a history of pica is infrequent.

A diagnosis of systemic toxocariasis should be considered in any child with persistent eosinophilic leukocytosis, especially given a history of pica. Laboratory and clinical findings are generally nonspecific and must be differentiated from other conditions with eosinophilia.

Ocular toxocariasis should be considered in any child with unilateral white or gray lesions in the fundus; it needs to be differentiated from retinoblastoma, congenital and developmental abnormalities, exudative retinitis, and other causes of uveitis.

Diagnostic confirmation is based on demonstration of the larvae in pathological specimens (biopsy or autopsy). Stool samples are not useful, as the larvae rarely if ever mature in human beings. Percutaneous liver biopsy infrequently yields evidence of the larvae; laparoscopic biopsy may be more useful.

Immunodiagnostic tests are available. A recent study showed that in 78 patients suspected of clinical toxocariasis an ELISA test for *T canis* was 91% sensitive and 86% specific (49).

The disease is usually self-limited and only in rare instances have there been fatalities resulting from an exaggerated immune response in the heart or CNS. The use of corticosteroids may be lifesaving in these patients and is indicated for actively inflamed eyes to prevent further changes leading to retinal detachment. Several antihelminthic drugs have been used clinically with variable response. Diethylcarbamazine greatly decreases the number of larvae recovered from tissues of experimentally treated mice; thiabendazole is less effective in this respect. Both drugs have been reported to lessen symptoms and shorten convalescent times in patients with VLM. The beneficial effects of thiabendazole may be more closely related to its antiinflammatory and analgesic properties than to its antihelminthic abilities.

The best treatment may be to increase prevention by reducing the frequency of accidental ingestion of infective eggs. This can be accomplished by reducing the exposure of children to infected dogs and puppies, treatment of infected dogs, and removing children with pica from environments thought to be contaminated.

Cutaneous Larva Migrans

The dog intestinal hookworms, *Ancylostoma caninum* and *A braziliense*, are the nematodes that cause human cutaneous larva migrans (creeping eruption).

Larvae enter human skin after direct contact in areas contaminated with canine feces such as beaches and playgrounds. The larvae do not possess the enzymes necessary to penetrate the dermis and remain confined to the epidermis.

About 2 weeks after exposure, skin eruptions occur manifested by serpiginous, pruritic, red tunnels which spread a few millimeters per day.

The skin appearance is diagnostic and infection is self-limited but may last for several weeks.

Thiabendazole is effective both orally (50) and as a topical suspension (51).

Echinococcosis

Echinococcus granulosus is a small tapeworm whose definitive host is the dog. The adult cestode is found in the small intestine of dogs and wolves; gravid segments release eggs which are shed in the stool and may remain viable for up to a year. Once ingested by human or other suitable intermediate host, the eggs make their way to the upper small intestine where they hatch and an oncosphere is released.

The released oncosphere penetrates the intestinal mucosa and obtains passage to the liver via portal veins. Here, most of the oncospheres are trapped; however, a few may pass through the liver and arrest in the lung. Those embryos that reach the systemic circulation may seed any organ. Wherever the parasite rests it is either destroyed by an inflammatory reaction or develops into a hydatid cyst, the latter being the culmination of a successful infection of the intermediate host. Cysts contain multiplying larvae and enlarge slowly over many years.

Upon death of the intermediate host, the larval hydatid may be eaten by a dog or another definitive host, whereupon the released scolices attach to the small intestinal mucosa. These scolices mature over a period of 6 to 8 weeks into an adult tapeworm 3 to 6 millimeters long, completing the life cycle (52,53).

Humans act as intermediate hosts, but the prevalence of human echinococcosis is dependent upon the direct association of man with infected canines. The frequency of infection is much higher in those regions where livestock is a major industry, especially in sheep raising areas, where dogs feed on uncooked offal (53). The two epidemiological patterns that have been established are domestic (or pastoral) and sylvatic (or wild). The sylvatic cycle is seen in the tundra zones and the coniferous forests of northern Alaska and Canada; intermediate hosts are reindeer and caribou (54).

The more common cycle is adapted to domesticated dogs that become infected when they eat the contaminated viscera of sheep, cattle, or pigs. The cycle of transmission continues when the eggs passed in the dogs' feces are consumed by the herbivorous intermediate host. Human echinococcosis in the United States is found in sheep ranchers in California, Arizona, New Mexico, and Utah.

The majority of infections with *E granulosus* are asymptomatic. Echinococcal cyst disease is indolent, and cysts enlarge slowly over many years. Some of the cysts die, shrink, become heavily calcified, and remain asymptomatic (55).

Symptomatic infections present with features of a space-occupying lesion and can involve almost any organ. Typical anatomical distribution is indicated by 1,802 cysts recorded in the Australasian Hydatid Registry: liver, 63%; lung, 25%; muscles, 5%; bone, 3%; kidney, 2%; spleen and brain, 1%; and heart, thyroid, breast, prostate, parotid, and pancreas all less than 1% (53).

The most important complications of hydatid cysts are rupture, infection, and problems caused by compression. Leaking cysts can precipitate a wide range of reactions from urticaria to anaphylaxis. Scolices that are released may lead to the establishment of secondary or metastatic hydatid infections elsewhere in the body. Bacterial infection of a cyst resembles an abscess of that organ (53,55).

A geographic history must be taken when suspecting hydatid disease, since the diagnosis is more likely in an area of the world where the disease is prevalent.

Plain x-rays of the abdomen may show calcification of the cyst rim. The chest film usually shows a round, uniformly dense lesion 1 to 20 centimeters in diameter, but calcification rarely occurs in lung cysts.

Skin testing for echinococcal antibody has a poor yield and false positives can be found in up to 40% of patients. Enzyme linked immunosorbent assay (ELISA), complement fixation, and indirect hemagglutination tests are better, but not all carriers have antibodies (90% with liver cysts; 75% with lung cysts). Aspiration of the cyst for diagnosis is contraindicated since leakage of contents or rupture of the cyst can lead to secondary infection or an anaphylactic reaction. Computerized axial tomography appears to be more helpful than ultrasound for pulmonary and extrahepatic cysts (55). The demonstration of intracystic septations, suggesting daughter cysts, is diagnostic of hydatid disease. Eosinophil counts or liver function tests may or may not be abnormal and should not be relied upon. Definitive diagnosis and treatment require surgery.

If the patient is asymptomatic and the cyst has been discovered by chance, then surgery can be delayed and the patient followed. Most authorities recommend surgery for all pulmonary cysts and hepatic cysts larger than 5 centimeters even if asymptomatic. Cysts that are densely calcified rarely expand. Surgery is indicated in all symptomatic patients.

Scolicidal agents for irrigation of the cyst prior to removal include hypertonic saline, 1% iodine solution, silver nitrate, or cetrimide (not available in the U.S.) (53,55,56).

Although albendazole shows promise as a chemotherapeutic agent for echinococcosis, especially with liver and peritoneal cysts (57), definitive therapy at present requires surgical resection of the cyst(s). Albendazole should be considered in cases where there is direct rupture and release of cyst contents (56), or when surgery is not possible.

Dipylidiasis

Dipylidium caninum is a common tapeworm of dogs. Larval cysticercoids of *D caninum* develop in fleas and biting lice that are the obligate intermediate hosts; dogs usually acquire this infection while nipping fleas. The ingested cysticercoid requires only 2 to 3 weeks to develop into an adult, proglottid shedding worm residing in the host intestine. Therefore, control of this parasite must include eradication of fleas and lice in addition to human antihelminthic therapy (58).

Human beings are infrequently parasitized, and most *Dipylidium* infections occur in children younger than 8 years, with one-third occurring in infants less than 6 months of age (59–62). Human infection begins when a flea or louse is accidentally ingested by a child while in contact with its pet. Symptoms are usually absent, but abdominal discomfort (61) or diarrhea and pruritis may occur (2). One case report describes a history of colic and feeding difficulties associated with dipylidiasis (62).

Diagnosis is made by isolating the proglottids from the feces or perineum. The parent usually notices the motile cucumber-seed-shaped proglottids, resembling maggots, in the stool. They can also migrate from the anus which can cause a misdiagnosis of pinworms by history.

Presently the treatment of choice is niclosamide, and the alternate therapy is paromycin sulfate.

Superficial Fungal Infections (Dermatophytosis)

Dermatophytosis is a common superficial fungal infection of dogs, cats, and man. Zoophilic dermatophytes are occasionally transmitted to humans causing tinea or ringworm. Dermatophytes rarely invade the skin, and produce disease by releasing allergens and creating an inflammatory reaction.

The most common fungi causing dermatophytosis in dogs are species of *Epidermophyton*, *Microsporum*, and *Trichophyton*. The cutaneous signs are variable and not characteristic for a specific dermatophyte. By far, the most common organism of dogs to cause skin infections of humans is *M canis*.

Diagnosis is established based on history, physical examination, Wood's lamp examination, KOH preparation, skin biopsy, and fungal cultures. Fungal culture is the most accurate way of confirming the diagnosis. Ten to thirty percent of human cases of tinea or ringworm, in urban settings, are estimated to be of animal origin (2).

In humans, treatment with topical antifungal agents is usually adequate; oral ketaconazole and fluconazole have also been shown to be effective.

Ectoparasite-Associated Illness

Dogs that frequent the out-of-doors may disseminate the flea and tick vectors responsible for such serious human diseases as plague, Rocky Mountain spotted fever, tularemia, and Lyme disease. Thus, a pet owner need not leave home to be exposed to these infections; his or her dog can bring the vectors right into the living room.

Other canine ectoparasites (mites, fleas) may cause vexing dermatoses in humans. The most common ectoparasite-induced dermatoses of dogs are scabies, cheyletiellosis, and fleas. It has been estimated that over 5% of the cases presenting to human dermatology clinics are directly attributable to animal ectoparasites (63).

Canine Scabies

Sarcoptes scabiei var. canis causes canine scabies (sarcoptic mange), a nonseasonal pruritic transmissible infestation of the skin of dogs which is transmissible to humans. The adult female mite penetrates to the level of the stratum granulosum where she feeds. She deposits her eggs in a burrow where they hatch and give rise to the larval form. These migrate to the surface and molt through nymphal and adult forms. Eggs develop into adult mites in 10 to 21 days.

Canine scabies has no age, sex, or breed preferences and is characterized by intense pruritis which is followed by an erythematous, nonfollicular papular dermatitis. These lesions, frequently found on the pinnae, face, limbs, and ventrolateral trunk, become excoriated and crusted. In the absence of early diagnosis or treatment, extension of these lesion may involve the entire animal with accompanying alopecia (64). It is thought that prolonged skin to skin exposure is important for transmission to take place from dog to human being; 30% to 50% of human contacts of a canine case may be affected.

Hypersensitivity appears to play a role in canine and human scabies. In both species, dermatological manifestations are out of proportion to the number of mites present. There is significant evidence that the immune system participates in the pathogenesis of this disease (65).

Diagnosis is generally established by history, clinical findings, or response to scabicides, since human skin scrapings frequently fail to demonstrate scabetic mites. Canine scrapings are more often positive, but in one study only 51% of canine scrapings were positive for ova or mites (65).

There is no correlation between the severity and duration of the canine disease and transmission to humans. The lesions in humans consist of vesicles, erythematous papules, wheals, crusts, and excoriations occurring in areas of pet contact. Therefore, it is seen especially on the arms, legs, abdomen, and chest. Unlike human scabies, there are no burrows, no involvement of the hands, finger webs, or genitalia. Human infestation often occurs in small epidemics (66).

The severity of the eruption, its extent and duration can vary considerably. Generally the lesions are self-limited without treatment after the infected animal has been separated.

Human scabies and papular urticaria are the main conditions to be differentiated from canine scabies in man. The history of exposure to an infested pet, the different distribution pattern, the lack of burrows, and demonstrating the causative organism on examination of the pet will aid in making the diagnosis.

Canine scabies is easily treated with weekly application of scabicidal dips (especially lindane or lime sulfur) until 2 weeks after clinical cure is achieved (65). All dogs in a household or in-contact dogs should be treated. In addition, a single washing of fomites in hot water and detergent is recommended.

Although many authors feel that human infestation is a self-limited disease, there have been some reports indicating this may not be the case (65). Successful treatment of humans has been achieved with a 24-hour application of gamma benzene hexachloride cream. Steroids are of value in those patients with severe inflammatory reactions, and antibiotics are indicated in those who develop secondary bacterial infections.

Cheyletiellosis

Cheyletiella dermatitis ("walking dandruff") is a nonseasonal, variably pruritic, transmissible infestation of the skin of dogs and cats caused by mites. In general, *C yasguri* is considered the species affecting dogs.

These mites do not burrow, but live in skin-surface keratin. They move about rapidly but occasionally pierce the skin with their hooks and become engorged with tissue fluids (65).

Like scabies, there is no apparent predilection for breed or sex. Pruritus is a variable finding, but there is usually some degree of dorsal scaling, crusting, and dermatitis (65). Adult dogs can be symptomatic carriers of mites, but puppies are most often clinically affected.

Skin lesions producd by *Cheyletiella* mites in human beings have been reported with human involvement occurring in 20% to 80% of canine cases. In man, the lesions begin as single or grouped erythematous macules which rapidly evolve into papules; these lesions frequently become vesicular or pustular. Old lesions develop a very characteristic central necrosis which is of diagnostic significance. The pruritus may be intense and involve any portion of the body, but rarely the face. Other eruptions which may be produced by these mites include bullae, urticaria, erythema multiforme, and generalized pruritus without dermatitis.

Diagnosis is based on historical and physical findings, positive skin scrapings or scotch tape preparations, and response to miticidal agents. Skin scrapings in man are rarely positive.

Human infestations are self-limited; *Cheyletiella* mites are unable to complete their life cycle on humans. The source of mites must be removed or treated with topical miticides. Dogs in contact with affected animals must be treated and their environment vigorously cleaned. The human dermatosis should resolve in 3 weeks without specific treatment.

Fleas

Fleas can cause asymptomatic infestation or severe hypersensitivity skin disease in dogs and humans. In the United States, the genera of most importance are *Ctenocephalides* and *Pulex* (65).

Hypersensitivity to flea salivary antigens plays a critical role in dermatoses. The typical lesion on human beings is an urticarial papule. Lesions favor exposed distal extremities and are extremely pruritic.

In diagnosing human flea bites it is important to demonstrate fleas in the environment. This is often done by having the patient walk through infested areas wearing white knee socks to better visualize the fleas.

Treatment involves flea control measures as well as topical or systemic antiinflammatory medication (if the reaction is severe). Effective flea control requires treatment of the affected pets, their areas, and other animal contacts. Flea bombs or sprays are needed to kill larval forms and prevent reinfection. Pets should not be allowed to forage in areas where *Yersinia pestis* is prevalent.

Measures to Minimize Dog-Associated Illness

Children should not be left unattended with dogs, unfamiliar dogs should be avoided, and feeding or sleeping dogs should not be startled.

Dogs should be vaccinated for rabies and possibly for leptospirosis.

Prophylaxis for dirofilariasis should be given in endemic areas.

Newly acquired puppies should be treated for intestinal parasites before being taken into the home.

Dogs should not be permitted to defecate on beaches or playgrounds, and animal feces on lawns should be removed at least weekly. Feces should not be used as fertilizer.

Dogs should not be allowed to eat offal.

Hands should be washed after handling animals, and diarrhea in pets should cause increased attention to hygiene.

Animals should be regularly inspected for fleas and ticks.

References

1. Friedmann E, Katcher AH, Lynch JJ, Thomas SA. Animal companions and one-year survival of patients after discharge from a coronary care unit. *Public Health Rep* 1980; 95:307–312.
2. Elliot DL, Tolle SW, Goldberg L, Miller JB. Pet-associated illness. *N Engl J Med* 1985; 313:985–995.
3. Weber DJ, Hansen AR. Infections resulting from animal bites. *Infect Dis Clin N Amer* 1991; 5:663–680.
4. Lauer EA, White WC, Lauer BA. Dog bites: a neglected problem in accident prevention. *Am J Dis Child* 1982; 136:202–204.
5. Aghababian RV, Conte JE Jr. Mammalian bite wounds. *Ann Emerg Med* 1980; 9:79–83.
6. Goldstein EJC, Citron DM, Wield B, Blachman V, Sutter VL, Miller TA, Finegold SM. Bacteriology of human and animal bite wounds. *J Clin Microbiol* 1978; 8:667–672.
7. Gnann JW, Bressler GS, Bodet CA, Avent CK. Human blastomycosis after a dog bite. *Ann Intern Med* 1983; 98:48–49.
8. Elenbaas RM, McNabney WK, Robinson WA. Prophylactic antibiotics and dog bite wounds. *JAMA* 1981; 246:833–834.
9. Hicklin H, Verghese A, Alvarez S. Dysgonic fermenter-2 septicemia. *Rev Infect Dis* 1987; 9:884–890.
10. Blaser MJ, Taylor DN, Feldman RA. Epidemiology of *Campylobacter jejuni* infections. *Epidemiol Rev* 1983; 5:157–176.
11. Blaser MJ, Cravens J, Powers BW, Wang WL. *Campylobacter* enteritis associated with canine infection. *Lancet* 1978; 2:979–981.
12. Salfield NJ, Pugh EJ. *Campylobacter* enteritis in young children living in households with puppies. *Brit Med J* 1987; 294:21–22.
13. Blaser MJ, Reller LB. *Campylobacter* enteritis. *N Engl J Med* 1981; 305:1444–1452.
14. Blaser MJ, Berkowitz ID, LaForce FM, Cravens J, Reller LB, Wang WLL. *Campylobacter* enteritis: clinical and epidemiologic features. *Ann Intern Med* 1979; 91:179–185.
15. Galton MM, Scatterday JE, Hardy AV. Salmonellosis in dogs. *J Infect Dis* 1952; 91:1–5.
16. Cook GC. Canine-associated zoonoses: an unacceptable hazard to human health. *Quart J Med* 1989; 70:5–26.
17. Willard MD, Sugarman B, Walker RD. Gastrointestinal zoonoses. *Vet Clin N Amer: Small Animal Practice* 1987; 17:145–178.
18. Feigin RD, Lober LA, Anderson D, Pickering L. Human leptospirosis from immunized dogs. *Ann Intern Med* 1973; 79:777–785.
19. Edwards GA, Domm BM. Human Leptospirosis. *Medicine* 1960; 39:117–156.

20. Goldstein EJC. Household pets and human infections. *Infect Dis Clin N Amer* 1991; 5:117–130.
21. McClain JB, Ballou WR, Harrison SM, Steinweg DL. Doxycycline for leptospirosis. *Ann Intern Med* 1984; 100:696–698.
22. Schmidt DR, Winn RE, Keefe TJ. Leptospirosis: epidemiologic features of a sporadic case. *Arch Int Med* 1989; 149:1878–1880.
23. Takafuji ET, Kirkpatrick JW, Miller RN, Karwacki JJ, Kelley PW, Gray MR, McNeil KM, Timboe HL, Kane RE, Sanchez JL. An efficacy trial of doxycycline chemoprophylaxis against leptospirosis. *N Engl J Med* 1984; 310:497–500.
24. Currier RW, Raithel WF, Martin RJ, Potter ME. Canine brucellosis. *J Am Vet Med Assoc* 1982; 180:132–133.
25. Polt SS, Dismukes WE, Flint A, Schaefer J. Human brucellosis caused by *Brucella canis*: clinical features and immune response. *Ann Intern Med* 1982; 97:717–719.
26. Hall WH. Modern chemotherapy for brucellosis in humans. *Rev Infect Dis* 1990; 12:1060–1099.
27. McDade JE. Ehrlichiosis—a disease of animals and humans. *J Infect Dis* 1990; 161:609–617.
28. Dawson JE, Anderson BE, Fishbein DB, Sanchez JL, Goldsmith CS, Wilson KH, Duntley CW. Isolation and characterization of an *Ehrlichia* sp. from a patient diagnosed with human ehrlichiosis. *J Clin Microbiol* 1991; 29:2741–2745.
29. Anderson BE, Dawson JE, Jones DL, Wilson KH. *Ehrlichia chaffeensis*, a new species associated with human ehrlichiosis. *J Clin Microbiol* 1991; 29:2838–2842.
30. Mayer G, VanOre S. Recurrent pharyngitis in family of four. *Postgrad Med* 1983; 74:277–279.
31. Hasi DK, Collins JA, Flick SC. Canine parasitism. *Canine Pract* 1978; 2:42–47.
32. Current WL, Reese NC, Ernest JV, Bailey WS, Heyman MB, Weinstein WM. Human cryptosporidiosis in immunocompetent and immunodeficient persons. *N Engl J Med* 1983; 308:1252–1286.
33. Current WL. The biology of *Cryptosporidium*. *ASM News* 1988; 54:605–611.
34. Fayer R, Ungar BLP. *Cryptosporidium* spp. and Cryptosporidiosis. *Microbiologic Reviews* 1986; 50:458–483.
35. Havin TR, Juranek DD. *Cryptosporidiosis*: clinical, epidemiologic and parasitologic reivew. *Rev Infect Dis* 1984; 6:313–327.
36. Tzipori S, Campbell I. Prevalence of *Cryptosporidium* antibodies in 10 animal species. *J Clin Micro* 1981; 14:455–456.
37. Fang G. Araujo V, Guerrant RL. Enteric infections associated with exposure to animals or animal products. *Infect Dis Clin N Amer* 1991; 5:681–700.
38. Stehr-Green JK, Murray G, Schantz PM, Wahlquist SP. Intestinal parasites in pet store puppies in Atlanta. *Am J Pub Health* 1987; 77:345–346.
39. Ciferri F. Human pulmonary dirofilariasis in the United States: a critical review. *Am J Trop Med Hyg* 1982; 31:302–303.
40. Dayal Y, Neafie RC. Human pulmonary dirofilariasis: a case report and review of the literature. *Am Rev Resp Dis* 1975; 112:437–443.

41. Tsung SH, Lin JI, Han D. Pulmonary dirofilariasis in man. *Am J Med Sci* 1982; 283:106–110.
42. Merrill JR, Otis J, Logan WD Jr, Davis B. The dog heartworm (*Dirofilaria immitis*) in man: a epidemic pending or in progress? *JAMA* 1980; 243:1066–1068.
43. Harrison EG Jr, Thompson JH. Dirofilariasis of human lung. *Am J Clin Path* 1965; 43:224–234.
44. Glickman LT, Schantz PM. Epidemiology and pathogenesis of zoonotic toxocariasis. *Epidemiol Rev* 1981; 3:230–250.
45. Schantz PM, Glickman LT. Toxocaral visceral larva migrans. *N Engl J Med* 1978; 298:436–439.
46. Glickman LT, Shofer FS. Zoonotic visceral and ocular larva migrans. *Vet Clin of N Amer: Small Animal Practice* 1987; 17:39–53.
47. Glickman LT, Schantz PM, Cypress RH. Canine and human toxocariasis: Review of transmission, pathogenesis and clinical disease. *J Amer Vet Med Assoc* 1979; 175:1265–1269.
48. Huntley CC, Costos MC, Lyerly A. Visceral larva migrans syndrome: clinical characteristics and immunologic studies in 51 patients. *Pediatrics* 1965; 36:523–536.
49. Jacquier P, Gottstein B, Stingelin Y, Eckert J. Immunodiagnosis of toxocarosis in humans: Evolution of a new enzyme-linked immunosorbent assay kit. *J Clin Micro* 1991; 29:1831–1835.
50. Katz R, Ziegler J, Blank H. The natural course of creeping eruption and treatment with thiabendazole. *Arch Dermatol* 1965; 91:420.
51. Whiting DA. The successful treatment of creeping eruption with topical thiabendazole. *S Afr Med J* 1976; 50:253–255.
52. Schieven BC, Brennan M, Hussain Z. *Echinococcus granulosus* hydatid disease. *ASM News* 1991; 57:407–410.
53. Grove DI, Warren KS, Mahmoud AAF. Algorithms in the diagnosis and management of exotic diseases X. Echinococcosis. *J Infect Dis* 1976; 133:354–358.
54. Wilson JF, Diddams AC, Rausch RL. Cystic hydatid disease in Alaska. *Amer Rev Resp Dis* 1968; 98:1–15.
55. Schaefer JW, Khan YM. Echinococcus (hydatid disease): Lessons from experience with 59 patients. *Rev Infect Dis* 1991; 13:243–247.
56. Scully R, Mark EJ, McNeely WF, McNeely BU. Case records of the Massachusetts General Hospital, Case 45-1987. *N Engl J Med* 1987; 317:1209–1218.
57. Todorov T, Vutoa K, Petkov D, Mechkov G, Kolev K. Albendazole treatment of human cystic echinococcosis. *Trans Roy Soc Trop Med Hyg* 1988; 82:453–459.
58. Georgi JR. Tapeworms. *Vet Clin N Amer: Small Animal Practice* 1987; 17:1285–1305.
59. Chappell CL, Penn HM. *Dipylidium caninum*, an underrecognized infection in infants and children. *Pediatr Infect Dis J* 1990; 9:745–747.
60. Margolis B. Dog tapeworm infestation in an infant. *Am J Dis Child* 1983; 137:702.
61. Bartsocas CS, Von Graevenitz A, Blodgett F. *Dipylidium* infection in 6-month-old infant. *J Pediatr* 1966; 69:814–815.
62. Turner JA. Human dipylidiasis (dog tapeworm infection) in the United States. *J Pediatr* 1962; 61:763–768.

63. Hewitt M, Walton GS, Waterhouse M. Pet animal infestations and human skin lesions. *Brit J Derm* 1971; 85:215–225.
64. Thomsett LR. Mite infestations of man contracted from dogs and cats. *Brit Med J* 1968; 3:93–95.
65. Scott DW, Horn RT Jr. Zoonotic dermatoses of dogs and cats. *Vet Clin N Amer: Small Animal Practice* 1987; 17:117–144.
66. Smith EB, Claypoole TF. Canine scabies in dogs and in humans. *JAMA* 1967; 199:95–100.

7
With Man's Worst Friend (The Rat)

JAMES G. FOX

Introduction

Historically, the rat has been considered a scourge to mankind. For example, the rat is a reservoir for plague called the Black Death Which accounted for millions of deaths in Europe during the Middle Ages. Pandemics of plague ravaged earlier civilizations and undoubtedly had "plagued" mankind prior to recorded history. Also, numerous other diseases are spread to man by the rat; thus Hans Zinsser's quote from his text *Rats, Mice and History*: "Man and rat will always be pitted against each other as implacable enemies," conveys the general revulsion that society holds for the wild rat (1).

Even though various methods have been used by countless countries attempting to eradicate the rat, it continues to successfully colonize both urban and rural settings on a global level. For example, during the early 1900s rodenticides containing live cultures of *Salmonella enteritidis* were distributed on a large-scale basis by commercial and public health organizations in an attempt to eliminate feral rats. These cultures were known as "rat viruses" and widely used in Europe, England, and the United States as 'rat poisons" (2). However, the enthusiasm for their use waned when it was discovered that the spread of the organisms couldn't be limited; predictably, the baiting program was implicated in several epidemics among exposed human populations (2). Surprisingly, as late as the 1950s in England, *S enteritidis* (serovar *danzy*) was isolated from adults living 4 miles apart. The source of infection was traced to contaminated cakes from a local bakery. Mice that had acquired the infection from living *S danzy* cultures in rodenticide baits had infected food in the bakery (3).

Another novel approach in England and the United States used domestic ferrets for rodent control. This practice became popular in the United States during the early part of the twentieth century, and tens of thousands of ferrets were raised and sold for this purpose. The Department of Agriculture distributed bulletins announcing the use of ferrets for rodent abatement (4). Because rodents are extremely fearful of ferrets and will flee even their scent, only a few ferrets were needed to disperse literally hundreds of rodents from granaries, barns, and warehouses. A ferretmeister would deploy his ferrets on an infested farm or granary, and the animal would then "ferret out" the rodents from their hiding places and nests. Men and terrier dogs, strategically located, would eradicate the rodents as they emerged from hiding. Alternatively, small farms or granaries would maintain ferrets and allow the territorial imperative for up to about 650 feet (200 m)—considered to be the ranging domain of a ferret—with an adequate food source. The introduction of commercially available rodenticides, however, has dramatically reduced the popularity of ferrets as rodent exterminators (4).

The black roof rat (*Rattus rattus*) which coexisted with man in the small, crowded, unsanitary environs of the medieval era, has been largely displaced by the more aggressive, larger brown Norway rat (*Rattus norvegicus*) (5–7). This species of rat lives farther from contemporary, better constructed urban domiciles, taking up residence in back yards, sewers, industrial buildings, dumps, or granaries. In this environment, the rat often competes for food and territory with other wild rodents and therefore can share zoonotically transmitted diseases. Fortunately, human fleas which accounted for widespread human-to-human transmission of plague have almost been eliminated from cities in the United States and thus the likelihood of epidemics initiated by rat zoonoses has been reduced. Nevertheless, zoonotic transmission of rat diseases still occurs and as major cities suffer from overcrowding, structural decay, and inadequate waste removal, the rat population will increase and the probability of transmission of these diseases to the homeless or underprivileged correspondingly increases.

Contrary to the image of the rat depicted by Zinsser, the laboratory rat, used extensively for decades in biomedical research, has provided immeasurable benefit to mankind's understanding of disease processes and disease control and elimination. However, the use of rats in research and the current popularity of rats as "pocket pets" also affords the opportunity for this segment of the population to become infected with rat-borne diseases. The purpose of this chapter, therefore, will be to highlight those zoonotic diseases of the rat, and in certain cases the same disease in the mouse, which have clinical relevance in the United States and its territories (8).

Rat Bites

Approximately 40,000 rat bites are reported annually according to one carefully researched report (5). Several studies indicate that over two-thirds of the rat bites occur in children under 10 years of age. Adult humans attacked by rats are usually debilitated or otherwise helpless. Most bites occur on hands and feet, but may also be present on the head and face of infants, sometimes with disfiguring consequences. Occasionally, deaths due to rat bites have been recorded in infants or debilitated adults (6). It has been estimated in one study that 2% of rodent bites in humans become infected (9). Several bacterial pathogens have been isolated from rat bites including *Leptospira interrogans*, *Pasteurella multocida*, and *Staphylococci*; however, the most commonly isolated microorganisms are *Streptobacillus moniliformis* and *Spirillum minus* (10,11).

Bacterial Diseases

Rat-Bite Fever

Rat-bite fever can be caused by either of two microorganisms: *Streptobacillus moniliformis* (Haverhill fever) or Sodoku caused by *Spirillum minus*. The bite of an infected rat is the usual source of infection. In some cases, other animal bites or rare traumatic injuries unassociated with animal contact cause the infection. Unless treated, both organisms can result in a serious human disease causing arthritis (not usually seen with Sodoku), pneumonia, hepatitis, enteritis, and endocarditis (12–20).

These organisms are present in the oral cavity and upper respiratory passages of asymptomatic rodents, usually rats (21). In one study, *Streptobacillus moniliformis* was isolated as the predominant microorganism from the upper trachea of laboratory rats (22). Other small surveys indicate isolation of the organism in 0:15, 7:10, 2:20, 7:14 laboratory rats and 4:6 wild rats (23). Surveys in wild rats indicate 0% to 25% infection with *Spirillum minus* (24). *Spirillum minus* does not grow in vitro and requires inoculation of culture specimens into laboratory animals with subsequent identification of the bacteria by dark-field microscopy. *Streptobacillus moniliformis* grows slowly on artificial media, but only in the presence of sera, usually 10% to 20% rabbit or horse serum incubated at reduced partial pressures of oxygen (25).

Rat-bite fever is not a reportable disease, which makes its prevalence, geographic location, racial data, and source of infection in humans difficult to assess. The disease, though uncommon in man, has nonetheless appeared among researchers working with laboratory rodents, particularly rats (12). Historically, wild rat bites and subsequent illness (usually in small children) relate to poor sanitation and overcrowding (24). One survey of rat bites in Baltimore tabulated rat-bite fever in 11 of 87 cases (26). Acute febrile diseases, especially if associated with animal bites, are routinely treated with penicillin or other antibiotics. Therefore, accurate data regarding prevalence is usually not provided.

Streptobacillus moniliformis incubation varies from a few hours to 1 to 3 days, whereas *Spirillum minus* incubation ranges from 1 to 6 weeks. Fever is present in either form. Inflammation associated with the bite and lymphadenopathy are frequently accompanied by headache, general malaise, myalgia, and chills (13–16). The discrete macular rash that often appears on the extremities may generalize into pustular or petechial sequelae. Arthritis occurs in 50% of all cases of *Streptobacillus moniliformis* but is less common in *Spirillum minus*. *Streptobacillus moniliformis* may be cultured from serous to purulent effusion which is recovered from affected larger joints.

If antibiotic treatment is not instituted early, complications such as pneumonia, hepatitis, pyelonephritis, enteritis, and endocarditis may develop (18,19). Death has occurred in cases of *Streptobacillus moniliformis* involving pre-existent valvular disease.

Plague

In the United States human infections due to *Yersinia pestis*, a gram-negative coccobacillus, are sporadic and limited, usually resulting from infected flea or rodent contact. Since 1924 to 1925, when a plague epidemic ravaged Los Angeles, neither urban plague nor rat-borne plague has been diagnosed in the United States (27). All reported cases since then have been reported in states located west of the 101st meridian.

Although wild rat populations still account for the primary reservoir of plague with transmission of *Y pestis* to humans via fleas, particularly *Xenopsylla cheopis*, in many parts of the world and they remain a continued threat in the U.S., sciurid rodents (rock squirrels, California ground squirrels, chipmunks, and prairie dogs) account for the primary plague reservoir in the western parts of the U.S. (28–30). Cricetid rodents, such as the woodrat, are occasionally cited as reservoir hosts. The oriental rat flea, *X cheopis*, the common vector of plague, is well established throughout the U.S., particularly in the southern U.S. and southern California. Plague is infrequently reported in the U.S., with a low of one case in 1972 and a high of 40 cases in 1983 (27). Ninety percent of the cases have been diagnosed in New Mexico, Colorado, and California. Urban development (particularly in New Mexico) encroached into plague-enzootic rodent habitats, placing these populations at increased risk of contracting the disease. In addition to rodent epidemics, dogs, and increasingly cats, have served as either passive transporters of the disease or have been actively infected (30,31). The disease occurs seasonally, with the highest proportion occurring during May through September.

Bubonic plague in humans is usually characterized by fever (2 to 7 days postexposure) and the formation of large, tender, swollen lymph nodes, or buboes. If untreated, the disease may progress to severe pneumonic or systemic plague. Inhaled infective particles, particularly from animals with plague pneumonia, may also result in the pneumonic form of the disease.

Human infection is usually the result of a bite from an infected flea, but can also occur via cuts or abrasions in the skin, or via infected aerosols coming in contact with the oropharyngeal mucous membrane.

Primary pneumonic plague historically occurred by inhalation of infectious droplets from a pneumonic plague patient. However, in the last several decades this form of the disease has occurred from exposure to infected animals (usually cats) that have developed secondary pneumonia due to septicemic spread of the organism (27,30,31). Owners or veterinarians attending these sick animals are then infected by inhaling infected aerosols generated by the plague bacteria.

A presumptive diagnosis can be made by visualizing bipolarstaining, ovoid, gram-negative rods on the microscopic examination of fluid from buboes, blood, sputum, or spinal fluid; confirmation can be made by culture. Complement fixation, passive hemagglutination, and immunofluorescence staining of specimens can be used for serologic confirmation.

Mortality without antibiotic therapy, particularly in cases of pneumonic plague can exceed 50% in untreated cases. Chloramphenicol is the drug of choice for treating plague meningitis and endophthalmitis (27,32).

An inactivated plague vaccine is available for laboratory personnel working with the organism and for high-risk individuals (e.g., wildlife management employees, Peace Corps volunteers) exposed to plague reservoirs in endemic areas.

Rodent and flea control, particularly in high endemic areas, is an indispensable part of containing exposure to plague, as is restricting certain locales for recreational use.

Yersinosis

Yersinia enterocolitica is now recognized as a cause of enteritis in humans. Pigs and dogs are considered natural reservoirs for *Y enterocolitica* serovar 3. Biovar 4, is a common cause of the disease in humans. This strain has also been isolated from *R norvegicus* and *R rattus* in Japan (33). It has been suggested that rats may play a role in the ecology of *Y enterocolitica* in swine herds. Control of wild rat populations among swine herds may reduce the potential transmission of this organism via pork products. More recently another pathogenic strain, serovar 08, was isolated from wild rodents: woodmice, geisha mice, and a vole (34). This strain, however, was not evident in random samples of brown or black rats taken from select locales in Japan (34). Further epidemiological studies are needed in the United States to determine the importance of wild rats as reservoirs for *Y enterocolitica*.

Leptospirosis

Leptospirosis is solely a zoonotic disease of livestock, pet and stray dogs, and wildlife, including wild rats. In addition to rats, rodent reservoir hosts of leptospirosis are mice, field moles, hedgehogs, gerbils, squirrels, rabbits, and hamsters (35,36). Human to human transmission is extremely rare. *Leptospira interrogans* (comprising >200 serovars) have been isolated worldwide. Although particular serotypes usually have distinct host species, most serotypes can be carried by several hosts. *Leptospira* are well adapted to a variety of mammals, particularly wild animals and rodents.

In the chronic form, the organism is carried and shed in the urine inconspicuously for long periods of time. Rodents are the only major animal species that can shed leptospires throughout their life span without clinical manifestations (35,36). Active shedding of leptospires by rodents can go unrecognized until personnel handling the animals become clinically infected, or are infected by exposure to water or food contaminated by urine.

Leptospira icterohaemorrhagiae was first recovered in 1918 in the U.S. from wild rats sampled in New York City. In one recent study in Detroit, more than 90% of adult brown Norway rats were infected with *L icterohaemorrhagiae* (37). In an earlier study conducted in Baltimore, 45.5% of 1,643 rats were infected with *Leptospira*; higher prevalence rates occurred in older rats (~60%) (38). Other studies confirm the high prevalence of this organism in wild rats inhabiting cities in the U.S. (39,40). Rats and mice are also common animal hosts for another serotype, *L ballum*, although it has been found in other wildlife as well. Water can oftem be contaminated with infected rat urine. The infection can persist unnoticed in laboratory rodents, though their carrier rates for laboratory maintained rodents in the United States are unknown, but probably low (23). Recently, however, there was a report of leptospirosis in a research colony of mice in the United States being housed in a large research institution (39).

Because leptospirosis in humans is often difficult to diagnose, the low incidence of reported infection in humans may be misleading. From 1974 to 1979 only 498 cases were reported, for an incidence of 0.05 per 100,000 people per year (40). Outbreaks have been documented in the United States from personnel working with laboratory mice (41,42). In one study, 8 of 58 employees handling the infected laboratory mice (80% of breeding females were excreting *L ballum* in their urine) contracted leptospirosis (41). In several European laboratories, personnel have been infected with leptospires from laboratory rats (23).

Infection with *Leptospira* sp. most frequently results from handling infected rodents (contaminating the hands with urine) or from aerosol exposure during cage cleaning (41,42,43). Skin abrasions or exposure to mucous membranes may serve as the portal of entry. All secretions and excretions from infected animals should be considered infective. In one instance, a father apparently was infected after his daughter used his toothbrush to clean a contaminated pet mouse cage (44). Handling infected wild rats also increases the risk of contracting leptospires (45). Recently, a young man died of acute leptospirosis by falling into a heavily polluted river contaminated with *L icterohaemorrhagiaes* (40). Rodent bits can also transmit the disease (46). In Detroit, children from the inner city had a significantly higher *L icterohaemorrhagiaes* antibody when compared to children living in the Detroit suburbs. Therefore, children living in rat infested tenements may be at increased risk of infection (47).

The disease may vary from unapparent infection to severe infection and death. Infected individuals experience a biphasic disease (40,41,48). They become suddenly ill with weakness, headache, myalgia, malaise, chills, and fever and usually exhibit leukocytosis. During the second phase of the disease, conjunctival suffusion and a rash may occur. Upon examination, renal, hepatic, pulmonary, and gastrointestinal findings may be abnormal. Penicillin is the drug of choice in treating early onset of leptospirosis infection (48,49). Ampicillin and doxycycline also have been effective in treating people with leptospirosis. Tetracycline has been used successfully to eradicate *L ballum* in a mouse colony (50).

Because of the variability in clinical symptoms and lack of pathognomonic pathological findings in humans and animals, serologic diagnosis or actual isolation of leptospires is imperative (48). As an aid to diagnosis, leptospires can sometimes be observed by examination or direct staining of body fluids or fresh tissue suspensions (51). The definitive diagnosis in humans or animals is made by culturing the organisms from tissue or fluid samples, or by animal inoculation (particularly in 3- to 4-week-old hamsters) and subsequent culture and isolation. Culture media with long-chain fatty acids with 1% bovine serum albumin are routinely used as a detoxicant (48). Serologic assessment is accomplished by indirect hemagglutination, agglutination analysis, complement fixation, microscopic agglutination, and fluorescent antibody techniques (48). The serologic test most frequently used is the modified microtiter agglutination test. Titers of 1:100 or greater are considered significant.

Borrelia species (Tick-borne Relapsing Fever)

Tick-borne relapsing fever occurs primarily in foci in the western part of the United States, as well as other parts of the world. The disease is caused by at least 15 *Borrelia* species and is transmitted to humans from a variety of rodents (chipmunks, squirrels, rats, mice, prairie dogs, hedgehogs) via soft ticks of the genus *Ornithodorus*. The rat has also been used experimentally to study the pathogenesis of the disease (52).

Salmonellosis

The genus *Salmonella* are gram-negative bacteria with approximately 2,000 serotypes. Nontyphoidal salmonellosis is caused by any of these serotypes. Other than *Salmonella typhi*, the causative agent of typhoid fever, salmonellosis occurs worldwide and is important in humans and animals. *S typhi* and *Salmonella choleraesuis* have only one serotype, whereas the remaining 2,000 serotypes are within the species *Salmonella enteritidis*. References to the *Salmonella enteritidis* serotypes are abbreviated such that "enteritidis" is dropped, e.g., *S enteritidis* serotype *typhimurium* is called *Salmonella typhimurium* (53). *Salmonella typhimurium* is the serotype most commonly associated with disease in both animals and man. Other serotypes most commonly reported from man and animal are *Salmonella heidelberg*, *Salmonella agona*, *Salmonella montevideo*, and *Salmonella newport*. Salmonellae are pathogenic to a variety of animals.

Rats are extremely susceptible to infection with *Salmonella* sp. In studies performed in the 1920s through 1940s, prevalence of *Salmonella* in wild rats surveyed in the U.S. varied from 1% to 18%, compared to 19% of wild rats in Europe (2,23,39,54). In experimental studies, when rats were dosed orally with *Salmonella*, 10% shed the organism in the 2 months after inoculation, and a few remained carriers when examined 5 months after experimental challenge. These rats, when placed with other naive rats, were capable of initiating new epizootics (55). Fortunately, the disease in laboratory rats, though common prior to 1939, has rarely been isolated in U.S. commercially reared rats since that time. However, because the rat is used experimentally to study *Salmonella* pathogenesis, personnel working with these animals must take appropriate precautions to prevent zoonotic transmission.

Salmonella are ubiquitous in nature and are routinely found in water or food contaminated with animal or human excreta. Fecal-oral transmission is the primary mode for spread of infection from animal to animal or to man. Rat feces can remain infective for 148 days when maintained at room temperature (56). Transmission is enhanced by crowding and poor sanitation.

As with other fecal-oral transmitted diseases, control depends on eliminating contact with feces, food, or water contaminated with *Salmonella*, or animal reservoirs excreting the organism (53). *Salmonella* survive for months in feces, and are readily cultured from sediments in ponds and streams previously contaminated with sewage or animal feces. Fat and moisture in food promote survival of *Salmonella*. Pasteurization of milk and proper cooking of food (56° C for 10 to 20 minutes) effectively destroys *Salmonella*. Municipal water supplies should be routinely monitored for coliform contamination (57).

Clinical signs of salmonellosis in humans include acute sudden gastroenteritis, abdominal pain, diarrhea, nausea, and fever. Diarrhea and anorexia may persist for several days. Organisms invading the intestine may create septicemia without severe intestinal involvement; most clinical signs are attributed to hematogenous spread of the organisms. As with other microbial infections, the disease's severity relates to the organism's serotype, the number of bacteria ingested, and the host's susceptibility. In experimental studies with volunteers, several serovars induced a spectrum of clinical disease from brief enteritis to serious debilitation. Incubation varied from 7 to 72 hours. Cases of asymptomatic carriers, persisting for several weeks, were common (24).

Salmonella are flagellated nonsporulating, aerobic gram-negative bacilli that can be readily isolated from feces on selective media designed to suppress bacterial growth of other enteric bacteria. *Salmonella* serotyping requires antigenic analysis (53).

Salmonella gastroenteritis is usually mild and self-limiting. With careful management of fluid and electrolyte balance, antimicrobial therapy is not necessary. In humans, antimicrobial therapy may prolong rather than shorten the period during which *Salmonella* is shed in the feces (57,58). In one double-blind placebo study of infants, oral antibiotics did not significantly affect the duration of *Salmonella* carriage. Bacteriological relapse after antibiotic treatment occurred in 53% of the patients and 33% of these suffered a recurrence of diarrhea, whereas none of the placebo group relapsed (58).

Other Possible Bacterial Infections

Campylobacteriosis, a common diarrheal disease in humans caused by *Campylobacter jejuni/coli*, is isolated from a variety of animals, including rats. Animals can be responsible for zoonotic spread of this organism; however, rats have not, to date, been incriminated (53,59). Another pocket pet, the hamster, has been suggested as possibly infecting homosexuals with *Campylobacter* (*Helicobacter*) *cinaedi* (60).

Recently, beta hemolytic Group G streptococci was isolated from rats with cervical lymphadenitis, as well as from the pharynx of normal laboratory rats (61). Streptococci Group G causes a wide variety of clinical diseases in humans, including septicemia, pharyngitis, endocarditis, pneumonia, and meningitis. Asymptomatic carriage of Group G streptococci also is common in humans. At present, however, there is no documented evidence that streptococci from rats are transmitted to, or acquired by, humans (62).

Pathogenic *Staphylococcus aureus* of human phage type can cause clinical disease in mice and rats. This organism has been introduced into SPF barrier-maintained mouse colonies and SPF rats and guinea pigs; the same phage type was isolated from their animal caretakers (63–65).

Colonization by normal *S aureus* strains in the nasopharyngeal area of humans presumably minimizes zoonotic potential of animal-originated *S aureus*.

Viral Diseases

Hemorrhagic Fever with Renal Syndrome, Nephropathia Epidemica (Hantaan Virus)

Hemorrhagic fever with renal syndrome (HFRS), and nephropathia epidemica are used to describe a group of rodent-borne diseases caused by several Hantaviruses (family Bunyaviridae) (36,66,67). In Southeast Asia the disease is endemic, whereas focal epidemics throughout the Eurasian continent and Japan have been recorded. American soldiers became infected with the disease during the Korean War. Severity of the disease will depend on the particular immunotype of the virus as well as the respective natural reservoir host.

Korean hemorrhagic fever occurs seasonally in agricultural workers, with bimodal population peaks of the reservoir host—the striped field mouse *Apodemus agragarius*—and its ectoparasites. HFRS is characterized by fever, headache, myalgia, and hemorrhagic manifestations that may lead to shock from massive capillary leakage of plasma protein. Previously significant, mortality has now been reduced to 6% with hospitalization and dialysis (68).

Nephropathia epidemica (NE), a less severe form, is encountered in Scandinavia, western Russia, and several other European countries. The etiological virus has been isolated and named Puumala virus by Finnish researchers. The natural reservoir is the bank vole *Clethrionom glareolus*. Infected persons, usually adult men with vole contact, exhibit sudden onset of fever, abdominal or low back pain, elevated serum creatinine levels, and polyuria; fatalities are rare.

In the late 1970s, a disease resembling HFRS was reported in laboratory workers in Japan, Belgium, and Korea. Retrospective epidemiological evaluation of the first laboratory-associated outbreak and additional urban outbreaks in Japan revealed that the reservoir of the disease was laboratory and wild rats. Over 100 cases of HFRS in man have been linked to exposure to laboratory rats infected with the virus (69,70). Persons infected exhibited a range of illness, from a nonspecific influenza-like episode to acute renal insufficiency and hemorrhagic diathesis. Because the worldwide distribution of infected laboratory rats or their tissues may have occurred, testing of potentially contaminated colonies and transplantable rat tumor banks was undertaken. One individual had serologic evidence of infection in the U.S., and in Britain a mild clinical case was diagnosed. Caesarian rederivation procedures employed for imported animals probably prevented or eliminated the spread of infection at most institutions.

Hantaan-related virus infection in wild rats, both *R rattus* and *R norvegicus*, raised concern regarding the potential spread of disease by international shipping. Sea ports throughout the world, including many in the United States, harbor rats infected with Hantaan or a related virus. To date, serologic evidence of disease in the United States has been noted but no human clinical cases have been associated with this type of exposure (71).

The Prospect Hill virus, another Hantavirus, has been isolated from meadow voles (*Microtus pennsylvanicus*) in Maryland; it has not been associated with human disease although serologic surveys indicate unapparent infection throughout the United States with a distribution of virus limited to the geographic distribution of the animal host. Recently, however an outbreak of acute respiratory illness, with significant mortality, has been linked to a newly recognized hantavirus (69a). The disease has been limited thus far to the Southwestern U.S. and the rodent host is suspected to be the deer mouse. Occurrence of this disease highlights the importance of preventive measures to limit exposure to rodents and their excreta (69b).

Hantaviruses do not cause disease in their respective rodent hosts, although virus can be detected in the salivary glands and numerous visceral organs of chronically infected animals. The virus is shed in the saliva, feces, and urine; transmission to humans is generally believed to be from aerosols generated from contaminated rodent excreta (69). There is also the potential for transmission via ectoparasites. Detection of infected rodents or infected rodent tissue prior to entry into the laboratory is crucial in preventing zoonotic disease. ELISA, IFA and hemagglutination inhibition tests are available for serodiagnosis.

Rabies

Rabies virus, a rhabdovirus, has been recognized as a clinical disease for centuries in both Europe and Asia. The virus, when inoculated into animals, usually via a bite, produces a fatal disease in all warm-blooded species with a high degree of probability; rats should therefore be listed as a susceptible host.

Rabies occurs on all continents except Australia. Other islands, such as Hawaii, New Zealand, and Great Britain are also fortunate in not having rabies in their domestic or wild animal populations. Rabies occurs infrequently in man, but its presence in natural reservoirs, such as wild carnivores, bats, and, rarely, certain rodents such as squirrels, is endemic in certain parts of the United States as well as other parts of the world. Rabies in skunks, raccoons, and bats has increased markedly in the last several decades and now accounts for more than 85% of all reported cases in the U.S. (72). From 1971 through 1989, woodchucks accounted for 68% of the 200 rodent cases reported in the U.S. (72). Other rodents, including rats, are almost never infected with rabies, and no human cases of rabies of rodent origin have been reported in the last 50 years. However, in the Federal Republic of Germany, from 1961 to 1967, nine Norway rats and eight muskrats were reportedly infected with rabies and had supposedly bitten humans (23).

Rickettsial Diseases

Murine Typhus (Endemic Typhus)

Murine typhus is caused by *Rickettsia typhi*. Although this disease has been recognized for centuries, it wasn't until the 1920s that it was distinguished from epidemic typhus. The absence of louse infestation in humans, and the disease's seasonal occurrence and sporadic nature help differentiate it from louse-borne typhus (i.e., epidemic typhus). Epidemic typhus is only seen in the eastern U.S. in association with flying squirrels (73).

Murine typhus is primarily a disease of rats with its principal vector being the oriental rat flea, *Xenopsylla cheopis* and another flea, *Nasopsyllus fasciatus*. These fleas will also naturally colonize the mouse, *Mus musculus*. The cat flea, *Ctenocephalides felis*, (as well as seven other species of fleas) has also been implicated in the spread of the disease. Rickettsia are ingested with a blood meal of the flea, they multiply in the gut, and are subsequently passed out in the dejecta of the flea. Infection in the rat and the human is the result of contamination of the puncture wound by flea feces (74). Recent experimental evidence indicates that a flea bite can also directly transmit the infection (74). *R typhi* are resistant to drying and remain infectious for up to 100 days in rat feces.

Murine typhus occurs worldwide, and in the United States it is usually diagnosed in southeastern or Gulf states, as well as in areas along the northern portion of the Mississippi River (76). It also is associated with human populations subjected to areas of high density wild rat colonies, such as ports, granaries, farms, or rat-infested buildings in inner cities. Laboratory personnel have been infected with this agent when inoculating rodents and handling infected animals (76).

After infection with the rickettsia, the incubation period is 7 to 14 days. Because murine typhus is difficult to diagnose either clinically or anatomically from other rickettsial diseases, specific serologic tests are extremely important in making the correct diagnosis (74). The acute febrile disease is usually characterized by general malaise, headache, rash, and chills, with signs ranging from mild to severe. An encephalitic syndrome can also occur (32). In one report, 25% of 180 patients with the disease had delirium, stupor, or coma (78). Fortunately, these findings resolve with lowering of the febrile response. Fatality rate for all ages is about 2%, but increases with age.

Recovery of rickettsial organisms or antigens from biological specimens is inconsistent and is not routinely done except in labs equipped to process and identify these samples. It must be remembered that rickettsia are hazardous and have accounted for numerous infections of laboratory personnel. Currently, serologic diagnosis is accomplished by ELISA and RIA; however, the IFA technique remains the most commonly used. Unfortunately, this test cannot distinguish epidemic from endemic typhus. The CDC considers a fourfold rise in titer detected by any technique (except Weil-Felix) as evidence of rickettsial infection. Complement fixation titer of 1:16 or greater in a single serum sample from a patient with clinically compatible signs is also considered diagnostic (72).

Proper antibiotic therapy is the most effective measure to prevent morbidity or mortality due to rickettsial infections. Tetracycline and chloramphenicol have proven to be effective in hastening recovery and preventing neurological sequelae, such as deafness due to XIII-cranial nerve involvement (32).

Fleas can be controlled by applying insecticides (organochlorines, as well as others) as residual powders or sprays in areas where rats nest or traverse. It is imperative that insecticides be applied prior to using rodenticides; this will prevent fleas from leaving the dead rodents and feeding on human hosts (75).

Rickettsial Pox

A variety of rodents are infected with other rickettsial diseases. *Mus musculus* is the natural host for the causative agent of rickettsial pox, *Rickettsia akari*, a member of the spotted fever group of rickettsia (76,77). This organism is also isolated from *R rattus* and *R norvegicus*, and the rat under certain circumstances may transmit the disease to humans. The disease is transmitted by the mite *Liponyssoides* (*Allodermanyssus*) *sanguineus*. The disease has been diagnosed in New York City and other eastern cities, as well as in Russia, Egypt, and South Africa (77). The incubation period is approximately 10 to 24 days, and the clinical disease is similar to that noted in murine typhus. The rash of rickettsial pox commences as a discrete maculopapular rash, which then becomes vesicular. The palms and soles are usually not involved. About 90% of affected persons develop an eschar, with a shallow ulcer covered by a brown scab (74,77). Although headaches are common and may be accompanied by stiff necks, lumbar CSF samples are normal. Pulmonary and gastrointestinal involvement also are almost never encountered. Diagnosis, treatment, and control are similar to those described for murine typhus.

Mycoses
Dermatophytes

In almost all rat- and mouse-associated ringworm infections in humans, *Trichophyton mentagrophytes* has been isolated as the etiological agent (Table 7.1) (78–83). Classic murine ringworm, reportedly caused by *Trichophyton quinckeanum*, is usually restricted to feral rodents, but successful crossing of cultures of this strain with tester strains of perfect state *T mentagrophytes* (*Arthroderma benhamiae*) proves that *T quinckeanum* is not a distinct species and is indistinguishable from *T mentagrophytes* (84).

Dermatophytes are distributed worldwide, with some species reportedly more common in certain geographic locations. From a study of 1,288 animals from 15 different species of small mammals in their natural habitats, 57 *T mentagrophytes* were isolated, most commonly from the bank vole (*Clethriomys glareolus*), followed by the common shrew (*Sorex araneum*) and house mouse (*M musculus*) (85). Agricultural workers exposed to these mammals in granaries and barns risked contracting *T mentagrophytes* infections; indeed, 77% of 137 agricultural workers were infected with ringworm. Only 23% of the workers showed sings of infection (85).

In laboratory mice and rats, ringworm infection is often asymptomatic, going unrecognized until laboratory personnel become infected (Table 7.1) (80). In one study, for the 8-month period before dermatophyte infected mice were treated, almost half the people handling the mice developed ringworm, although less than 1% of the mice showed any signs of disease (81).

Transmission occurs via direct or indirect contact with asymptomatic carrier animals, with the skin lesions of infected rodents, with contaminated grain, or with animal bedding. Causal fungi present in air, dust, or on surfaces of animal holding rooms are also transmittal sources (78).

Ringworm is in many cases nonfatal, usually self-limiting, and, because it is sometimes asymptomatic, often ignored by the affected person. The dermatophytes cause scaling, erythema, and occasionally vesicles and fissures; the fungi cause thickening and discoloration of the nails. On the skin of the trunk and extremities, lesions may be circular with a central clearing. The locations of the fungus signifies the clinical categories, for example, tinea capitis or tinea unguium. When humans are infected by one of the dermatophytes recovered from mice or rats, the fungus appears on the body and/or extremities, most commonly on the arms and hands.

Zoophilic *T mentagrophytes* produce an acute inflammatory response which often undergoes rapid resolution; the infection may produce furunculosis, widespread tinea corporis, and deep involvement of the hair follicles.

TABLE 7.1. *Trichophyton mentagrophytes* infections associated with laboratory mice, rats, or pet mice.

Probable source of infection	Number of persons infected	Lesions appearing on infected mice or rats	References
Pet white mice; inbred albino laboratory mice (VSBS, A2G)	7 children; 2 lab technicians	2 or 104, diffuse alopecia	78a
Laboratory mice	6 lab technicians		79
Laboratory mice	2 lab technicians	0 of 96 (222 cultured), survey of commercial stock	80
BALB/c C3H/Bl mice	6 lab technicians	<1% of all mice, carrier rate 90%	81
White mice	1 lab worker	% not determined, alopecia, increased scaling on head and back, 10 mice	82
White mice	1 bacteriologist	60 of 400, crusted or crustless plaques, circular with prominent periphery; general alopecia; mortality in some mice	83
Wistar rats	1 technician	20% colony with alopecia and scaly skin	80
Rats	1 technician	Alopecia with crusting and erythema	84

Topical fungicides or griseofulvin per os is effective in eradicating dermatophytes from animals and humans. Strict environmental and personal hygiene help lower the incidence of ringworm. Personnel should wear rubber gloves when touching infected rodents.

Helminth Diseases

Roundworms

Angiostrongylus (*Parastrongulus*) *cantonensis* (Rat Lung Worm)

A clinical syndrome known as eosinophilic meningitis results in humans who accidentally ingest raw aquatic animals, e.g., prawns (transport hosts) and snails or slugs (intermediate hosts), harboring infective larvae of the lungworm or by eating larvae which have contaminated vegetables. In humans, the infective larvae migrate to the central nervous system, and may undergo 1 to 2 molts, but do not develop into adult worms— thus the human is a dead end host. The rat serves as the reservoir host where the adult worm develops and passes infective eggs in rat feces, which are then ingested by the intermediate host. Spread of the organism to rats has been linked to dispersal of the African land snail (*Achatina fulica*) (75,86).

Historically, this disease was restricted to the Far East and the Pacific Rim, including Hawaii and Tahiti. Recently, the disease has been reported in Cuba and the lungworm has been recovered in rats in Puerto Rico and New Orleans (75,86). It is therefore likely that the disease will be more commonly diagnosed in the Americas in the future.

The disease may often be subclinical or have an indistinct 2 to 4 month prepatent period. The distinguishing clinical feature of the disease is the presence of elevated eosinophils (>10%) of the leukocytes found in abnormal CSF. Other CNS signs can also be present, such as severe headache, meningeal irritation (nuchal rigidity), and increased intracranial pressure. Visual impairment may occur if there is ocular involvement. A febrile response is usually mild to absent. Only the most severe infections result in permanent impairment or, in some cases, death (87).

Occasionally in <10% of the cases, larval or young adult worms can be recovered from the CSF. The infection must be distinguished from other helminth CNS infections, such as paragonimiasis, fascioliasis, trichinosis, strongyloidiasis, cysticercosis, echinococcosis, and ascarids. A microenzyme-linked immunosorbent assay for antibodies directed against the antigens of the parasite either in serum or CSF has been recently developed and is helpful in confirming the diagnosis (86).

Effective anthelmintic regimens have not been developed, (although ivermectin shows promise in animal trials), and potential therapeutic intervention designed to kill the parasite may indeed exacerbate the inflammatory response and clinical signs. Clinical treatment is usually supportive to relieve headache and nausea. In some cases corticosteroids have been used. Thiabendazole has been used with some success during the first week of infection (87). Prevention of the infection is obviously preferred. This is accomplished by avoidance of eating raw vegetables and underwashed or unfrozen snails and aquatic crustaceans in endemic areas.

Tapeworms

Hymenolepsis nana: The Dwarf Tapeworm of Man

The dwarf tapeworm is a common parasite for both rats and mice. The infection in humans occurs most frequently in children who live in warm climates. Its presence in humans is noted worldwide and it is the most frequently detected tapeworm in the United States (76). *Hymenolepsis nana* is unique among tapeworms because it does not require an intermediate host to complete its life cycle. The adult tapeworm develops after the egg is ingested; the hooked oncosphere invades the intestinal mucosa, develops into a cysticeroid larvae, and 2 weeks later the larvae mature into adult worms. The *Hymenolepsis nana* eggs can contaminate hands, eating utensils, food, or aerosolized dust, and then be accidentally ingested. Internal autoinfection may also occur. The tapeworm can also use fleas and beetles for the development of its life cycle; these in turn are then accidently ingested by humans. Personal hygiene, sanitation, and rodent control are important in preventing transmission. Humans with mild infection and in a good nutritional state usually have no symptoms, or it may cause diarrhea, anorexia, vomiting, pruritis of nose and anus, or uticaria. In severe infections, signs are consistently present and include diarrhea, abdominal pain, anorexia, and CNS signs (76). Niclosamide for 5 to 7 days is the treatment of choice after demonstration of the characteristic eggs in the feces.

Hymenolepsis diminuta: The Rat Tapeworm

This tapeworm is especially common in the Norway rat and the black rat; however, it is rarely diagnosed in humans (88), though it has been seen in patients from several parts of the United States (76).

The rat tapeworm requires an intermediate host for larval development. This is usually the larval stage of rat fleas, but other arthropods such as many beetle species, earwigs, and meal moths can serve as intermediate hosts.

Symptoms of the infection are usually not noted and diagnosis is made by recovery of the eggs in feces. The eggs are distinguished from *Hymenolepsis nana* by the lack of polar filaments.

Treatment with niclosamide, similar to the regimen used to treat *Hymenolepsis nana*, is recommended. Control is dependent on elimination of rodents from the premises.

Arthropod Infestations

Mites

Several arthropods found on rats, mice, and other wild rodents are vectors of human disease, and some cause allergic dermatitis as well (Table 7.2) (89). Fleas are seldom found on laboratory rodents but are common parasites of feral rodents. The Oriental rat flea *Xenopsylla cheopis*, and another flea, *Nasopsyllus fasciatus*, naturally infest both mice and rats; they are vectors for murine typhus. That *X cheopis* easily establishes itself in animal facilities can be demonstrated by the flea bites two students received while working in animal rooms housing mice (89).

TABLE 7.2. Selected ectoparasites of rodents with zoonotic potential.*

Species	Disease in humans	Host	Agent Transmitted
Mites			
Obligate skin mites			
Sarcoptes scabiei subspecies	Scabies	Mammals	
Trixacarus caviae	Dermatitis	Guinea pigs	
Nest inhabiting parasites			
Ornithonyssus bacoti	Dermatitis, murine typhus, rickettsialpox	Rodents and other vertebrates	Coxsackie, WEE,** SLE† virus, Rickettsia typhi, Rickettsia akari, Francisella tularensis
Liponyssoides sanguineus	Dermititis, rickettsialpox	Rodents, particularly Mus musculus	Rickettsia akari
Haemogamasus pontiger	Dermatitis	Rodents, insectivores, straw bedding	
Haemolaelaps casalis	Dermatitis	Birds, mammals, straw, hay	
Eulaelaps stabularis	Dermatitis, tularemia	Small mammals, straw bedding	F tularensis
Ixodids (ticks)			
Dermacentor variabilis	Irritation, RMSF,†† tularemia, tick paralysis, other diseases	Wild rodents, cottontail rabbits, dogs from endemic areas	Rickettsia rickettsia, F tularensis
Amblyomma americanum	Irritation, RMSF,†† tularemia	Wild rodents, dogs	
Ixodes scapularis	Irritation, possible tularemia	Dogs, wild rodents	
Ixodes dammini	Human babesiosis, Lyme disease	Wild rodents, especially Peromyscus sp.	Borrelia burgdorferi, Babesia microti
Fleas			
Xenopsylla cheopis	Dermatitis, plague, murine typhus, H. nana, H diminuta	Rat, mouse, wild rodents	Rodent tapeworms, Yersinia pestis, Rickettsia typhi
Nasopsyllus fasciatus	Dermatitis, plague, H nana, H diminuta, murine typhus	Rat, mouse, wild rodents	Rodent tapeworms, Yersinia pestis, Rickettsia typhi
Leptopsylla segnis	H diminuta, H nana, murine typhus	Rat	Rodent tapeworms, harbors salmonella, Rickettsia typhi

*Found in laboratory animals that causes allergic dermatitis or from which zoonotic agents have been recovered in nature. (See Reference 89)

**WEE, western equine encephalitis

†SLE, St. Louis equine encephalitis

††RMSF, Rocky Mountain spotted fever

TABLE 7.3. Reports of *ornithonyssus bacoti*-induced dermatitis in man: United States, 1931 through 1982.

Host	Person(s) afflicted	Environment	Lesions	Anatomical Location	References
Rat	200 adults and children	Residence, Theatre	Adults: urticarial wheals, papules / Children: papules, urticarial wheals, vesicles	Adults: ankles, trunk, back, neck / Children: beltline, upper part of shoulders	90
Rat	4 women, 1 man	Department store	Wheals, papules, few wheals with central puncture	Women: arms, forearms / Man: hands, ankles, legs, beltline, shoulders, neck	91
Rat Mice	Employees	Department store	Macular skin eruptions	—	92
Rat	Infants, Adult occupants	Founding home	Papular urticaria, grouping of bites	—	93
Rat	8-yr-old boy; 5 siblings and both parents affected with milder symptoms	Residence	Excoriated urticarial papules	Trunk, upper part of arms, buttocks	94
Norway rat	60-yr-old	Residence	1- to 4-mm papules, excoriated macules	Neck, shoulders, back, scalp, forearm, arms, abdomen	95
Rat	56-yr-old father and 2 sons; 73-yr-old woman	Residence (apartment over food store)	"Insect bites," papular excoriated dermatitis	Thorax, extremities, buttocks, genitalia, entire body	96
Rat	69-yr-old woman	Residence	Papules with erythema	Breast, shoulders, arm	97
Rat Mice	3 female adults, 3 children	Residences	Papular urticaria, erythematous papules, excoriated papules	Neck, shoulders, arms, legs, abdomen, back	98
Mice	5 research personnel 2 animal care technicians	Animal research laboratory	Several millimeters to >1 cm raised erythematous papules and nodules	Wrists, arms, abdomen, chest	99

Ornithonyssus bacoti: Tropical Rat Mite

Ornithonyssus bacoti can be found on many rodents; the brown Norway rat and the black roof rat are probably the primary host species (75). Since the time of the first report of human *Ornithonyssus bacoti*-associated dermatitis in Australia in 1913, and a 1923 report in man in the United States, many other cases have been described throughout the world (Table 7.3) (90–99).

Ornithonyssus bacoti is an obligate blood-sucking parasite, usually tan, but red when engorged with blood. Both the male and female feed on a rodent as their preferred host. The female is 700 µm to 1 mm in length; the male is smaller. Eggs are laid in bedding or wall crevices by the female, which survives for about 70 days and feeds about every 2 days during this period. The mite has five developmental stages: adult, egg, nonfeeding larva, blood-sucking protonymph, and nonfeeding deutonymph. After feeding, the adults and protonymphs leave their host and seek refuge in cracks and crevices. The life cycle from adult to egg requires 7 to 16 days at room temperature. Unfed protonymphs have survived for 43 days (76).

The mite often gains access to human premises on wild rodents, and lives in crevices. If wild rodents are not readily available, the mite will seek blood elsewhere, either from the laboratory rodent (if in an animal research facility) and/or humans. In some infestations, the rodent shows no clinical signs. However in more chronic cases, dermatitis and anemia may develop. In the past, this mite has been a troublesome parasite in certain laboratory animals, especially rats, mice, and hamsters (100).

Tropical rat mites produce painful, pruritic lesions on man. Examination of patients often discloses papular lesions on the wrists, arms, abdomen, and chest. Raised erythematous papules and nodules several millimeters to greater than 1 cm in size occur singly or in linear configuration. Epidemiologically, cases usually occur in clusters that involve a common source of exposure to the mite. Experimentally, cases have been shown to be a vector of pathogens. In the laboratory, mite transmission of various rickettsial species, *Pasteurella tularensis*, and Coxsackievirus between different laboratory animals has been shown (101–104).

Affected individuals are treated with topical lindane. Papular dermatitis will regress after a period of 7 to 10 days posttherapy. Recurrence of *Ornithonyssus* infestations is common unless the premises and laboratory animals have been treated with an appropriate insecticide, and any feral rodents eradicated. Lindane can also be used to eradicate the mites from research rodent colonies (105).

References

1. Zinsser H. *Rats, Mice and History*. Boston, Little, Brown and Co., 1935.
2. Weisbroth SH. Bacterial and Mycotic Diseases. In: Baker HJ, Lindsey JR, Weisbroth SH (eds): *The Laboratory Rat*, Vol. I. New York, Academic Press, 1979: pp. 194–230.
3. Brown CM, Parker MT. *Salmonella* infection in rodents in Manchester. *Lancet* 1957; 273:1277–1279.
4. Fox JG. *Biology and Diseases of the Ferret*. Philadelphia, Lea and Febiger, 1988.
5. Committee on Urban Pest Management. *Urban Pest Management*. Washington D.C., National Academy Press, National Academy of Sciences, 1980.
6. Pratt HD, Bjornson BF, Littig KS. Control of domestic rats and mice. *US Dept HEW, Publication No (CDC) 76-8141*, Atlanta, GA, 1976.
7. Schwartz E. Notes on commensal rats. *Am J Trop Med* 1942; 22:577–579.
8. Fox JG, Brayton JB. Zoonoses and other human health hazards. In: Foster HL, Small JD, Fox JG (eds): *Biology of the Laboratory Mouse*, Vol. II. New York, Academic Press, 1982: pp. 403–423.
9. Ordog GJ. Rat bites: fifty cases. *Ann Emerg Med* 1985; 14:126.
10. Weber DJ, Hansen AR. Infections resulting from animal bites. In: Weinberg A, Weber D (eds): *Inf Dis Clin NA*. Philadelphia, W.B. Saunders, 1991; 5:663–677.
11. Weber DJ, Wolfson JS, Swartz MN. *Pasteurella multocida* infections: report of 34 cases and review of the literature. *Medicine* 1984; 63:133.
12. Anderson LC, Leary SL, Manning PJ. Rat-bite fever in animal research laboratory personnel. *Lab Anim Sci* 1983; 33:292.
13. Arkless HA. Rat-bite fever at Albert Einstein Medical Center. *Penn Med J* 1970; 73:49.
14. Cole JS, Stoll RW, Bulger RJ. Rat-bite fever: report of three cases. *Ann Intern Med* 1969; 71:979.
15. Gilbert GL, Cassidy JF, Bennett NM. Rat-bite fever. *Med J Aust* 1971; 2:1131–1134.
16. McGill RC, Martin AM, Edmunds PN. Rat-bite fever due to *Streptobacillus moniliformis*. *British Med J* 1966; 1:1213.
17. Raffin BJ, Freemark M. Streptobacillary rat-bite fever: a pediatric problem. *Pediatrics* 1979; 64:214.
18. Richter CP. Incidence of rat-bites and rat-bite fever in Baltimore. *JAMA* 1954; 128:324.
19. Roughgarden JW. Antimicrobial therapy of ratbite fever. *Arch Intern Med* 1965; 116:39.
20. Taylor AF, Stephenson TG, Giese HA, et al. Rat bite fever in a college student. *MMWR* 1984; 33:318.
21. Wilkins EGL, Millar JGB, Cockcroft PM, et al. Rat-bite fever in a gerbil breeder. *J Infect* 1988; 16:177.
22. Paegle RD, Tweari RP, Bernhard WN, et al. Microbial flora of the larynx, trachea and large intestine of the rat after long term inhalation of 100 percent oxygen. *Anesthesiology* 1976; 44:287–290.
23. Geller EH. Health hazards for man. In: Baker HJ, Lindsey JR, Weisbroth SH (eds): *The Laboratory Rat*, vol 1. New York, Academic Press, 1979: pp. 402.

24. Hull TG. *Diseases Transmitted from Animals to Man*, 4th ed. Springfield, IL, Charles C. Thomas, 1955.

25. Fox JG, Newcomer CE. Rodent-associated zoonoses and health hazards. In: Arnold DC, Grice H, Krewski D (eds): *Handbook of in vivo Toxicity Testing*. Orlando, Academic Press, 1990: pp. 72–102.

26. Brooks JE. A review of commensal rodents and their control. *Rev of Environ Control* 1973; 3:405–453.

27. Craven RB, Barnes AM. Plague and tularemia in animal associated human infections. In: Weinberg AN, Weber DJ (eds): Inf Dis Clinics North Am. 1991; 5:165–177.

28. Kaufman AF, Boyce JM, Martone WJ. Trends in human plague in the United States. *J Infect Dis* 1980; 141:522.

29. Mann JB, Martone WJ, Boyce JM. Endemic human plague in New Mexico: Risk factors associated with infection. *J Inf Dis* 1979; 140:397–401.

30. Rosner WW: Bubonic plague. *J Am Vet Med Assoc* 1987; 191:406–409.

31. Rollag OJ, Skeels MR, Nims LJ, et al. Feline plague in New Mexico: report of five cases. *J Am Vet Med Assoc* 1981; 179:1381–1383.

32. Mushatt DM, Hyslop NE Jr. Neurologic aspects of North American zoonoses. Weinberg A, Weber DJ, ed. Inf Dis N America 1991; 5:703–731.

33. Kaneko K, Hamada S, Kasai Y, et al. Occurrence of *Yersinia enterocolitica* in house rats. *Applied Environ Micro* 1978; 36:314–318.

34. Iinuma Y, Hayashidani H, Kaneko K, et al. Isolation of *Yersinia enterocolitica* serovar 08 from free-living small rodents in Japan. *J Clin Micro* 1992; 30:240–242.

35. Torten M. Leptospirosis. In: Steele JH (ed): *CRC Handbook Series in Zoonoses*. Cleveland, CRC Press, 1979; 1:363–421.

36. Fox JG, Lipman NS. Infections transmitted from large and small laboratory animals. In: Weinberg A, Weber D (eds): *Infectious Diseases of North America*. Philadelphia, W.B. Saunders, 1991; 5:131–163.

37. Thiermann AB. Incidence of leptospirosis in the Detroit rat population. *Am J Trop Med & Hyg* 1977; 26:970–974.

38. Li H, Davis DE. The prevalence of carriers of leptospira and salmonella in Norway rats of Baltimore. *Am J Hyg* 1952; 56:90–100.

39. Alexander AD. Leptospirosis in laboratory mice. *Science* 1984; 224:1158.

40. Sanger JG, Thiermann AB. Leptospirosis. *J Am Vet Med Assn* 1988; 193: 1250–1254.

41. Stoenner HG, Maclean D. Leptospirosis (ballum) contracted from Swiss albino mice. *Arch Intern Med* 1958; 101:706–710.

42. Barkin RM, Guckian JC, Glosser JW. Infections by *Leptospira ballum*: A laboratory-associated case. *South Med J* 1974; 67:155–176.

43. Friedmann CTH, Spiegel EL, Aaron E, McIntyre R. *Leptospirosis ballum* contracted from pet mice. *Calif Med* 1973; 118:51–52.

44. Boak RA, Linscott WD, Bodfish RE. A case of *Leptospirosis ballum* in California. *Calif Med* 1960; 93:163–165.

45. Luzzi GA, Milne LW, Waitkins SA. Rat-bite acquired leptospirosis. *J Infect* 1987; 15:57.

46. Looke DFM. Weil's syndrome in a zoologist. *Med J Aust* 1986; 144:597–601.

47. Demers RY, Thiermann A, Demers P, et al. Exposure to *Leptospira icterohaemorrhagiae* in inner-city and suburban children: a serologic comparison. *J Family Practice* 1983; 17:1007–1011.

48. Faine S. Leptospirosis. In: Bacterial Infections of Humans Evans AS, Brachman PS (eds): New York, Plenum Medical Book Co, 1991: pp. 367–393.

49. Taber E, Feigin RD. Spirochetal infections. *Pediatr Clin North Am* 1979; 26:377.

50. Stoenner HG, Grimes EF, Thraikill FB, Davis E. Elimination of *Leptospira ballum* from a colony of Swiss albino mice by use of chlortetracycline hydrochloride *Am J Trop Med Hyg* 1958; 7:423–426.

51. Sulzer CR, Harvey TW, Galton MM. Comparison of diagnostic techniques for the detection of leptospirosis in rats. *Health Lab Sci* 1968; 5:171–173.

52. Coffey EM, Eveland WC. Experimental relapsing fever initiated by *Borrelia hermsii* I. Identification of major serotypes in the rat. *J Inf Dis* 1971; 117:23.

53. Fox JG. Zoonotic diseases. Campylobacter infections and salmonellosis. *Seminars Vet Med Surg* (small animals). 1991; 6:212–218.

54. Bartram JT, Welsh H, Ostroleur M. Incidence of members of the *Salmonella* group in rats. *J Inf Dis* 1940; 67:222–226.

55. Price-Jones C. Infection of Rats by Gärtner's Bacillus. *J Path and Bact* 1927; 30:45.

56. Welch H, Ostrolenk M, Bartram MT. Role of Rats in the Spread of Food Poisoning Bacteria in *Salmonella* Group. *Am J Pub Health* 1941; 31:332–340.

57. Pavia AT, Tauxe RV. Salmonellosis: Nontyphoidal. In: Evans AS, Brachman PS (eds): *Bacterial Infections of Humans. Epidemiology and Control* 2nd ed. New York, Plenum, 1991: pp. 573–592.

58. Nelson JD, Kusmiesz H, Jackson LH, et al. Treatment of *Salmonella* gastroenteritis with ampicillin, amoxicillin, and placebo. *Pediatrics* 1980; 65: 1125–1130.

59. Fox JG. In vivo models of enteric campylobacteriosis: natural and experimental infections. In: Nachaminkin I, Blaser M, Tompkins L (eds): *NIH Symposium on Compylobacter jejuni*; Washington, D.C., Am Soc Microbiology Press 1992: pp. 131–138.

60. Gebhart CH, Ferrell CL, Murtaugh MP, et al. *Campylobacter cinaedi* is normal intestine flora in hamsters. *J Clin Microbiol* 1989; 27:1692–1694.

61. Corning BF, Murphy JC, Fox JG. Group G *Streptococcal* lymphadenitis in rats. *J Clin Micro* 1991; 29:2720–2722.

62. Rolston KVI. Group G streptococcal infections. *Arch Int Med* 1986; 146: 857–858.

63. Davey DG. The use of pathogen free animals. *Proc R Soc Med* 1962; 55:256–262.

64. Blackmore DK, Francis RA. The apparent transmission of staphylococci of human origin to laboratory animals. *J Comp Pathol* 1970; 80:645–651.

65. Shults FS, Estes PC, Franklin JA, et al. Staphylococcal botrymomycosis in a specific-pathogen-free mouse colony. *Lab Anim Sci* 1973; 23:36–42.

66. LeDuc JW. Epidemiology of hantaan and related viruses. *Lab Anim Sci* 1987; 37:413.

67. Yanagihara R. Hantavirus infection in the United States: epizootiology and epidemiology. *Rev Infect Dis* 1990; 12:449.

68. Tsai, TF. Hemorrhagic fever with renal syndrome: clinical aspects. *Lab Anim Sci* 1987; 37:419.

69. Tsai, TF. Hemorrhagic fever with renal syndrome: mode of transmission to humans. *Lab Anim Sci* 1987; 37:428.

69a. Komatsu K, et al. Update: Hantavirus disease Southwestern U.S., 1993. *MMWR* 1993; 42:570–572.

69b. CDC. Hantavirus infection—southwestern United States interim recommendations for risk reduction 42 (no. RR-12) in press.

70. Umenai T, Lee PW, Toyoda T, Yoshinaga K, Horiuchi T, Lee HW, Saito T, Hongo M, Nobunga T, Ishida N. Korean hemorrhagic fever in staff in an animal laboratory. *Lancet* 1979; i:1314–1315.

71. Childs JE, Glass GE, Korch GW, et al. Evidence of human infection with a rat associated hantavirus in Baltimore, Maryland. *Am J Epidemiol* 1988; 127:875–878.

72. McDade JE, Fishbein DB. Rickettsiaceae: The Rickettsiae in Laboratory Diagnosis of Infectious Disease, Principles and Practice vol II. Lennette EH, Halonen P, Murphy FA (eds): New York, Springer-Verlag, 1988: pp. 864–890.

73. Duma RJ, Sonenshine DE, Bozeman FM, et al. Epidemic typhus in the United States associated with flying squirrels. *JAMA* 1981; 245:2318–2323.

74. Farhang-Azad A, Traub R, Baqar S. Transovarial transmission of murine typhus, rickettsiae in *Xenopsylla cheopsis* fleas. *Science* 1985; 227:543–545.

75. Beaver PC, Jung RC. *Animal Agents and Vectors of Human Disease*, 5th ed. Philadelphia, Lea & Febiger, 1985.

76. Brettman LR, Lewin S, Holzman RS, et al. Rickettsial pox: report of an outbreak and a contemporary review. *Medicine* 1981; 60:363–372.

77. Benenson AS (ed). *Control of Communicable Disease in Man* 14th ed. Washington, D.C., American Public Health Association, 1985.

78. Stuart BM, Pullen RL. Endemic (murine) typhus fever: clinical observations of 180 cases. *Ann Int Med* 1945; 23:520–525.

78a. MacKenzie DWR. *Trichophyton mentagrophytes* in mice: Infections of humans and incidence amongst laboratory animals. *Sabouraudia* 1961; 1:178–182.

79. Alteras I. Human infection from laboratory animals. *Sabouraudia* 1965; 3:143–145.

80. Dolan MM, Klingman AM, Kobylinski PG, et al. Ringworm epizootics in laboratory mice and rats: experimental and accidental transmission of infection. *J Inves Derm* 1958; 23–5.

81. Davies RR, Shewell J. Control of mouse ringworm. *Nature* 1964; 202:406–407.

82. Booth BH. Mouse ringworm. *Arch Dermatol Syphilol* 1952; 66:65–69.

83. Cetin ET, Tahsinoglu M, Volkan S. Epizootic of *Trichophyton mentagrophytes* (*interdigitale*) in white mice. *Pathol Microbiol* 1965; 28:839–846.

84. Povar ML. Ringworm (*Trichophyton mentagrophytes*) infection in a colony of albino Norway rats. *Lab Anim Care* 1965; 15:264–265.

85. Chmel L, Buchvald L, Valentova M. Spread of *Trichophyton mentagrophytes* var. Gran. infection to man. *Int J Dermatol* 1975; 14:269–272.

86. Kliks MM, Lau WK, Palumbo NE. Neurologic Angiostrongyliasis: Parasitic Eosinophilic Menigoencephalitis. In: Balows, et al (eds): *Laboratory Dia-*

gnosis of Infectious Diseases: Principles and Practice. Vol. 1. New York, Springer-Verlag, 1988: pp. 754–767.

87. Kliks MM, Kroenke K, Hardman JM. Eosinophilic radiculomyeloencephalitis: an angiostrongyliasis outbreak in American Somoa related to ingestion of *Achatina fulica* snails. *Am J Trop Med Hyg* 1982; 31:1114–1112.

88. Faust EL, Russell PF. *Craig & Faust Clinical Parasitology,* 8th ed. Philadelphia, Lea & Febiger, 1970.

89. Yunker CE. Infections of laboratory animals potentially dangerous to man: Ectoparasites and other arthropods, with emphasis on mites. *Lab Anim Care* 1964; 14:455–465.

90. Dove WE, Shelmire B. The tropical rat mite, *Liponyssus bacoti* Hirst 1914: The cause of a skin eruption of man, and a possible vector of endemic typhus fever. *JAMA* 1931; 96:579–584.

91. Weber LF. Rat mite dermatitis. *JAMA* 1940; 114:1442.

92. Riley WA. Rat mite dermatitis in Minnesota. *Minn Med* 1940; 23:423–424.

93. Haggard CN: Rat mite dermatitis in children. *Pediatrics* 1955; 15:322–324.

94. Dowlati Y, Maguire HC. Rat mite dermatitis: a family affair. *Arch Dermatol* 1970; 101:617–618.

95. Hetherington GW, Holder WR, Smith DB. Rat mite dermatitis. *JAMA* 1971; 215:1499–1500.

96. Wainschel J. Rat mite bite. *JAMA* 1971; 216:1964.

97. Charlesworth EN, Clegern RW. Tropical rat mite dermatitis. *Arch Dermatol* 1977; 113:937–938.

98. Theis J, Lavoipierre MM, LaPerriere R, et al. Tropical rat mite dermatitis. *Arch Dermatol* 1981; 117:341–343.

99. Fox JG. Outbreak of tropical rat mite dermatitis in laboratory personnel. *Arch Dermatol* 1982; 118:676–679.

100. Keefe TJ, Scanlon JE, Wetherald LD. *Ornithonyssus bacoti* (Hirst) infestation in mouse and hamster colonies. *Lab Anim Care* 1964; 14:366–369.

101. Petrov VG. On the role of the mite *Ornithonyssus bacoti* Hirst as a reservoir and vector of the agent of tularemia. *Parazitologiia* 1971; 1:7–14.

102. Schwab MR, Allen R, Sulkin SE. The tropical rat mite (*Liponyssus bacoti*) as an experimental vector of coxsackie virus. *Am J Trop Med Hyg* 1952; 1:982–986.

103. Hopla CE. Experimental transmission of tularemia by the tropical rat mite. *Am J Trop Med Hyg* 1951; 31:768–782.

104. Philip CB, Hughes LE. The tropical rat mite, *Liponyssus bacoti,* as an experimental vector of rickettsial pox. *Am J Trop Med Hyg.* 1948; 28:697–705.

105. Harris JM, Stockton JJ. Eradication of the tropical rat mite *Ornithonyssus bacoti* (Hirst 1913) from a colony of mice. *Am J Vet Res* 1960; 21:316–318.

8
Around Cats

ELLIE J.C. GOLDSTEIN and CRAIG E. GREENE

The origins of the domestic cat are unknown. However, mummified cats have been found in the treasure rooms of the Egyptian pyramids and their images inscribed in the royal hieroglyphics. The genis *Felis* includes both the modern domestic house cat as well as the puma, cougar, golden cats, jaguarundi, ocelot, serval, lynx, and bobcat. Today, it is estimated that more than 56 million cats are kept as household pets in the United States and that 30.5% of households own cats (1–3). There are numerous diseases which may be transmitted from cats to humans or that cats and people acquire from common sources (2), some of which are described in this chapter. However, it is likely that the domestic cat may act as a reservoir to many other zoonoses that are as yet unrecognized.

Anthrax

Anthrax is caused by *Bacillus anthracis*, a gram-positive spore-forming rod. Infection in humans is almost always a result of contact with infected animals or their byproducts (especially goat hair). The alkaline soil of many tropical and subtropical regions allows vegetative spore growth resulting in a soil-borne systemic disease of domestic animals including cats. Soil may remain contaminated for many years. In cats, anthrax is manifested by inflammation, edema, and necrosis of the upper gastro-intestinal tract. Spread to regional lymph nodes and liver and spleen are frequent. Human infection usually results from handling infected tissues or carcasses or the animal skin. Inhalation anthrax is a rare phenomenon in humans in the United States.

In humans, cutaneous lesions are the most common clinical presentation. Twenty-four to 48 hours after exposure, a small and often pruritic papule forms at the inoculation site. The area, although painless, develops brawny edema; the lesion enlarges and the center becomes necrotic. Regional adenopathy and lymphangitis may be associated with the skin lesion. The differential diagnosis includes brown recluse spider bite, orf, tularemia, and plague.

Diagnosis is by gram-stain of the exudate and isolation of the organism. Therapy with intravenous penicillin G and subsequent oral penicillin for 7 to 10 days is generally effective for cutaneous anthrax. Inhalation anthrax is difficult to diagnose and is therefore usually fatal.

Cat Scratch Disease

The etiology of cat scratch disease (CSD) remains controversial. In 1988, English et al. (3a) reported the isolation of an aerobic gram-negative bacteria, subsequently named *Afipia felis* (4), from the lymph nodes of 10 patients with CSD. The organism is motile by a single flagellum, oxidase-positive, nonfermentative, and urease positive. It may be grown on buffered charcoal-yeast extract agar and nutrient broth, but rarely on McConkey agar, at 25° and 30°C (4). It can also be seen on tissue sections using a modified Warthin-Starry silver stain. CSD bacillus, or closely related members of the genus *Afipia*, may also be transmitted by dogs, monkeys, and even porcupines. However, *A felis* specific antibodies were found in only a minority of CSD patients in a subsequent serologic survey (4a). This study found approximately 88% of CSD patient's sera did show antibodies to *Rochalamaea henselae*, the agent associated with bacillary angiomatosis (4a). *R henselae* is a small, curved, pleomorphic gram-negative rod that grows slowly (13–33 days) on CDC anaerobic blood agar, has non-hemolytic colonies, and is oxidase-negative and X-factor dependent (4b). Recently it has been isolated from immunocompetent patients with CSD-like adenitis (4b). This report and other evidence (4c) adds to the support the important role of *R henselae* as the more usual agent of CSD. The relationship and importance of *A felis* and *R henselae* in CSD is currently under study.

CSD is worldwide in distribution, and in temperate climates there is a fall and winter prevalence. It often affects children and persons <21 years old (80% of cases). Exposure is usually associated with a young, newly acquired, or stray cat, and not usually with long-time pets. Injury may be a bite, scratch, or lick. Approximately 1 week after injury (range 3 to 10 days), a primary inoculation papule, which often goes unnoticed, may appear at the site of injury. Subsequently, 5 to 120 days later (average, 2 weeks) tender, regional adenopathy may develop. Adenopathy, which often lasts >3 weeks, may be the only symptom in half the cases and suppurates in approximately 15% of cases. Since this is a benign and usually self-limited disease in immunocompetent individuals, this too often goes unnoticed or unreported. Some healthy patients experience a "flu-like" illness. Most patients will present because of the adenopathy, especially if it involves the head and neck area. Consequently, the differential diagnosis often centers around this problem. Depending on the area of the adenopathy, various diseases should be excluded including streptococcal pharyngitis, infectious mononucleosis, toxoplasmosis, cytomegalovirus infection, syphilis, lymphogranuloma venerum, cellulitis, Hodgkins' disease, dental abscess, etc.

Other symptoms include fatigue and malaise (28%); fever (101°–106°F) (31%); splenomegaly (12%); exanthem (4%); parotid swelling (2%); and seizures (1% to 2%). Other symptoms include ocular granuloma, erythema nodosum, osteomyelitis, pneumonia, and liver abscesses. The most serious complication is the development of acute encephalopathy and altered consciousness. Spontaneous recovery is usual with encephalopathy as well, usually within 2 weeks.

Diagnosis requires three or more of the following criteria:

1. History of animal contact, usually an immature cat, and, if possible, the identification of an inoculation site
2. Exclusion of other diagnostic possibilities
3. A node biopsy showing granulomatous formation, preferably with stellate microabscesses
4. A positive CSD skin test
5. Isolation of the organism or serologic evidence of recent infection with either *Afipia felis* or *Rochalimaea henselaea*.

There are also atypical cases and cases in immunocompromised patients which may have diverse and unusual manifestations.

Therapy at this time is supportive. If needed, aspiration of a necrotic node is preferable to excision, which may be necessary in some cases. Chronic sinus tracts can develop. The role of antimicrobial therapy remains undetermined. Susceptibility studies have suggested that both organisms are variably susceptible to antibiotics, with much strain to strain variation. Clinical success and failure have been attributed to the same antimicrobial agents, including gentamicin, tetracyclines, ciprofloxacin, and sulfamethoxazole-trimethoprim. Corresponding conflicting results occur from studies of in vitro susceptibility. Dolan et al. (4b) have noted in vitro resistance of *R. henselae* to first generation cephalosporins correlated with clinical therapeutic failure.

Bacillary (Epithelioid) Angiomatosis

Patients with HIV infection have been reported to develop Kaposi's sarcoma-like lesions after cat scratch. Lesions contain a distinctive pattern of vascular proliferation on histopathological sections. Both CSD and bacillary angiomatosis have organisms that appear similar on Warthin-Starry stain. Lesions were often multiple and appeared on a variety of body surfaces. Osseous lesions of the fibula, radius, femur, and tibia, as well as hepatic abscesses, splenic involvement, and extensive bone marrow infiltration have been described. Systemic symptoms including fever, night sweats, and weight loss may also be associated with the disease. This disease was originally thought to be a variant of CSD in an immunocompromised patient population, and it is difficult to differentiate it from CSD on clinical grounds. More recently, the causative agent, currently called BA-TF, was found to be closely related to but distinct from *Bartonella bacilliformis* and *Rochalimaea quintana* (5,6). More recently, *Rochalimaea henselae* and *Rochalamaea quintana* have been isolated from pateints with bacillary angiomatosis and bacillary peliosis and are shown to be the etiologic agents of these diseases (6a,6b,6c) as well as many cases of Cat Scratch Disease. Some investigators have reported successful therapy with agents such as doxycycline (7) as well as diverse other agents. What role antimicrobial therapy plays in this disease also remains to be determined.

Campylobacteriosis

Campylobacter jejuni has emerged as one of the most frequent bacterial causes of diarrheal diseases in the United States. The organism is a motile, curved, microaerophilic gram-negative rod that inhabits the gastrointestinal tract of animals and has been isolated from cat feces. Newly acquired, young cats are more likely to be carriers. Those cats with diarrhea pose a greater zooenotic risk. Most human infection is acquired from contaminated food, especially undercooked poultry, and water.

In humans, a "flu-like" illness with fever and malaise, etc., will precede the development of cramping diarrhea. Infection is usually self-limiting; however, colitis, bacteremia, and metastatic infections may result. A reactive arthritis may also occur after resolution of the diarrheal illness.

Prevention of infection by hand washing after cat contact and prior to eating should be common sense. Therapy is with symptomatic treatment. Antimicrobial agents such as erythromycin or the new fluoroquinolones (norfloxacin, ciprofloxacin, and ofloxacin) have proven effective.

Cryptosporidiosis

Human cryptosporidiosis was first reported in 1976 (8,9) and has become recognized as an important cause of gastrointestinal illness in AIDS patients, causing not only diarrhea but also cholecystitis. The diarrhea is often profuse and watery associated with cramping abdominal pain, fever, and emesis. Immunocompetent patients will sometimes have a milder and self-limited form of illness, while immunocompromised patients will have prolonged and severe courses that will warrant attempts at therapeutic intervention. Weight loss and volume depletion with electrolyte imbalance may even require hospitalization. Infection is often in the small intestine (ilium) and may be focal in nature. Cryptosporidial cholecystitis may be manifested by right upper quadrant pain and emesis; ultrasound may reveal a thickened gallbladder wall and dilated ducts. In AIDS patients it must also be differentiated from CMV acalculous cholecystitis. Cryptosporidia have also been isolated in sputum and lung tissue from immunocompromised hosts, although its role in pulmonary disease is less well defined.

Cats and many other species of mammals, birds, and reptiles may act as the definitive host for cryptosporidia. It is thought that there are two species and that *C parvum* causes disease in mammals and man. After ingestion, the sporozoite excysts and enters the villous intestinal border. Several asexual developmental forms ensue. Ultimately, thin-walled oocysts may invade other cells, while thick-walled oocysts are excreted into the feces. These oocysts are quite hardy and difficult to destroy. Crowding in either animal or human environments (e.g., day care centers, underdeveloped countries) and unsanitary practices are associated with an increased risk of acquisition of cryptosporidiosis. Infection has been transmitted between species, e.g., from animal to human, as well as from human to human. In cats, infection with feline leukemia virus or the presence of other intestinal pathogens is associated with more severe disease and increased shedding.

Diagnosis is by demonstrating the organism in stool specimens or tissue biopsies. In stool specimens, special stains are required to identify the organism and, consequently, they must be specifically ordered. Definitive therapy remains imperfect. Many drugs, such as spiramycin and paromomycin (Humatin), have met limited success. Patients often turn to alternative nonallopathic treatment modalities which also meet with limited success. Several new agents are about to begin clinical trials in 1993.

Histoplasmosis

Histoplasma capsulatum is an imperfect dimorphic fungus that is endemic in the central United States and may be found in other temperate and tropical climates. The freeliving mycelial stage of *H capulatum* grows in the soil and produces both micro- and macroconidia. Inhalation of the microconidia leads to conversion to the yeast phase in the body and subsequent pulmonary infection which, in turn, may lead to dissemination. While bird droppings are the most frequent cause of human disease, cats are also susceptible to histoplasmosis that can lead to human transmission, albeit infrequently. Most infected cats develop disseminated disease and usually die, but they may develop ulcerated skin lesions. A further description may be found in the "Feathered Friends" chapter.

Pasteurella multocida Infection

Most people associate *Pasteurella multocida* with infected dog and cat bite wounds; indeed, almost all feline species commonly carry this organism in their oropharynx as normal flora. Additionally, when cats lick their paws, they are in effect inoculating *P multocida* onto their claws.

It is estimated that 400,000 persons are bitten or severely scratched by cats annually in the United States. Many of these wounds never become infected and are trivial in severity.

However, the problem of infection resulting from cat bites and scratches is an important and frequent medical problem. Most people are bitten or scratched while handling cats known to the victims. A variety of studies show that cat bites become infected more frequently than do dog bites (10–12). Cats' teeth are small but sharp, and when the bite is to the hand it can easily penetrate the joints, bones, and tendons. Infections following cat bite are usually a cellulitis, often with a gray malodorous discharge but without lymphangitis or regional adenopathy; septic arthritis, tenosynovitis, and osteomyelitis may also occur.

Consequently, the use of antimicrobial therapy as "prophylactic" therapy is warranted to reduce the incidence of infection in cases of moderate to severe wounds, wounds to the hands, and especially wounds near a joint or those causing pain. Other organisms, both aerobic and anaerobic feline oral flora, can be cultured from many wounds (13). The complete bacteriology of cat bite wounds remains incomplete.

Most wounds can be treated with out-patient management. If there is any edema, then the affected part should be elevated. Failure to adequately elevate the injured part is one of the most common causes of therapeutic failure. The location of punctures, especially in relation to the bones and joints of the hand, should be noted. Prophylactic therapy with an antimicrobial agent such as penicillin or amoxicillin-clavulanic acid is inexpensive and prudent. Alternative agents could include sulfamethoxazole-trimethoprim, doxycycline, fluoroquinolones (ciprofloxacin, ofloxacin, etc.) and possibly cefuroxime axetil. The duration of therapy for "prophylaxis" is 3 to 5 days, while that for established infection such as cellulitis often requires 10 to 14 days. More serious complications such as septic arthritis and osteomyelitis will require prolonged courses of antimicrobials. Occasionally, anti-inflamatory agents will reduce the post-traumatic arthritis that subsequently develops in a minority of cases. In some areas, rabies prophylaxis may be considered (see Rabies Chapter). Tetanus toxoid should be administered if the patient is not current on immunizations.

Plague

Plague is caused by *Yersinia pestis*, a gram-negative coccobacillus. While cat fleas are considered poor vectors for transmission, domestic and wild cats may contract this disease, usually in the summer months. Cats will be exposed via ingestion of an infected rodent or via its fleas. Cats manifest disease in the same way as humans, with either bubonic, septicemic, or pneumonic plague. This illness is covered in the chapter "Man's Worst Friend (The Rat).

Q Fever

Cats may occasionally be infected with *Coxiella burnetii*, the rickettsia causing Q fever. Cat infection may ensue from ingestion or inhalation of organisms from the environment. Most cats are asymptomatic. Humans may occasionally become infected from cats by direct exposure to or inhalation of infected material from parturient or aborted tissue from infected cats. This illness is covered in the chapter On-the-Farm.

Rabies

Approximately 5,000 animals per year are proven positive rabid in the United States. While domestic animals account for less than 20% of all rabid animals, over the past 10 years rabid cats have been more common than rabid dogs. Cats acquire rabies from exposure to infected wildlife. Rabid cats may develop frenzied rabies, but more often become reclusive. This disease is covered in Chapter 11.

Salmonellosis

There has been a continuous increase in the number of cases of salmonellosis reported in the United States over the past several years. A small number of these approximately 50,000 annual cases may come from exposure to household pets. In these instances the victims are usually children, and disease results from direct fecal-oral exposure. Cats may acquire infection from infected foods, especially uncooked meat or fish-meal, or contaminated water. Up to 14% of normal and healthy appearing cats may be infected or may be carriers that can shed organisms orally as well as fecally. They may manifest illness as a gastroenterological disease with diarrhea, excessive salivation or emesis, or as a systemic illness with fevers, etc.

The characteristics of human salmonellosis can be divided into asymptomatic (most usual), enterocolitis, enteric fever with bacteremia, metastatic complications, and chronic carrier state. Enterocolitis must be differentiated from other infectious diarrheal illnesses such as campylobacteriosis, shigellosis, viral disease, and noninfectious diarrheal diseases. The incubation period is 6 to 48 hours. Cramping abdominal pain, emesis, nausea, and diarrhea are common. Occasionally, salmonellosis must be differentiated from appendicitis and other conditions of the acute abdomen requiring surgery.

Diagnosis is by isolation of the organism from stool cultures or blood cultures. Most infections are asymptomatic or mild and self-limited and do not require antimicrobial therapy. However, in patients with serious infection, such as enteric fever, bacteremia, or metastatic complications, or in the immunocompromised host, antimicrobial therapy is advocated. The choice of an antimicrobial must be determined by considering local resistance patterns for empiric therapy. Agents used have included ampicillin, chloramphenicol, and trimethoprim-sulfamethoxazole. Recently, the fluoroquinolones (norfloxacin, ciprofloxacin, ofloxacin) have shown efficacy in salmonellosis. They are an attractive choice since they are active against almost all other enteric bacterial pathogens as well. However, resistance has developed, albeit rarely to date, and they are contraindicated in pregnant women and children whose epiphiseal plates have not yet closed. Some studies have also utilized some parenterally administered third generation cephalosporins. Prevention by practicing good handwashing after petting cats or changing litter boxes is prudent.

Anaerobiospirillum Diarrhea

Anaerobiosporillum species are anaerobic spiral bacteria with bipolar tufts of flagella that have been associated with cases of human diarrhea. Human disease included 3 to 7 days of diarrhea, fever, abdominal pain, and emesis. Malnick et al (14) developed a selective medium that allowed its detection in the feces of 7 of 10 asymptomatic cats sampled during elective surgery. Consequently, cats may act as a vector in human disease.

Yersinia pseudotuberculosis Gastroenteritis

Yersinia pseudotuberculosis is a well-established cause of human diarrheal disease, diffuse abdominal illness sometimes mimicking acute appendicitis, and sepsis. Recently, Fukushima et al (15) used serotyping, endonuclease restriction analysis to prove that two young children had become infected and symptomatic after having drunk water from puddles in a garden that was contaminated by feces from cats. Cats may also exhibit clinical infection with anorexia, vomiting, and severe diarrhea.

Toxocariasis

Toxocara cati is a helminthic parasite that affects cats and may incidentally infect humans. Cats may be infected transplacentally or may become infected via oral intake of infected feces. After ingestion, the ova hatch in the small intestine and migrate to other body organs, including the liver and lungs. Organisms that are coughed up or subsequently swallowed will then mature in the small intestinal lumen. Excreted ova subsequently develop in the soil, taking weeks to mature. Human infection results from ingestion of infected soil or animal feces and is most usual in toddlers with pica and playing in areas where cats defecate.

Most human infection is asymptomatic. Some patients will develop a cough or wheezing or an asthmatic presentation from the parasite's pulmonary migration. Some patients will present with hepatomegaly, abdominal pain, and eosinophilia. This must be differentiated from other parasitic diseases such as strongylodiasis, trichinosis, ascariasis, anisakiasis, schistosomiasis, and echinococcosis. The organism may migrate to any part of the body and localize in the retina causing blindness.

Diagnosis is usually by clinical grounds. Serologic studies are available but are not specific. The organism is occasionally found incidentally in tissue biopsy. Therapy for this form of disease is usually symptomatic, as the disease is usually self-limited.

Occasionally, *T cati* can cause cutaneous larva migrans or the creeping eruption. More commonly, cats are infected with *Ancyclostoma braziliense* and subsequently shed ova. This is also a disease of children who play in areas where cats defecate. It is more common in the southeastern United States and in areas with a temperate climate and sandy or shady soil. Larvae come into contact with human skin and burrow under it to cause itching and paresthesias. The lesion can become erythematous along a serpiginous tract. Eosinophilia may be present. Disease is usually self-limited, but may be treated with thiobendazole, orally or topically.

Toxoplasmosis

Toxoplasma gondii, the causative agent of toxoplasmosis, is a ubiquitous, obligate intracellular protozoan that can affect almost all warm-blooded animals, including humans. Domestic cats and their relatives are the definitive hosts of *T gondii*. Millions of oocysts are excreted in the feces daily, and ingestion of infested food or water may cause disease in cats. Cat excretion of oocysts is self-limited and occurs for only 1 to 3 weeks after initial infection. However, approximately 1% (~560,000) of cats in the United States are thought to be infected and excreting oocysts on any given day. Congenital transmission in cats and ingestion of tissue cysts (bradyzoites) in contaminated meats (most common) can also lead to feline disease.

Bradyzoites are released from the infected muscle and penetrate the epithelium of the cat small intestine. Subsequently, the parasite matures and goes through a variety of stages until it disseminates into tissues, and unsporulated and uninfective oocysts are passed in the feces. This process may take between 3 days and 3 weeks to be completed. Uninfective oocysts will begin to sporulate, depending on climate and temperature factors, as soon as 2 to 3 days after deposition, and may remain infective and viable for 1 year in the soil. They do not sporulate at $<4°C$ or $>37°C$. Consequently, the incidence of disease will be lower in cold and arid climates.

Human infection may occur after ingesting uncooked or undercooked meat of livestock that contains tissue cysts; this is probably the most usual method of zoonotic transmission. A single tissue cyst may contain thousands of organisms; they are common in skeletal muscle, heart muscle, and brain tissue. However, infection may develop from exposure to fecal oocysts when changing cat litter or gardening in areas where cat feces has been deposited.

The clinical spectrum of human disease is variable and includes asymptomatic forms (common) and acute or chronic symptomatic forms. Human congenital transmission occurs when a woman becomes acutely infected, usually asymptomatically, during pregnancy. This may result in spontaneous abortion or stillbirth. A variable percentage of infants born after such exposure may develop a wide variety of sequelae including mental and psychomotor retardation, cerebral calcifications, chorioretinitis, jaundice, hepatosplenomegaly, anemia, and pneumonia. Each presentation must be differentiated from other causes of similar problems such as the other etiological agents of the TORCH syndrome complex (Toxoplasmosis, Other [syphilis, sepsis, listeriosis, etc.], Rubella, Cytomegalovirus, Herpes).

Approximately 10% to 20% of immunocompetent individuals manifest symptomatic toxoplasmosis, usually with cervical adenopathy, but do not require therapy. This regional adenopathy needs to be differentiated from that due to streptococcal pharyngitis, infectious mononucleosis, Hodgkin's Disease, CSD, sarcoidosis, and cytomegalovirus infection. The disease manifestations are both protean and nonspecific. Other symptoms may include fever, malaise, fatigue, myalgias, sore throat, and rash. While most disease is self-limited, rarely lasting more than 3 to 6 months, some patients will have prolonged symptoms including depression, and some infections will disseminate with development of myocarditis, pneumonia, retinal disease, or encephalitis. A disseminated form of acute cutaneous toxoplasmosis may occur. Patients with disseminated disease often benefit from therapy. The immunocompromised host, including AIDS patients, HIV infected patients, and cancer patients (especially those on chemotherapy), may develop more serious disease manifestations including brain abscess, retinitis, encephalopathy, pneumonia, and hepatitis. The immunocompromised patient always requires therapy for acute toxoplasmosis or any complication of recurrent (reactivation) disease.

Diagnosis is by serologic studies or by isolation or cytological demonstration of the organism from blood or body fluids or by histological demonstration of the trophozoite. Most cases are diagnosed by serologic studies. However, a high prevalence rate of antibodies, sometimes even at high levels ($>1:512$), in the general population may make this difficult. Both false-positive and false-negative tests can occur. However, a negative serologic test result virtually excludes the diagnosis in an immunocompetent individual.

The need for therapy will depend on the immune status of the host, the host's defenses, and the location of infection. The standard therapy has been sulfadiazine and pyrimethamine. Duration of therapy will depend on specific host factors and site of infection. AIDS patients with cerebral toxoplasmosis will require a prolonged, perhaps lifelong, course. Trimethoprim-sulfamethoxazole has been used instead of sulfadiazine. Alternative therapy with clindamycin plus pyrithamine has been advocated in sulfa allergic patients. Spiramycin has been used in therapy of pregnant women and infants with congenital infection.

Prevention of infection should be advocated for immunocompromised patients at risk of disease. They should be instructed not to change cat litter or to do so daily so that the oocysts do not have a chance to sporulate prior to exposure. In addition they should not garden in areas where cats may have defecated, nor should they beat-clean rugs which may be contaminated.

Tularemia

Tularemia is caused by a small, gram-negative coccobacillus, *Francisella tularensis*, that grows poorly on routine culture media. It is ubiquitous and most often found in wild mammals such as rabbits, but may affect cats. Cat infection usually results from a bite by an infected tick, which may serve as both reservoir and vector, or by hunting or ingestion of infected rabbits. Young cats may die from disseminated infection. Older cats may develop draining abscesses as well as fever and adenopathy. Cat-associated human tularemia has occurred in conjunction with bite wounds. Consequently, the local endemicity of infected animals and appropriate vectors should alert the physician to this possibility.

The ulceroglandular form of tularemia is most common and causes regional adenopathy and ulcerative skin lesions. This manifestation must be differentiated from other causes of skin infections including staphylococcal, streptococcal, and bite wound infection due to *P multocida* and Cat Scratch Disease. Pneumonia, without sputum production, may develop in ~15% of ulceroglandular disease patients. Most cases are diagnosed by a compatible clinical picture and antibody titers, since isolation of the organism is difficult and, if accomplished, may pose health risks to the laboratory technologists.

Standard therapy is with streptomycin 10 to 20 mg/kg/day, IM for 7 to 14 days. Tetracyclines and chloramphenicol have been used successfully but may be associated with increased rate of relapse.

Dermatophilosis

Cats may become infected with *Dermatophilus congolensis*, an actinomycete, that causes abscesses in muscles, lymph nodes, and fistulas tracts. Humans handling infected cats may become accidentally infected. Human infection is manifested by an exudative, pustular dermatitis at the site of contact. The lesions will spontaneously resolve within 2 weeks and do not usually require antimicrobial therapy.

Dipylidiasis

Dipylidium canium is a common cat tapeworm that may infect humans, usually children. Fleas ingest eggs which then develop into the cystercus stage. When fleas are ingested, the tapeworm subsequently develops in the intestinal tract; humans become infected when they ingest fleas. The patient may develop eosinophilia and mild gastrointestinal discomfort. Diagnosis is by demonstration of proglottids in a stool sample. Therapy is with niclosamide. This disease needs to be distinguished from other parasitic causes of eosinophilia.

Opisthorchiasis

Opisthorchias felineus is a common liver fluke of cats that can occasionally be transmitted to humans. It is a disease of fish-eating mammals, such as cats, and is endemic in Southeast Asia and Eastern Europe, but not the United States. Embryonated eggs are excreted by the definitive host in the feces. The eggs are ingested by specific snail species and develop until they are released as cercariae into fresh water where they penetrate into the fish host. Human infection comes from ingestion of rare or raw infected fish. The parasites mature into adults in the bile ducts. Most patients are asymptomatic; however, signs of cholangitis and hepatitis may develop. Diagnosis is by finding eggs in a fecal sample. Therapy is with praziquantel.

Scabies

Sarcoptes scabiei, also known as the "seven-year itch," can infect cats and be transmitted to humans. Scabies mites cause hypersensitivity in human hosts, often manifested by pruritic, papular lesions at areas where they burrow into the skin. The itching increases at night. Cat scabies burrow into human skin but are unable to complete their life cycle, and so a cutaneous scraping test will not be diagnostic. Rather, diagnosis is by clinical presentation. Therapy consists of ridding the offending pet of mites and laundering clothes and bedding.

Cheyletiella Species

Cheyletiella species consist of animal mites, some of which can infest cats and may occasionally cause human infestation.

Dermatophytoses

Domestic cats can harbor a wide variety of molds and yeasts in the hair of their coats and on their skin. Both symptomatic disease and asymptomatic carriage may occur. These include *Epidermophyton floccosum*, *Microsporum* species, and *Trichophyton* species. These dermatophytes spread between animals and potentially from animals to humans and also humans to animals. Infections often involve the hair shaft and follicle from which infectious arthrospores are disseminated to the local environment and remain viable for months. Up to 89% of cats may harbor dermatophytes of which *M canis* is the most common.

In cats, the most common manifestation is a patchy alopecia, but scaling or granulomatous dermatitis may also be evident. Since transmission is possible, cats should be treated with topical antifungal agents, and some may require oral antifungal agents as well. Additionally, areas must be cleaned of hairs and dander to stop transmission. Approximately 50% of humans exposed to cat dermatophytes will develop symptomatic infection, including ringworm and tinea capitis. In humans the infection can manifest as alopecia, scaling or crusting lesions and ulcers, and nodules. Secondary bacterial infection may also occur.

Diagnosis is by culture of skin scrapings, examination of scrapings using potassium hydroxide digestion or by using a Woods lamp. As in cats, human therapy is usually topical antifungals such as clotrimazole, miconazole, etc., or in severe cases oral agents such as ketoconazole, fluconazole, or griseofulvin. Again, cleaning the environment of cat hairs and dander from carpets, bedding, clothing, etc., is essential for control. Air conditioning and heating filters must also be changed regularly. Pets may need to be restricted from bedrooms.

References

1. Barnham M. Once bitten twice shy: the microbiology of bites. *Rev Medical Microbiol* 1991; 2:31–36.
2. Greene CE (ed): *Infectious Diseases of the Dog and Cat*. Philadelphia, W. B. Saunders Co., 1990.
3. Statistical Abstracts of the United States, 1990. Washington D.C., U.S. Department of Commerce, p. 234.
3a. English CK, Wear DJ, Margileth AM, Lissner CR, Walsh GP. Cat scratch disease: isolation and culture of the bacterial agent. *JAMA* 1988; 259: 1347–52.
4. Brenner DJ, Hollis DG, Moss CW, et al. Proposal of *Afipia* gen. nov., with *Afipia felis* sp. nov. (Formerly the cat scratch disease bacillus), *Afipia clevlandensis* sp. nov. (Formerly the Cleveland Clinic Foundation strain), *Afipia broomeae* sp. nov., and three unnamed genospecies. *J Clin Microbiol* 1991; 29:2450–2460.
4a. Regnery RL, Olson JG, Perkins BA, Bibb W. Serological response to *Rochalimaea henselae* antigen in suspected cat scratch disease. *Lancet* 1992; 339:1443–5.
4b. Dolan MJ, Wong MT, Regnery RL, Jorgensen JH, Garcia M, Peters J, Drehner D. Syndrome of *Rochalimaea henselae* adenitis suggesting cat scratch disease. *An Intern Med* 1993; 118:331–6.
4c. Schwartzman, WA. Infections due to *Rochalimaea*: the expanding clinical spectrum. *Clin Infect Dis* 1992; 15:893–902.
5. Relman DA, Loutit JS, Schmidt TM, et al. The agent of bacillary angiomatosis. *N Engl J Med* 1990; 323:1575–1580.
6. Birtles RJ, Harrison TG, Taylor AG. The causative agent of bacillary angiomatosis. (letter) *N Engl J Med* 1991; 325:1447.
6a. Koehler JE, Quinn FD, Berger TG, LeBoit PE, Tappero JW. Isolation of *Rochalamaea* species from cutaneous and osseous lesions of bacillary angiomatosis. *N Engl J Med* 1992; 327:1625–31.
6b. Tappero JW, Mohle-Boetani J, Koehler JE, et al. The epidemiology of bacillary angiomatosis and bacillary peliosis. *JAMA* 1993; 269:770–5.
6c. Welch DF, Pickett DA, Slater LN, Steiger AG, Brenner DJ. Rochalimaea henselae sp. nov., a cause of septicemia, bacillary angiomatosis, and parenchymal bacillary peliosis. *J Clin Microbiol* 1992; 30:275–80.
7. Mui BSK, Mulligan ME, George WL. Response of HIV-associated disseminated cat scratch disease to treatment with doxycycline. *Am J Med* 1990; 89:229–231.

8. Nime FA, Burek JD, Page DL, et al. Acute enterocolitis in a human being infected with the protozoan *Cryptosporidium*. *Gastroenterol* 1976; 70: 592–598.

9. Meisel JL, Perea DR, Meligro C, et al. Overwhelming watery diarrhea associated with *Cryptosporidium* in an immunosuppressed patient. *Gastroenterol* 1976; 70:1156–1160.

10. Douglas LG. Bite wounds. *Am Fam Phys* 1975; 11:93–99.

11. Elenbaas RM, McNabey WK, Robinson WA. Evaluation of prophylactic oxacillin in cat bite wounds. *Ann Emerg Med* 1984; 13:155–157.

12. Tindall JP, Harrison CM. *Pasteurella multocida* infections following animal injuries, especially cat bites. *Arch Derm* 1972; 105:412–416.

13. Goldstein EJC, Citron DM, Wield B, et al. Bacteriology of human and animal bite wounds. *J Clin Microbiol* 1978; 8:667–672.

14. Malnick H, Williams K, Phil-Eboise J, Levy AS. Description of a medium for isolating *Anaerobiospirillum* spp., a possible cause of zoonotic disease, from diarrheal feces and blood of humans and use of the medium in a survey of human, canine and feline feces. *J Clin Microbiol* 1990; 28:1380–1384.

15. Fukushima H, Gomyoda M, Ishikura S, et al. Cat-contaminated environmental substances lead to *Yersinia pseudotuberculosis* infection in children. *J Clin Microbiol* 1989; 27:2706–2709.

9
And Other House Pets

Bruno B. Chomel

Many infectious diseases in humans can be acquired through contact with pets. Dogs and cats may be the most frequent household pets around the world, but there are also many other vertebrates that share our household environment. At least 55% of all households in the United States have a dog or a cat, and 15% to 20% have pet birds (1), but the pet population is also composed of millions of rodents, reptiles, or aquarium fish, not to mention less common species such as wild carnivores, monkeys, or, more recently, the miniature pig. It is estimated that 20 million American homes have aquariums at any given time (2).

The objective in this chapter is not to cover every species that can be pets and every disease, especially the rare and exotic ones that can be transmitted to us, but rather to focus on the most common "other house pets," and the potential health threats they can represent. Only a few lines and summary tables at the end of this chapter will be devoted to more uncommon pets, especially ferrets and primates. Zoonoses that have involved confirmed house pet transmission are presented in more detail. If one excludes gastrointestinal zoonoses, especially salmonellosis, most of the zoonoses potentially transmitted by these animals are usually rare events.

Pet Rabbits and Rodents

Zoonoses transmitted by pet rabbits and rodents are quite rare. Very few zoonoses affect rabbits, thus making them good pets that can be house trained. Most of the health problems encountered with rabbits and rodents are related to allergies or bites. A distinction should be made between the domestic pets (rabbits, guinea pigs, hamsters, mice, or rats) and wild rodents kept as pets. Although the first group is rarely involved in transmitting zoonoses, a special warning should be made for wild animals; for example, woodchucks could transmit rabies, and squirrels can transmit tularemia, rat bite fever, or leptospirosis. As a general rule, wildlife should not be kept as pets because of the health risk. Any wild animal should be handled with caution and referred to wildlife specialists. Zoonoses of pet rabbits and rodents are reviewed in Table 9.1.

TABLE 9.1. Zoonoses potentially transmitted by pet rabbits and Rodents.

Animal Species	Zoonoses			
	Viral	Bacterial	Parasitic	Mycotic
Rabbit	None known	**Pasteurellosis*** **Salmonellosis** Yersiniosis [tuberculosis]** [tularemia] [Listeriosis]	**Cheyletellosis**	**Dermatophytosis** (Trichophyton mentagrophytes) (Microsporum)
Mouse	**LCM** [HFRS]	**Salmonellosis** Pasteurellosis Yersiniosis Mycoplasmosis [Rat bite fever] [Leptospirosis]	**Teniasis** (Hymenolepis nana) (H diminuta) [Giardiasis] [Cryptosporidiosis]	**Dermatophytosis** (T mentagrophytes)
Rat	**HFRS Encephalo myocarditis** [Rabies]	**Salmonellosis** **Pasteurellosis** Yersiniosis **Rat-bite fever** [Leptospirosis]	**Teniasis (H nana)** (H diminuta) Sarcoptic mange (Trixacarus diversus)	**Dermatophytosis** (T quinckeanum)
Guinea pig	LCM?	**Salmonellosis** **Yersiniosis** Campylobacteriosis **Pasteurellosis** [Leptospirosis]	**Sarcoptic mange** (Trixacarus caviae) [Crytosporidiosis]	**Dermatophytosis** (T mentagrophytes)
Hamster	**LCM**	**Campylobacteriosis** **Salmonellosis** Yersiniosis **Pasteurellosis** [Leptospirosis]	**Sarcoptic mange** **Tapeworm** (H nana)	**Dermatophytosis**
Gerbils	None known	**Salmonellosis** [Leptospirosis]	**Teniasis (H nana)** [cutaneous Leishmaniasis]	None Known
Squirrel	[Rabies]	**Pasteurellosis** **Rat-bite fever** **Tularemia** [Relapsing fever] [RMSF] [Plague]	None Known	None Known

* Boldface used for most common zoonoses
** Brackets used for rare zoonoses

Rabbits

The domestic or European rabbit is certainly an excellent pet for children, as diseases of major public health importance in domestic rabbits are rarely encountered. Biting is uncommon, but rabbits can inflict painful scratches with their rear limbs if improperly restrained (3). Among rabbit infectious diseases, *Pasteurella multocida* may cause cutaneous infection in susceptible persons (4). Other diseases to which rabbits are susceptible, e.g., salmonellosis and tularemia, are extremely rare and are more commonly transmitted to humans by wild animals. More commonly, some external parasites of the rabbit may be transmitted to humans, including fur mite acariasis (*Cheyletiella*) and dermatophytosis (*Trichophyton*).

Cheyletiella Infestation (Rabbit Fur Mite)

The rabbit fur mite, *Cheleytiella parasitivorax*, is uncommon in the domestic rabbit. It is an external parasite of the skin and hair that does not excavate tunnels or furrows in the skin. The life cycle is completed in about 35 days. Adult females and eggs can survive 10 days off the animal body, but the larvae, nymphs, and adult males are not very resistant and die in about 2 days in the environment (5). Lesions in rabbits involve hair loss and a mild scaly, oily dermatitis. In humans, the disease consists of a papular and pruritic eruption on the arms, thorax, waist, and thighs. Human infestation is transitory, as the mites do not reproduce on human skin. To prevent human infestation, infested rabbits should be treated with insecticides such as methyl carbamate once a week for 3 to 4 weeks.

Fungal Skin Infections (Ringworm)

Fungal skin infections due to *Trichophyton mentagrophytes* are rare. In rabbits, irritation and inflammation of skin areas occur with crusts, scabs, and hair loss. Affected animals should be isolated. Antifungal treatment with topical or systemic griseofulvin (25 mg/kg/day) for 4 weeks is effective. The spectrum of ringworm in humans varies from subclinical colonization to an inflammatory scaly eruption which spreads peripherally and causes localized alopecia. Diagnosis is made by identifying hyphae in skin scrapings on a potassium hydroxide slide or by isolation in fungal culture media, the only method that allows identification of the species. In humans, topical treatment with clotrimazole (Lotrimin, Mycelex) or miconazole (Monistatderm), twice a day for 2 to 4 weeks, is usually sufficient. When extensive lesions are observed, oral griseofulvin (Fulvicin, Grifulvin V, Grisactin) should be used. In adults, the dosage is 500 mg twice a day for 4 weeks, at least (6).

Rodents

Although rodents, especially mice and rats, are definitively associated with transmission to humans of major fatal diseases such as plague, typhus, and leptospirosis, they can be very good pets. The albino rat, a domestic variety of the brown rat (*Rattus norvegicus*) and the albino domestic mouse (*Mus musculus*) are kept by many people. However, guinea pigs, hamsters, and gerbils are the most common house pets among the rodent group.

As mentioned by Wagner (7), the most important concerns about rodents for pet owners are bites and allergies.

Human allergies to rodent dander are common. Symptoms are characterized by cutaneous (reddening, itching, hives) and respiratory problems.

Infectious diseases from pet rodents are rare events. Among these, salmonellosis and lymphocytic choriomeningitis are of major concern.

Salmonellosis

Guinea pigs are highly susceptible to salmonella infection and develop severe clinical disease (septicemia). In guinea pigs, high mortality is the rule. Mice and rats are also very susceptible and may carry subclinical infections for long periods. These infections are usually caused by *Salmonella typhimurium* or *S enteritidis*. If salmonellosis occurs in a child who has a pet rodent, the pet's feces should be cultured for *Salmonella*. However, shedding may be only intermittent.

Lymphocytic Choriomeningitis

Lymphocytic choriomeningitis (LCM) virus is found in many rodent species and spreads to humans through contact with infected aerosols, direct animal contact, or rodent bites. The natural reservoir of the disease is the domestic mouse (*Mus musculus*), which usually does not present any signs (3,5,6,8).

Epidemiology. The LCM virus, (an RNA virus of the Arenaviridae family) is transmitted among rodents horizontally through secretions (urine, saliva, feces) and vertically to the embryos, especially in mice. Infected offspring develop a persistent infection and shed the virus during most of their lifespan. Outbreaks have been reported in laboratory mice, and human cases occurred in houses where infected mice were caught. In man, the disease is sporadic, but outbreaks may occasionally occur. Such outbreaks of LCM occurred in the late 1960s and early 1970s in Germany and the United States, and were associated with the use of hamsters as pets. In Germany, 47 human cases associated with pet hamsters were reported within a 2-year period (9). In the United States, a nationwide epidemic occurred in late 1973 and early 1974 totalling at least 181 cases in 12 states with 57 cases in New York

State (10) and in California. All were associated with pet hamsters from a single breeder in Birmingham, Alabama. This breeder was an employee of a biological products firm whose tumor cell lines were found positive for LCM. This same cell source was also incriminated in a prior outbreak at the University of Rochester Medical Center in New York (11). Since suspending the sale of these pet hamsters by the Birmingham breeder and of the distribution of positive tumor cell lines by the biological products firm, no further outbreaks have been reported in the United States.

Symptoms. In hamsters, LCM virus infection is usually not associated with signs of illness (12) and can only be detected by laboratory tests. In humans, the course of infection varies from clinically inapparent to a flu-like infection with fever, headache, and severe myalgia occurring 5 to 10 days after infection. A small number of patients progress to aseptic meningitis, which is characterized by a very high lymphocyte count in the cerebrospinal fluid. On rare occasions, there may be meningoencephalitis. Chronic sequelae are not common and fatal cases are rare.

Diagnosis. Diagnosis of infection in humans is based on viral isolation from blood, nasopharynx, or cerebrospinal fluid samples taken early in the attack and inoculated onto tissue cultures or injected intracerebrally into LCM-free adult mice. Indirect immunofluorescence testing or rising titers of Complement Fixation (CF) antibodies, which appear during the first or second week of the disease, on paired sera reveal a recent infection. Serum neutralization tests can also be used.

Treatment. Since the disease is self-limiting, treatment is for symptomatic relief only.

Dermatophytosis

Tinea favus of rats and mice, caused by *Trichophyton quinckeanum*, is widespread (3). In laboratory mice and guinea pigs, infection is mainly due to *T mentagrophytes*. The lesion, localized on the head or trunk, is white and scabby; but rodents often have no noticeable lesions. The infection is transmitted to humans and dogs. (For diagnosis and treatment, see specific paragraph in zoonoses of the rabbit).

Bites: Pasteurellosis, Rat-Bite Fever, Tularemia, and Rabies

Pasteurellosis

Among bite transmitted zoonoses, infection by *Pasteurella multocida* is certainly the most common among domestic pets. If most of the cases occur from cat and dog bites, nevertheless rodents harbor *P multocida* in their oral cavity and can at times transmit the organism through a bite wound. *Pasteurella multocida* is likely to be the pathogen if cellulitis develops within a few hours after the bite. Swelling, reddening, and intense pain in the region are the main signs and symptoms. If the incubation period is longer, staphyloccocal or streptococcal infection is more likely. Appropriate treatment for pasteurellosis is penicillin. Cultures should always be obtained from infected bite wounds in order to administer the appropriate antibiotics. Alternatively, therapy should be started with amoxicillin/clavulanate potassium (Augmentin), 500 mg 3 times daily for 5 to 7 days.

Rat-Bite Fever (RBF)

Rat-bite fever is a rare disease that can be transmitted by healthy rats, which can carry *Streptobacillus moniliformis* or *Spirillum morsus muris* in their nasopharynx.

Streptobacillary RBF is a rare disease in the United States. Of 14 cases of rat-bite fever on record since 1958, seven originated from the bite of laboratory rats (13,14). Bites by wild rodents (rats, squirrels) can also transmit the infectious agent (14). Infection has also followed consumption of contaminated raw milk (13). Streptobacillary RBF has an incubation period of 3 to 10 days, a rapidly healing point of inoculation, and abrupt onset of irregularly relapsing fever, shaking chills, vomiting, headache, arthralgia, myalgia, and regional lymphadenopathy. Shortly after onset, a maculopapular rash appears on the extremities. Endocarditis is a possible complication. Diagnosis of rat-bite fever is made by culture of the organism from blood or joint fluid (6). Recommended therapy for RBF is penicillin [parenteral procaine penicillin G 600,000 u twice daily for 7 days] (13). Alternatively, streptomycin or tetracycline can be used (14).

Spirillary RBF is even rarer and has an incubation period of 1 to 6 weeks (5). Clinically, *Spirillum morsus minor* differs from streptobacillary fever in the rarity of arthritic symptoms, a distinctive rash, and a common reactivation of the healed wound when symptoms appear.

Tularemia

Tularemia, also know as "rabbit fever," is an acute febrile illness caused by *Francisella tularensis*. Rodents are very susceptible to the disease which usually causes a fatal septicemia. Because the disease is mainly transmitted by ticks and fleas from rodent to rodent, pet rabbits or rodents *should not be* a major risk for transmission of tularemia. There have been documented cases of transmission from domestic cats and, more recently, from the bite of a squirrel kept as a household pet which died minutes after biting a child (15). In humans, the commonly accepted drug of choice for treatment of tularemia is streptomycin (8).

Rabies

Because bites from pet rodents are frequent events, one must be concerned with rabies. No case of rabies has ever been reported from bites by pet rodents. However, one should be very careful any time a wild rodent kept as a pet has bitten a person. Cases of rabies have been reported in woodchucks, squirrels, and even in a rat (16).

Yersiniosis

Infections by *Yersinia pseudotuberculosis* and *Y enterocolitica* may be contracted from pet rodents. Guinea pigs are very commonly infected with *Y pseudotuberculosis* (17). The course of the disease in these animals is usually subacute. Loss of weight and diarrhea are often the only clinical signs. Healthy carriers are common. In rats and mice, the infection is common but usually without clinical signs. Children can be infected by fecal-oral contamination. In humans, the disease is mainly observed in children, adolescents, and young adults. The most common clinical form, after 1 to 3 weeks of incubation, is mesenteric adenitis or pseudoappendicitis, with acute abdominal pain in the right iliac fossa, fever, and vomiting. The disease is usually more common in young males. Diagnosis requires the isolation and identification of the etiological agent. Serologic tests, such as Enzyme Linked Immuno Sorbent Assay (ELISA) are also available. When the disease is mild (uncomplicated pseudoappendicular syndrome), antimicrobial chemotherapy is not useful (18). *Yersinia pseudotuberculosis* is usually sensitive to ampicillin, aminoglycosides, or tetracycline (19). *Yersinia enterocolitica* is also found in rodents, which are usually healthy carriers (20). Chinchillas are very susceptible to the infection, and several epizootics occurred in Europe and the United States (5). Guinea pigs also are commonly infected by *Y enterocolitica*. Usually serotypes found in rodents do not affect humans. In humans, *Y enterocolitica* affects mainly young children. The major symptoms are an acute enteritis with watery and sometimes bloody diarrhea of 3 to 14 days duration, and abdominal pain. Diagnosis is based on isolation of the agent from feces of patients. An ELISA test on paired sera is also useful to determine infection. Aminoglycosides and trimethoprim-sulfamethoxazole are the most appropriate antibiotics (19).

Campylobacteriosis

Campylobacter infection can occur in some rodent species. Proliferative ileitis, a specific enteric syndrome of hamsters is probably caused by a strain of *Campylobacter* sp. Hamsters certainly represent a potential source of human infection, but no hamster-associated cases have been reported to date (8). In humans, campylobacter infection is characterized by diarrhea, abdominal pain, cramps, fever, and vomiting. The diarrhea is frequently bloody. The incubation period is 2 to 5 days, and the disease usually does not last more than a week. Treatment is usually limited to fluid replacement therapy.

Some Rare Viral Diseases

Hemorrhagic Fever with Renal Syndrome (HFRS) or Korean Hemorrhagic Fever

HFRS describes a group of rodent-borne viral diseases (Hantaan virus) which are endemic or occur as focal epidemics on the Eurasian continent and Japan. In general, Hantaan virus isolates from Asia are considered more pathogenic to humans than European and North American strains. Wild rodents in rural areas or wild rats in cities (21) are the reservoirs of the virus which they can shed for several weeks. Several outbreaks have been reported in Japan and Europe in laboratory personnel (22) infected by laboratory rats. Hantaan viruses cause chronic, apparently asymptomatic, infections of their rodent hosts, but associated human cases may reveal the animal infection. The disease in laboratory personnel has been characterized by fever and a "flu-like" syndrome, with fever, myalgia, and, few days later oliguria, proteinuria, and hematuria. Usually, patients will recover without sequelae. Infection is contracted by handling infected animals or from contaminated aerosols. Most laboratory rat suppliers employ a screening test and then destroy infected colonies. The diagnosis of infection is based on viral isolation and, more often, on serodiagnosis by indirect immunofluorescence (IFA) or ELISA.

Encephalomyocarditis

This is a rare disease in humans caused by a Picornaviridae (RNA). Sporadic cases have been reported and the virus isolated from children in Germany, the Netherlands, and the United States; epizootics have occurred in pigs (5). Rodents, especially the genus *Rattus*, have been considered the main reservoir of the virus, and transmit the virus to rats and other species through bites. However, no human case has been identified from a rodent source.

Cestodiasis (Tapeworm)

Cestodes, or tapeworms, infect a wide range of species including rabbits and rodents. *Hymenolepis nana*, the dwarf tapeworm, is found in rodents, especially hamsters. *H diminuta* is the rat tapeworm, but may also be found in other rodents. Hymenolepiasis occurs primarily in children. The prepatent period is 15 to 30 days. Usually the infestation is asymptomatic in humans, but if parasites are present in large numbers gastrointestinal disorders such as abdominal pain, nausea, vomiting, and diarrhea may occur. Eggs of some *Hymenolepis* sp. are infective to the definitive host when passed in the feces. Infection in humans from infected rodents may be acquired either by ingestion of eggs from fecally contaminated fingers, or from contaminated food or water. When eggs of the directly transmitted *Hymenolepis* sp. are ingested, they hatch in the intestine, liberating an oncosphere that enters a mucosal villus and develops into a cysticercoid larva within 5 days. The cysticercoid ruptures the villus, migrates into the lumen, and attaches to the lower small intestine. It reaches the adult phase in 2 weeks and starts to release eggs. Diagnosis of infection is made by microscopic identification of the eggs in the feces. Praziquantel (Biltricide) and niclosamide (Yomesan, Niclocide) are effective for treatment of hymenolepis infection (3–5,19). Treatment of infected rodents can be done with 1 mg of niclosamide per 10 g of body weight given at 7-day intervals or with 0.3% active ingredient in the feed for 7 days (7).

Acariasis (*Trixacarus caviae*)

Several external parasites can infest rodents. Among these, *Trixacarus caviae*, a parasite mainly found in guinea pigs, can be transmitted to humans. In guinea pigs, the infection is usually asymptomatic. Stress, and/or poor care can lead to severe alopecia, dermatitis, and pruritus on the body and legs. The skin is thickened, dry, and scaly. Treatment is based on a solution of 1:40 lime sulfur in water applied to the skin and repeated weekly for 6 weeks, or a once a week application of 10% lindane for 3 weeks. Ivermectin injected at 200 mg/kg SQ is a useful treatment for ectoparasitism (17). In humans, pruritic skin lesions on the hands, arms, or neck can be observed in children. Diagnosis may be established by recovering the mite from its burrow and identifying it microscopically. Treatment of infected children with crotamiton (Eurax) in one application per day for 2 to 5 days is the most common treatment, or lindane (1% gamma benzene hexachloride: Kwell) can be used (3,19).

Turtles, Lizards, Snakes and Aquarium Fish

Today reptiles are commonplace pets, residing in approximately 453,000 households in the United States. One of every 200 households has turtles, lizards, snakes, or crocodiles as pets (23). Zoonoses of reptiles and aquarium fishes are reviewed in Table 9.2.

Salmonellosis

Salmonellosis is certainly the most frequent and major zoonosis transmitted by reptiles, especially turtles (24,25). Of all zoonoses, *Salmonella* infections present the most significant hazard to children; they are at greater risk of disease than are adults because children and animals are

TABLE 9.2. Zoonoses potentially transmitted by reptiles and aquarium fishes.

Animal Species	Zoonoses			
	Viral	Bacterial	Parasitic	Mycotic
Turtle	None Known	**Salmonellosis*** Yersiniosis Campylobacter [Aeromonas]	None Known	None Known
lizards, snakes	None known	**Salmonellosis** **Yersiniosis** [Edwarsiella tarda] [Plesiomonas]	Pentastomiasis	None Known
Fish	None Known	**Mycobacteriosis** [Erysipelothrix] [Melioidosis]	None Known	None Known

* Boldface used for most common zoonoses
** Brackets used for rare zoonoses

frequently in close contact with each other, and handwashing practices in children are often not well developed (26).

Pet turtles have been recognized as a major source of human salmonellosis since Hershey and Mason isolated *S hartford* from the pet turtle of a 7-month-old infant with *S hartford* gastroenteritis (27). Subsequent investigations established that 14% of the estimated two million cases of human salmonellosis in the United States between 1970 and 1971 were linked to pet turtles, mainly the red eared turtle (*Pseudemys scripta elegans*) (28). With an annual sale of 15 million turtles, zoonotic salmonellosis was a growing problem. By 1975, commercial distribution of turtles less than 4 inches long was banned within the United States by the Food and Drug Administration. A 77% decrease in turtle-associated salmonellosis was noted following enactment (29,30). Nevertheless, an estimated 3 to 4 million turtles are shipped annually from the United States and sold all around the world. Several outbreaks have been reported in Japan (31), Great Britain (32,33), Puerto Rico (34), Israel (35), and France (36). Turtles are usually healthy carriers of *Salmonella* and shedding is very irregular, but they may shed *Salmonella* for up to 11 months. The problem of *Salmonella* infection in turtles arises from the widespread contamination and persistence of the microorganism in turtle breeding ponds and nesting areas. Turtles can acquire the organism in ovo or after hatching (37). Use of antibiotics for attempted control of *Salmonella* in pet turtle husbandry has been widely practiced. In their attempt to eradicate *Salmonella* with gentamycin sulfate, turtle farmers have created an even greater health hazard through selection of antibiotic-resistant strains (38). Treatment of pet turtles is not recommended, and infected reptiles should be destroyed. However, knowledge of the potential health hazards, along with proper sanitation, is usually sufficient to prevent human infection. Pet turtles should not be displayed in classrooms where children can handle them or have contact with their container. Identification of the microorganism from stool culture and an antibiogram should be performed when salmonellosis is suspected. Similarly, culture should be performed from the pet reptile or from its aquarium. In humans, primary treatment of salmonellosis consists of fluid and electrolyte replacement. Antibiotics are not recommended, except in severe froms, as they not only fail to shorten the duration of the illness but also may prolong the carrier state.

Salmonella infection can be acquired not only from pet turtles, but also from other reptiles such as lizards or snakes (39), from frogs (40), or aquarium fish (41).

Other Gastrointestinal Bacterial Infections

Edwardsiella

Human infection with *Edwardsiella tarda* is uncommon. This organism can be found in cold-blooded animals, reptiles, and fish (goldfish, catfish, bass). In humans, the organism may cause gastroenteritis resembling *Salmonella* infections. At least one case was reported in the United States, associated with a pet turtle (42).

Plesiomonas

Plesiomonas (Aeromonas) shigelloides is a gram-negative rod that causes progressive ulcerative stomatitis in snakes ("mouth-rot disease"). It may cause gastroenteritis in humans. A case of acute gastroenteritis has been reported from a zoo animal keeper infected after handling a sick boa constrictor (43). Diagnosis is made by stool culture. In humans, treatment with trimethoprim/sulfamethoxazole (Bactrim, Septra) for 5 days is usually effective.

Yersiniosis

Yersinia enterocolitica has been found in water and on cold-blooded animals (frogs, fish) (44,45). However, the serotypes involved are not usually found in humans.

In the United States, more than 20 million household aquariums are maintained, accommodating an annual sale of approximately 600 million pet fish (46), mostly coming from foreign countries (south East Asia, South America) and from Florida. However, very few cases of zoonoses are reported, and no major outbreaks of human disease for which diseased fish were directly responsible have been reported recently (46). Among the bacterial diseases, mycobacteriosis is certainly of major concern.

Mycobacteriosis

Mycobacterial infections are certainly among the major zoonoses that can be transmitted by aquarium fish (47,48). *Mycobacterium marinum, M fortuitum and M platypolcitis* have been associated with both fish and human disease for many years. Skin ulcers due to *M marinum*, contracted from fish tanks, were reported. In two cases, a cut in the hand had preceded the cleaning of a home fish aquarium (49). Infection by *M marinum*, also known as "swimming pool granuloma," is characterized, after several weeks of incubation, by papular lesions, usually on the fingers or hands, which evolve into dark suppurative lesions. In infected fish, granulomatous lesions are usually observed. A diagnosis can be made by isolating and identifying the organism. Infected fish should be destroyed, and the aquarium disinfected with 5% calcium hypochlorite solution before other fish are added (50). In humans, infection resolves following treatment with minocycline (Minocin), 100 mg twice daily for 6 to 8 weeks (6). Use of rifampin (Rifadin, Rimactane) has also been very successful (51), although indications for therapy are controversial (V. chap.).

Melioidosis and Exotic Fish

Melioidosis is an uncommon disease in humans with a wide range of clinical manifestations from inapparent infection to a rapid fatal septicemia. *Pseudomonas pseudomallei*, the infectious agent, is endemic in Southeast Asia where it is saprophytic in certain soils and waters. Recent studies have shown that the water in tanks which contained exotic, imported aquarium fishes was contaminated with this bacillus. Disinfection of aquariums with bleach between water changes should be recommended in pet stores to prevent spread of infection (52).

Erysipelothrix Infection

Erysipelothrix insidiosa has been reported in humans contaminated by handling fish. It is mainly an occupational disease affecting fishermen. The organism can be found on the surface of the fish and produces skin lesions in man known as "fish rose." *Erysipelothrix* infection is almost invariably introduced through minor skin wounds. Local erysipeloid most commonly occurs on the hands and, sometimes, local lymphangitis and lymphadenitis may occur. Despite the potential of this organism to infect aquarium owners, no human cases have been reported from aquarium fish contamination. Penicillin is the appropriate treatment for erysipeloid (53).

Pentastomiasis

Pentastomes (*Armillifer* sp.) are annulate metazoa that are almost exclusively parasites of the reptilian respiratory system. Snakes are the definitive hosts, and many wild rodents, on which snakes feed, are the intermediate hosts. The female parasite deposits eggs in the respiratory cavities of the reptiles. The eggs are expectorated or swallowed and then eliminated with the feces. Humans can be accidental hosts by handling infected reptiles and then placing contaminated hands to the mouth. In humans, the infection is usually asymptomatic. The encapsulated larvae might be found during laparotomies or can be diagnosed by radiographic examination (5,54).

Wild Carnivores

Among the large variety of house pets, wild carnivores, especially ferrets, have experienced increasing popularity, with an estimated 6,000 ferrets sold annually (55). According to Rupprecht et al (56), there are currently 5 to 7 million pet ferrets in approximately 4 to 5 million households in the United States. Despite the fact that ferrets are enjoyable pets, much concern has been raised following severe injuries to children by ferrets kept as house pets. The state of California does not allow ferrets nor several other exotic animals as house pets (55). As pets, ferrets can also represent a health hazard by transmitting several disease agents to humans. Zoonoses of ferrets are reviewed in Table 9.3.

Like other carnivores, ferrets are susceptible to rabies. In the United States, rabies has been reported 13 times in ferrets since 1958, most often from pet ferrets, of which some were acquired from pet shops (57). Rabies immunization of ferrets with an inactivated vaccine has been shown to be effective for at least a year (56). The USDA granted approval on February 8, 1990, for the use of this vaccine in ferrets of 3 or more months of age. Annual booster vaccinations are required. However, the Centers for Disease Control recommends that ferrets that have bitten humans be destroyed and their brains examined for rabies.

Influenza

Ferrets are very susceptible to influenza viruses, and have served for years as an animal model in the laboratory (55,57). In ferrets, flu is

TABLE 9.3. Zoonoses potentially transmitted by ferrets.

Zoonoses:	Viral	Bacterial	Parasitic	Mycotic
	Influenza* Rabies	**Campylobacteriosis** **Salmonellosis** Tuberculosis [Leptospirosis] [Listeriosis]	Cryptosporidiosis Toxocariasis Giardiasis	Dermatophytosis

*Boldface used for most common zoonoses

characterized by sneezing, fever, lethargy, mucoserous nasal discharge, conjunctivitis, and photophobia. The course of the influenza infection usually lasts less than a week. The disease can be severe in young ferrets. Human cases of influenza have occurred from contamination by aerosols from infected ferrets (57). Similarly, ferrets can be infected by humans shedding the virus.

Other Potential Zoonotic Pathogens

Ferrets can harbor several pathogenic microorganisms in their digestive tract, especially *Salmonella*, and *Campylobacter*. In a 9-month survey of ferrets used in biomedical research, 4% had *Salmonella* and 18% had *Campylobacter jejuni/coli* isolated from their feces (58). Although no human cases have been reported from ferret contamination, ferrets must be considered possible reservoirs for *Campylobacter* and *Salmonella* organisms. Ferrets should not be allowed to roam freely, and their feces should be discarded in a hygienic manner (57). Ferrets can harbor many other zoonoses, including cryptosporidiosis, tuberculosis, and listeriosis. They share many parasites with dogs and cats (*Toxocara*, *Ancylostoma*), as well as dermatophytosis (*Microsporum canis*, *Trichophyton mentagrophytes*). A complete description of these infections has been recently documented by Marini et al (57).

Nonhuman Primates

During the last 17 years, laws restricting importation of nonhuman primates into the United States have considerably reduced the number of primates appearing in the pet trade. However, nonhuman primates sometimes find their way into the hands of pet owners. Until the 1974 prohibition, New World primates were used extensively in the pet trade, especially the squirrel monkey (59). Because of close phylogenic ties between humans and nonhuman primates, zoonoses transmitted by monkeys are numerous, some of them being particularly severe in humans. For public health reasons, as well as animal welfare and environment protection, the author strongly supports the policy that monkeys should not be kept as pets. It is not the purpose of this chapter to present all the zoonoses that can be transmitted by primates, as excellent reviews have been recently published (59–62). A short table of the major and most severe zoonoses is given for information (Table 9.4).

Among the major zoonoses, salmonellosis and shigellosis are certainly the most frequent in monkeys, as gastrointestinal illnesses are very common. Nonhuman primates are also very susceptible to respiratory infections, and tuberculosis must be considered as a major risk for monkeys and their owners or caretakers. Monkeys are very susceptible to

TABLE 9.4. Zoonoses potentially transmitted by nonhuman primates.

Zoonoses:	Viral	Bacterial	Parasitic	Mycotic
	Hepatitis A*	**Salmonellosis**	**Amoebiasis**	Dermatophytosis
	Measles	**Shigellosis**	**Balantidoisis**	(T mentagrophytes)
	Herpes B	**Tuberculosis**	Hymenolepis	(Microsporum spp)
	[Rabies]	Campylobacteriosis	Strongyloides	
	[Marburg]	Yersiniosis	Giardiosis	
	[Monkeypox]	Klebsiellosis		
		[Tularemia]		

* Boldface used for most common zoonoses
** Brackets used for rare zoonoses

Mycobacterium tuberculosis, *M bovis*, and *M avium*, and suspect animals should not be treated. Monkeys are also very susceptible to some viral diseases, such as measles. Infected children can easily transmit the virus to pet monkeys. Some viral diseases of the nonhuman primates may be deadly to infected humans. An example is the Herpes B virus, which may be shed by healthy monkeys (mainly macaques) in their saliva. In monkeys, rabies is a rare disease, but cases have been reported from pet monkeys vaccinated with live modified strains; also, only *inactivated rabies vaccines* should be used to immunize monkeys.

References

1. Stehr-green JK, Schantz P. The impact of zoonotic diseases transmitted by pets on the human health and the economy. *Vet Clin North Am [Small An Pract]* 1987; 17:1–15.
2. Gratzeck JB. Tropical fish: keeping a giant industry healthy, In Animal Health, 1984 yearbook of Agriculture:347–357.
3. Harkness JE, Wagner JE. *The Biology and Medicine of Rabbits and Rodents*, 2nd ed. Philadelphia, Lea & Febiger, 1983: p. 2104.
4. Harkness JE. Rabbit husbandry and medicine. *Vet Clin North Am [Small An Pract]* 1987; 17(5):1019–1044.
5. Acha P, Szyfres B. *Zoonoses and Communicable Diseases Common to Man and Animals*, 2nd ed. Washington D.C., Pan American Health Organization, 1987.
6. Chretien JH, Garagusi VF. Infections associated with pets. *Am Fam Pract* 1990; 41:831–845.
7. Wagner JE, Farrar PL. Husbandry and Medicine of small rodents. *Vet Clin North Am [Small An Pract]* 1987; 17:1061–1087.
8. Goscienski PJ. Zoonoses. *Pediatr Infect Dis* 1983; 2:69–81.
9. Ackermann R, Stille W, Blumenthal W, et al. Syrische goldhamster als unbertrager von lymphozytaren choriomeningitis. *Dtsch Med Wochenschr* 1972; 97:1725–1731.
10. Biggar RJ, Woodall JP, Walter PD, Haughie GE. Lymphocytic choriomeningitis outbreak associated with pet hamsters. Fifty-seven cases from New York State. *JAMA* 1975; 232:494–500.

11. Gregg MB. Recent outbreaks of lymphocytic choriomeningitis in the United States of America. *Bull World Health Org* 1975; 52:549–553.

12. Deibel R, Woodall JP, Decher WJ, Schryver GD. Lymphocytic Chorio-meningitis virus in man. Serologic evidence of association with pet hamsters. *JAMA* 1975; 232:501–504.

13. Anderson LC, Leary SL, Manning PJ. Rat bite fever in animal research laboratory personnel. *Lab An Sci* 1983; 33:292–294.

14. Rat bite fever in a college student, California. *MMWR* 1984; 33:318–320.

15. Magee JS, Steele RW, Kelly NR, Jacobs RF. Tularemia transmitted by a squirrel bite. *Pediatr Infect Dis J* 1989; 8:123–125.

16. Moro MH, Horman JT, Fischman HR, et al. The epidemiology of rodent and lagomorph rabies in Maryland, 1981 to 1986. *J Wild Dis* 1991; 27:452–456.

17. Anderson LC. Guinea pig husbandry and medicine. *Vet Clin North Am [Small An Pract]* 1987; 17:1045–1060.

18. Carniel E, Mollaret HH. Yersiniosis. *Comp Immun Microbiol Infect Dis* 1990; 13:51–58.

19. Benenson A. *Control of Communicable Diseases in Man*, 15th ed. Washington D.C., Am Public Health Assoc., 1990.

20. Seguin B, Boucaud-Maitre Y, Quenin P, Lorgue G. Recherche de *Yersinia enterocolitica* et des espèces apparentées chez le rat d'égout: présence d'une souche pathogène humaine. *Méd Mal Infect* 1986; 16:28–30.

21. Childs JE, Glass GE, Ksiazek TG, et al. Human-rodent contact and infection with lymphocytic choriomeningitis and seoul viruses in an inner-city population. *Am J Trop Med Hyg* 1991; 44(2):117–121.

22. LeDuc JW. Epidemiology of Hantaan and related viruses. *Lab An Sci* 1987; 37:413–418.

23. *The Veterinary Services Market*, Vols I, II. Prepared for the AVMA. Overland Park, KS, Charles, Charles and Associates, 1983, pp. 44–47.

24. Lamm SH, Taylor Jr A, Gangarosa EJ, et al. Turtle associated salmonellosis. I. An estimation of the magnitude of the problem in the United States, 1970–1971. *Am J Epidemiol* 1972; 95:511–517.

25. Turtle-associated salmonellosis—Ohio. *MMWR* 1986; 35:733–734, 739.

26. Altman R, Gorman JC, Bernhardt LL, Goldfield M. Turtle-associated salmonellosis. II. The relationship of pet turtles to salmonellosis in children in New Jersey. *Am J Epidemiol* 1972; 95:518–520.

27. Salmonella Surveillance Report No 10. Atlanta, Centers for Disease Control, 1963: pp. 22–24.

28. Chiodini RJ, Sundberg JP. Salmonellosis in reptiles: A review. *Am J Epidemiol* 1981; 113:494–499.

29. Cohen ML, Potter M, Pollard R, Feldman RA. Turtle-associated salmonellosis in the United States. Effect of Public Health action, 1970–1976. *JAMA* 1980; 243:1247–1249.

30. D'Aoust JY, Lior H. Pet turtle regulations and abatement of human salmonellosis. *Can J Public Health* 1978; 69:107–108.

31. Fujita K, Murono KI, Yoshioka H. Pet-linked salmonellosis. *Lancet* 1981; ii:525.

32. Anonymous: Reptilian salmonellosis. *Lancet* 1981; ii:130–131.

33. Borland ED. Salmonella infection in dogs, cats, tortoises and terrapins. *Vet Rec* 1975; 96:401–402.

260   B.B. Chomel

34. Tauxe RV, Rigau-Pérez JG, Wells JG, Blake PA. Turtle-associated salmonellosis in Puerto Rico. *JAMA* 1985; 254:237–239.
35. Chassis G, Groos EM, Greenberg Z, et al. Salmonella in turtles imported to Israel from Lousiana. *JAMA* 1986; 256:1003.
36. Sanchez R, Martin A, Bailly A, Dirat MF. Salmonellose digestive associée à une tortue domestique. A propos d'un cas. *Méd Mal Infect* 1988; 18(10): 458–459.
37. Kaufmann AF, Fox MD, Morris GK, et al. Turtle-associated salmonellosis. III. The effects of environmental salmonellae in commercial turtle breeding ponds. *Am J Epidemiol* 1972; 95:521–528.
38. D'Aoust JY, Daley E, Crozier M, Sewell AM. Pet turtles: A continuing international threat to public health. *Am J Epidemiol* 1990; 132:233–238.
39. Richard Y, Martel JL, Prave M, Deschanel JP, Borges E, Oudar J. Animaux exotiques, parcs zoologiques et salmonelloses. *Sci Vét Méd Comp* 1984; 86:135–144.
40. Barlett KH, Trust TJ, Lior H. Small pet aquarium frog as source of salmonella. *Appl Environ Microbiol* 1977; 1026–1029.
41. Mokhayer B et Tadjbakhche H. Isolement de *Salmonella havana* d'une épizootie sévissant sur les poissons rouges (queue de voile et comète). *Bull Soc Sci Vét Méd Comp* 1978; 80:147–150.
42. Nagel P, Serritella A, Layden TJ. Edwardsiella tarda gastroenteritis associated with a pet turtle. *Gastroenterology* 1982; 82:1436–1437.
43. Davis WA II, Chretien JH, Garagusi VF, Goldstein MA. Snake-to-human transmission of *Aeromonas (Pl) shigelloides* resulting in gastroenteritis. *South Med J* 1978; 71:474–476.
44. Harvey S, Greenwood R, Pickett MJ, Mah RH. Recovery of Yersinia enterocolitica from stream and lakes of California. *Appl Environ Microbiol* 1976; 32:352–354.
45. Zamora J, Enriquez R. Yersinia enterocolitica, Y. frederiksenii and Y. intermedia in Cyprinus carpio. *J Vet Med* 1987; 34:155–159.
46. Shotts EB. Bacteria associated with fish and their relative importance. In: JH Steele (ed). *CRC Handbook Series in Zoonoses*, Section A, Vol II. Boca Raton, Florida, CRC Press, 1980: pp. 517–525.
47. Thoen CO, Karlson AG, Himes EM. Mycobacterial infections in animals. *Rev Infect Dis* 1981; 3:960–972.
48. de German E, Shotts EB. Bacterial culture and evaluation of diseases of fish. *Vet Clin North Am [Small An Pract]* 1988; 18:365–374.
49. Kleeburg HH. Tuberculosis and other mycobacterioses. In: Hubbert WT, McCulloch WF, Schnurrenberger PR (eds): *Diseases Transmitted from Animals to Man*, 6th ed. Springfield, Il, C. Thomas Publisher, 1975: pp. 303–360.
50. Leibovitz L. Fish tuberculosis (Mycobacteriosis). *J Am Vet Med Assoc* 1980; 176:415.
51. Donta ST, Smith PW, Levitz RE, Quintiliani R. Therapy of *Mycobacterium marinum* infections. Use of tetracyclines vs rifampin. *Arch Intern Med* 1986; 146:902–904.
52. Dodin A, Galimand M. La mélioidose: maladie de pathologie comparée. *Bull Soc Sci Vét et Méd Comp* 1981; 83:255–258.
53. Shotts EB. Bacterial diseases of fish associated with human health. *Vet Clin North Am [Small An Pract]* 1987; 17:241–247.

54. Hendrix CM, Blagburn BL. Reptilian pentastomiasis: a possible emerging zoonosis. *Compendium Small An* 1988; 10:46–51.
55. Besch-Williford CL. Biology and medicine of the ferret. *Vet Clin N America [Small An Pract]* 1987; 17:1155–1183.
56. Rupprecht CE, Gilbert J, Pitts R, et al. Evaluation of an inactivated rabies virus vaccine in domestic ferrets. *J Am Vet Med Assoc* 1990; 196:1614–1616.
57. Marini RP, Adkins JA, Fox JG. Proven or potential zoonotic diseases of ferrets. *J Am Vet Med Assoc* 1989; 195:990–994.
58. Fox JG, Adkins JA, Maxwell KO. Zoonoses in ferrets. *Lab Anim Sci* 1988; 38:500–501.
59. Renquist DM, Whitney RA. Zoonoses acquired from pet primates. *Vet Clin N Am [Small An Pract]* 1987; 17:219–240.
60. Soave O. Viral infections common to human and nonhuman primates. *J Am Vet Med Assoc* 1981; 179:1385–1388.
61. Parrott TY. An introduction to diseases of nonhuman primates. *Compendium Small An* 1986; 8:733–738.
62. Satterfield WC, Voss WR. Nonhuman primates and the practitioner. *Vet Clin N Am [Small An Pract]* 1987; 17:1185–1202.

10
Fine Feathered Friends

Matthew E. Levison

Although many people these days "work" at leisure time activities, diseases are most commonly acquired from birds during the course of work, in the usual sense of the term, not leisure. However travel to highly endemic areas for pleasure puts people at risk of acquiring some of these bird-related diseases (histoplasmosis and togavirus infections), as does ownership of birds as pets (psittacosis).

Infectious diseases can be transmitted to humans from birds by one of several different mechanisms (Table 10.1): In group 1 infections, birds are the natural reservoir for the infectious agent, which causes illness among birds. The diseased birds then disseminate the infectious agent into the environment, and humans become infected as accidental hosts. Examples of such infections include: psittacosis, Newcastle disease, and yersinosis. In group 2 and 3 infections, birds are the natural reservoir for the infectious agent without causing them illness. The infectious agents disseminate from the colonized birds into the environment directly (for example, salmonellosis and mites) in group 2 or by means of insect vectors (for example, eastern, St. Louis, and western equine encephalitis and Japanese B encephalitis) in group 3 to involve humans as accidental hosts. In group 4 infections, birds are not the natural reservoir, but they facilitate growth of the organisms in the environment by means of their fecal matter: examples of this last category include the fungal diseases, histoplasmosis, and cryptococcosis (1).

Psittacosis

Pathogen

Chlamydia psittaci is an obligate intracellular bacterial parasite.

Source of Infection

The natural reservoirs of *C psittaci* are wild and domestic birds. Infection in birds is usually latent, but may become apparent when resistance

TABLE 10.1. Bird-related diseases.

Natural reservoir	Disease	Illness in Birds	Illness in Humans	Mode of spread
Group 1				
Bird	Psittacosis	Intestinal, respiratory	Respiratory	Aerosolized Bird feces
Domestic and wild fowl	Newcastle	Respiratory, neurological	Conjunctivitis	Aerosols, contaminated hands
Domestic and wild turkeys	Yersinosis	Intestinal	Intestinal	Contaminated food
Group 2				
Domestic and wild birds	Mites	None	Pruritic rash	Indirect and direct contact
Domestic Fowl	Salmonellosis	None	Diarrhea	Contaminated food
Group 3				
Domestic and wild birds	Togavirus infections	None	Encephalitis, polyarthritis, rash	Insect vector
Group 4				
Soil fertilized by bird droppings	Histoplasmosis	None	Respiratory	Aerosols
Soil fertilized by bird droppings	Cryptococcosis	None	Respiratory, neurological	Aerosols

is compromised by conditions such as crowding, prolonged transport, nutritional deficiencies, etc. In birds the infection is primarily gastro-intestinal and respiratory and results in diarrhea, fever, conjunctival congestion, and respiratory distress. The agent is shed in the liquid feces to contaminate the environment and feathers. As the fecal matter dries, the *Chlamydiae* become airborne, facilitated by motion of the feathers. In addition to coprophagia and cannibalism, birds acquire the disease by inhalation of infectious aerosols (i.e., airborne particles less than 5 microns in diameter). Airborne particles of this size do not settle out by gravity, but remain suspended; only ventilation and filtration by the lungs removes these particles from the atmosphere. Humans acquire the disease by inhalation of infectious aerosols.

Human Activity

Psittacosis is mainly an occupational disease among workers in turkey processing plants (2,3), duck or geese pluckers, pigeon breeders, and pet store employees.

Human Disease

C psittaci causes atypical pneumonia, that is, pneumonia usually characterized by an insidious onset, predominance of constitutional symptoms (such as fever, headache, and myalgias), shortness of breath, and a nonproductive hacking cough. Chest x-ray will show focal infiltrates, usually at the lung bases. More severe illness may be accompanied by nausea, vomiting, diarrhea, delirium, and hepatosplenomegaly. The illness, nevertheless, is usually self-limited and lasts 1 to 2 weeks, but the course can be shortened by the use of antibiotic therapy, e.g., doxycycline. The case-fatality ratio is less than 1% with appropriate therapy, except for the rare cases acquired from other people, when the disease has been noted to be more severe, with high mortality. The organisms can be recovered in culture from sputum and blood. Isolation of the organism should only be attempted in laboratories that use strict isolation techniques. Diagnosis is usually confirmed by a fourfold rise between onset and convalescence in serum complement fixing antibody titers.

Treatment in the adult consist of 2 weeks of doxycycline, 100 mg orally every 12 hours. A new macrolide, azithromycin, which may prove to be equally or more efficacious, achieves high intracellular concentration of the antibiotic, is bactericidal, has a long half-life that allows single daily dosing, and is well tolerated after oral administration.

Control

Chemoprophylaxis of psittacine birds with 0.5% chlortetracycline for 3 to 4 weeks prior to shipment or after arrival, or mass treatment and quarantine of flocks that are identified as being infected by serologic screening, have been used successfully to control the disease (4).

Newcastle Disease

Pathogen

The Newcastle agent is an RNA virus that is related to the mumps virus. In birds, the virus produces a variable clinical picture, usually with respiratory and neurological findings; more virulent strains produce hemorrhagic lesions in the digestive tract, associated with high mortality.

Source of Infection

Domestic fowl, especially poultry, and wild fowl are the natural reservoirs of the virus, and the virus is spread among the birds by the respiratory route as an aerosol and by the oral route by direct contact or from the contaminated environment.

Human Activity

The disease occurs primarily in poultry slaughterhouse workers, laboratory personnel, and vaccinators of the live virus vaccines, by rubbing eyes with contaminated hands or by inhalation of infectious aerosols (5).

Human Disease

After an incubation period of several days, patients usually develop conjunctivitis with minimal constitutional symptoms; some patients will develop an influenza-like illness, thought to be the consequence of aerosol exposure.

Control

The disease has been controlled by the routine use of vaccines in the poultry industry.

Yersinosis

Pathogen

Yersinia pseudotuberculosis is an enteric facultatively anaerobic gram-negative bacillus in the family of Enterobacteriaceae, like *Escherichia coli*, *Proteus mirabilis*, *Klebsiella pneumoniae*, etc. *Yersinia* grow well at refrigerator temperature, unlike other enteric pathogens, and also at 37° C on routine media. So-called cold enrichment is used to differentially isolate *Yersinia* from clinical material.

Source of Infection

The natural reservoir is believed to be domestic and wild animals, including turkeys, guinea pigs, sheep, cats, and rabbits (6,7).

Human Activity

The mechanisms by which the disease is transmitted to humans are unknown, but contamination of food from the animal reservoir is thought to be an important factor. Humans acquire the disease by the fecal-oral route.

Human Disease

Yersinosis presents as an acute abdomen, that simulates acute appendicitis, with fever, right lower quadrant pain, and vomiting. The course is usually benign and lasts for about 1 week, unless interrupted by surgery for suspected acute appendicitis; however, symptoms may persist for months (8).

Although not subjected to critical analysis, effective treatment in the adult is thought to consist of a 2 week course of either doxycycline or a fluoroquinolone, e.g., ciprofloxacin, 750 mg every 12 hours.

Control

In view of the obscure modes of transmission to man, control is problematic, but should involve protection of food and water against fecal contamination by fowl and other animals.

Mites

Pathogen

Mites that infest wild and domestic birds have four stages (egg, larva, nymph, and adult) in their life cycle, which can be completed within 1 week under favorable circumstances.

Source of Infection

The natural reservoir for these mites are birds. Humans are the accidental hosts. The adult of the species *Dermanyssus gallinae* feeds on birds at night, and during the day infests the buildings that house the birds, where the female mites lay eggs after feeding on the host's blood. Other species of mites, e.g., *Ornithonyssus bursa* and *O sylviarum* complete their entire life cycle on birds.

Human Activity

People who work during the day in buildings that house infested birds can become accidental hosts of *Dermanyssus*, whereas human infestation by *Ornithonyssus* occurs mainly from handling birds.

Human Disease

Intensely pruritic papular urticaria develop at sites on the skin where the mites have bitten.

Control

The most effective method to control mite bites is spraying clothing with insect repellent, such as products that contain dimethylphthalate.

Salmonellosis

Pathogen

Nontyphi *Salmonellae* are enteric facultatively anaerobic gram-negative bacilli in the family of Enterobacteriaceae. Identification is based on serotyping. Over 1,000 serotypes are known to infect humans. The majority of these strains can be grouped with polyvalent antisera into groups A to E. Definitive identification of serotype depends on reactivity to antisera directed against somatic O and flagellar H antigens. The relative frequencies with which specific serotypes are isolated varies among different geographic areas. *Salmonella typhimurium* is the most frequent *Salmonella* serotype isolated in the U.S.

Source of Infection

Whereas *S typhi* is a parasite specific for humans, the natural reservoir of nontyphi *Salmonellae* is a large variety of both wild and domestic animals (9). Animal to animal transmission can be facilitated by contamination of animal feed whose main ingredients are meal made from bone and meat. The most common source of human disease is poultry products such as eggs, chicken, turkey, and ducks, but meat from other animals is also involved. *Salmonella* on raw meat can contaminate utensils and surfaces where food is prepared and then be transferred to previously uncontaminated food. Cooking temperatures may not be high enough to lower the bacterial count sufficiently; in fact, the cooking temperatures found, for example, in the center of a stuffed turkey or soft-boiled or quick-scrambled egg, may actually foster bacterial growth.

Human Activity

Salmonellosis is acquired by ingestion of food or water contaminated by large numbers of organisms, e.g., $>10^5$ CFU/mL, when eating out or at home. Travelers' diarrhea is usually caused by any one of a variety of enteric pathogens, but is most commonly caused by enteropathogenic *Escherichia coli*, rather than nontyphi *Salmonella*. Direct transmission from person to person without food or water as the intervening vehicle does occur, usually by means of the fecal-oral route during male homosexual activity. Person to person spread has also been implicated in nursery and hospital outbreaks which involved patients in whom host defenses in the gastrointestinal tract, such as gastric acidity, small intestinal motility, and colonic bacterial flora are compromised, and lower inocula, i.e., $<10^5$ CFU/mL, are able to colonize the bowel and subsequently induce disease. Gastrointestinal defenses may be compromised by antacids, gastrectomy, agents that slow intestinal motility, and antibiotics. Some diseases, such as cirrhosis, lymphoma, and human immunodeficiency virus

(HIV) infection, which impair systemic host defenses, also increase susceptibility to salmonellosis. *Salmonella* that colonize and invade the intestinal mucosa may gain access to the bloodstream and produce transient bacteremia. Metastatic infection, usually in tissues that are previously diseased such as in hematomas, neoplasms, bone infarcts, degenerative arthritis, or even atherosclerotic abdominal aneurysms, may follow episodes of transient bacteremia. Control of *Salmonella* bacteremia is impaired in patients with an underlying hemolytic condition, such as sickle cell anemia. In fact, in patients with sickle cell anemia, *Salmonella*, rather than *Staphylococcus aureus*, is the most common cause of osteomyelitis in areas of bone compromised by ischemia or necrosis. Non typhoid salmonellosis is one of the most important bacterial infections in HIV-infected patients who are at risk for severe, recurrent bacteremic salmonella infection.

Human Disease

Non typhi *Salmonellae* cause an acute, self-limited, febrile, diarrheal disease of about 1 week's duration. Patients can carry *Salmonella* in the intestinal tract for several weeks, and more rarely for up to several months, during convalescence. Transient bacteremia is rarely detected in adult patients, but is more frequently detected in infancy (up to 50% in patients during the first week of life), as well as in elderly patients, and it is more common with some *Salmonella* species, such as *S cholerasuis*.

Control

Control is currently based on education of cooks at home and in commercial establishments about appropriate methods that will reduce contamination of food. Antibiotic therapy of infected patients, even with new potent agents such as the fluoroquinolones, does not shorten the course of the illness or ameliorate the symptoms, and fails to shorten the duration of the convalescent carrier state (10). Methods recommended for prevention of travelers' diarrhea applies to that of salmonellosis: use no ice in drinks; drink only bottled, carbonated beverages, hot tea or coffee, or beer; brush teeth with any of the aforementioned; eat only cooked, hot food; and eat no raw vegetables (e.g., salads), undercooked meats or fish, or peeled fruits (see section on travel-related illnesses).

Insect-Borne Togaviruses

Pathogens

Insect-borne encephalitis is caused by one of a group of related RNA viruses belonging to the family of Togaviruses that include the eastern equine and western equine encephalitis, St. Louis (11,12), Murray Valley, and Japanese B encephalitis agents (13,14). Sindbis and Ross River viruses are insect-borne Togaviruses that cause a nonencephalitic clinical picture (15).

Source of Infection

The distribution of western, eastern, and St. Louis encephalitis viruses overlaps extensively. For example, eastern equine virus has been isolated from eastern Canada, the Gulf and Atlantic coasts of the U.S., the Caribbean islands, and Central and South America. Western equine encephalitis and St. Louis equine encephalitis viruses also are distributed from Canada to Argentina. Japanese B encephalitis is found in most countries of the Far East and India. Sindbis virus is distributed in Africa, Asia, Australia, and the Philippines. The Ross River virus is distributed in northern and eastern Australia, and the Murray Valley virus in southern Australia and New Guinea. The natural reservoir of these viruses are native wild birds, among which the virus is spread by mosquitoes. Viral amplification in other birds or mammals may lead to epidemic outbreaks that involve domestic animals and humans, who are the accidental hosts. Epidemic outbreaks of encephalitis occur in late summer. With the equine encephalitis agents, outbreaks appear in horses prior to outbreaks of encephalitis in humans.

Human Activity

Habitation or travel in an area where insect-borne Togaviruses are endemic places a person at risk.

Human Disease

All these viruses, except for the Sindbis and Ross River viruses, produce an acute illness, with sudden onset of fever, headache, decreased sensorium, and stiff neck. More severe cases are complicated by progressive delirium, convulsions, coma, death, or residual neurological deficits in those who recover. Although eastern equine encephalitis occurs less frequently than St. Louis or western equine encephalitis, it has greater morbidity and mortality. Most cases of St. Louis encephalitis occur in those above 60 years of age, in whom the disease is particularly severe, whereas Murray Valley virus is more frequent and especially severe in children. Sindbis and Ross Valley viruses produce a mild illness characterized by fever, polyarthritis, jaundice, and a maculopapular or vesicular rash.

Control

Effective vaccines are available against Japanese B and western and eastern equine encephalitis. However, only the vaccine for Japanese

B encephalitis has been extensively used in humans. Mass vaccination programs have been carried out in several countries in the Far East, including Japan, Korea, and China, with good results in Japan. The vaccine is now available in the U.S. for prolonged travel to endemic regions. Prevention of these infections is usually limited to avoidance of mosquito bites through use of protective clothing, insect repellents on the body and clothing, and mosquito netting in dwellings in endemic areas. Eradication of the insect vectors has been effective, but costly.

Histoplasmosis

Pathogen

Histoplasmosis capsulatum is a dimorphic fungus: the yeast form grows in vitro at 37°C and in tissues; the mycelial form grows in vitro at room temperature. One variety of the organism (var. *duboisii*) has only been isolated in central Africa. The other variety is distributed worldwide, usually in major river valleys. In the U.S., infection is concentrated in the Mississippi, Missouri, and Ohio River valleys (16,17). Histoplasmosis is endemic in most of Latin America.

Source of Infection

The natural reservoir is soil, especially soils fertilized by bird or bat guano. Birds themselves are not infected, although some bats are infected and eliminate the fungus in their droppings. When contaminated soil is disturbed, for example, by bulldozing or razing old buildings, infectious aerosols of microconidia may be created; in poorly ventilated caves, tunnels, and mines inhabited by bats, the air may become heavily laden with infectious aerosols when disturbed by human activity (18,19).

Human Activity

Infection occurs in humans by inhalation of infectious aerosols when working at construction sites, or when visiting caves, tunnels, and abandoned mines in which bat droppings have accumulated.

Human Disease

In endemic areas infection is common, although the precise prevalence may vary from area to area. From 20% to over 81% of the population in endemic areas has a positive hypersensitivity reaction to the histoplasmin skin test, which indicates fast or current infection with *H capsulatum*.

The pathogenesis of histoplasmosis is thought to be identical to that of tuberculosis. The inhaled aerosols, particles less than 3 microns in diameter which may consist of only one or two infectious microconidia, easily bypass respiratory defense mechanisms in the upper respiratory tract and airways to lodge in the alveolus. In the lung, the microconidia may begin to grow and divide. Some particles may be engulfed by macrophages, which are eventually carried to regional lymph nodes. From there the intracellular pathogens are disseminated via lymphatics into the bloodstream, and then throughout the body to lodge in other reticuloendothelial organs such as the bone marrow, liver, and spleen (primary dissemination).

Clinical disease presents in a variety of ways. Acute pulmonary histoplasmosis resembles atypical pneumonia, the severity of which will depend on the number of infectious particles inhaled. Fever, headache, myalgias, and a dry, hacking cough develop initially. Several weeks after exposure to the infectious aerosol some patients develop erythema nodosum and arthralgias, probably at a time when the immune response first develops. With the onset of the immune response, further growth of the organisms is curtailed and the balance between the patient and the fungus is then temporarily cast in favor of the patient. Not all the organisms are killed, however; residual foci of latent infection remain, which can reactivate at any time in the future if host defenses should fail. In most patients acute pulmonary histoplasmosis is a self-limited process, and the only residual signs of this initial encounter with histoplasma microconidia are diffusely scattered foci of fine pulmonary or splenic calcifications.

Progressive pulmonary disease develops in a few patients. The initial pulmonary infiltrates develop into a fibronodular pattern and cavities that enlarge over months to years, but may become quiescent in some patients. Progressive pulmonary histoplasmosis is seen in older men with prior pulmonary disease.

Progressive dissemination with involvement primarily of the lung, liver, and bone marrow occurs rarely. Most of these patients have defects in cell-mediated immunity, e.g., patients with AIDS, severe debility, the very young or very old. The tempo of the illness may be acute or chronic, and is invariably fatal if untreated. It is manifest by hepatosplenomegaly, fever, night sweats, and mucosal ulcerations. Involvement of the bone marrow may produce anemia, leukopenia, and thrombocytopenia.

The var. *duboisii* produces granulomatous lesions in skin, subcutaneous soft tissue, and bone, in the form of abscesses and ulcerations.

A positive histoplasmin skin test indicates the presence of cellular immunity, but may be negative early in the course of disease or in patients with disseminated disease. It is used only for epidemiological purposes, not to diagnose a specific individual's illness. Indeed, the skin test may itself elicit an antibody response and confound the results of subsequent serologic testing. Serologic response, sputum culture, and culture and histology of biopsied tissues, e.g., bone marrow, liver, mucosal lesions, etc., are the main diagnostic methods.

Treatment is reserved for those patients with severe acute pulmonary, chronic progressive, and disseminated disease. Amphotericin B, 0.5 to 0.7 mg/kg intravenously daily for a total dose of 2 to 2.5 g has been standard therapy. Ketoconozole in doses of 400 mg orally daily for 6 or more months has proven equally effective (20).

Control

Control of the organism in the environment is difficult. Spraying of the ground with 3% formalin has been recommended, as has been the use of face masks when disturbing dirt or buildings where birds have roosted.

Cryptococcosis

Pathogen

Cryptococcus neoformans is a urease-positive yeast which has worldwide distribution. The organism exists in tissues in an encapsulated form, and in soil in an unencapsulated form. It reproduces both asexually as a yeast and sexually as a basidiomycete. *Cryptococcus* is identified in clinical specimens by detection of its polysaccharide capsule by mean of the India ink preparation, by use of mucicarmine stain of the polysaccharide capsule around the organism in tissue sections, or by means of an antibody to the capsular polysaccharide antigen in serum and other body fluids.

Source of Infection

Birds carry the organism in their intestinal tract without becoming ill. The organism is isolated from bird feces and soil contaminated with bird feces. The creatinine in the feces serves as a source of nitrogen for the organisms. Inhalation of an infectious aerosol, which is generated from contaminated dust or soil, is thought to be the mode of infection for humans. However the exact form of the infectious agent is unknown. The size of the encapsulated yeast (4 to 7 microns in diameter) may be too large to be an efficient aerosol. However, the unencapsulated yeast or the basidiospore, which measures 2 microns in diameter, may be a more appropriate size for the infectious particle.

Human Activity

Work in areas where pigeons roost or where soil is contaminated with pigeon feces poses a danger.

Human Disease

The portal of infection is thought to be the respiratory tract, although a minority of patients develop clinical manifestations of a respiratory illness. At the time most patients present with clinical cryptococcosis, they have extrapulmonary involvement, usually of the central nervous system, the asymptomatic primary pulmonary infection either having resolved spontaneously or left a residual pulmonary nodule (cryptococcoma). In the few patients with symptomatic pulmonary infection, the patients complain of fever, chest pain, cough, and hemoptysis, and, unless the patient is immunocompromised, the disease has not disseminated to extrapulmonary sites. Dissemination is likely in patients with AIDS, lymphoma, diabetes mellitus, cirrhosis, and those being treated with corticosteroids. Involvement of the central nervous system presents insidiously over weeks, with severe headache and progressive deterioration in mental status. The patient may have a stiff neck and focal cranial nerve signs. The cerebrospinal fluid will have a lymphocytic pleocytosis (5 to 500 white blood cell/cmm), low glucose concentration (<45 mg %), and high protein concentration (>45 mg %). In AIDS patients, but less so in others, the organisms are so numerous in the cerebrospinal fluid that they are readily visible on India ink preparation. In any case, the test for capsular polysaccharide antigen in the cerebrospinal fluid and serum, is positive in over 95% of patients, and is rarely falsely positive. In fact, the test in serum is more sensitive than that in cerebrospinal fluid in patients with AIDS. Patients may have focal neurological involvement as a consequence of cerebral cryptococcomas. Other sites for the development of disseminated disease include bone, skin, and prostate. The prostate has been implicated as a frequent site for relapsing infection after a course of antibiotic therapy.

Effective treatment for cryptococcal meningitis in patients without AIDS has been shown to be amphotericin B, 0.3 mg/kg intravenously daily combined with 5-flucytocine, 150 mg/kg in four divided oral doses daily for 6 weeks (21). In patients with AIDS, 5-flucytocine has been associated with an excessive bone marrow suppressive effect, and amphotericin B alone fails to eradicate the disease. After an initial course of 0.4 to 0.6 mg/kg of amphotericin B for at least 6 weeks, relapse of cryptococcal meningitis can be prevented in most patients with AIDS by giving 0.6 mg/kg intravenously weekly. Almost equally effective is fluconozole, 200 to 400 mg daily for 10 to 12 weeks after the last culture-positive cerebrospinal fluid culture. However, because of a slower initial response in clearance of cryptococci from the cerebrospinal fluid and excessive early mortality with fluconozole as compared to amphotericin B therapy, it is recommended that patients with AIDS be treated initially with amphotericin B, 0.6 mg/kg intravenously daily for 2 weeks, followed by fluconozole, 200 mg daily for the rest of the patient's life.

Control

Control of pigeon populations in areas of human habitation have been attempted for esthetic and health reasons with varying success.

References

1. Acha PN, Szyfres B. *Zoonoses and Communicable Diseases Common to Man and Animals*, 2nd ed. Pan American Health Organization, 1987.
2. Centers for Disease Control. Follow-up on turkey-associated psittacosis. *MMWR* 1974; 23:309–310.
3. Centers for Disease Control. Psittacosis associated with turkey processing—Ohio. *MMWR* 1982; 30:638–640.
4. Armstein P, Eddie B, Meyer KF. Control of psittacosis by group chemotherapy of infected parrots. *Am J Vet Res* 1968; 29:2213–2227.
5. Brandly CA. The occupational hazard of Newcastle disease to man. *Lab An Care* 1964; 14:433–440.
6. Wallner-Pendleton E, Cooper G. Several outbreaks of *Yersinia pseudotuberculosis* in California turkey flocks. *Avian Dis* 1983: 27:524–526.
7. World Health Organization Scientific Working Group. Enteric infections due to *Campylobacter, Yersina, Salmonella*, and *Shigella*. *Bull WHO* 1980; 58: 519–537.
8. Tertti R, Granfors K, Lehtonen O-P, et al. An outbreak of *Yersinia pseudotuberculosis* infection. *J Infect Dis* 1984; 149:245–250.
9. Bryan FL. Current trends in food-borne salmonellosis in the United States and Canada. *J Food Protect* 1981; 44:394–402.
10. Neill MA, Opal SM, Heelan J, et al. Failure of ciprofloxacin to eradicate convalescent fecal excretion after acute salmonellosis: Experience during an outbreak in health care workers. *Ann Intern Med* 1991; 114:195–199.
11. Centers for Disease Control. Arboviral infections of the central nervous systems—United States, 1986. *MMWR* 1987; 36(27):450–455.
12. Luby JP, Sulkin SE, Sanford JP. The epidemiology of St. Louis encephalitis: a review. *Annu Rev Med* 1969; 20:329–350.
13. Gatus BJ, Rose MR. Japanese B encephalitis; epidemiological, clinical and pathological aspects. *J Infect* 1983; 6:213–218.
14. Rosen L. The natural history of Japanese encephalitis virus. *Annu Rev Microbiol* 1986; 40:395–414.
15. Tesh RB. Arthritides caused by mosquito-borne viruses. *Annu Rev Med* 1982; 33:31–40.
16. Ajello L. Comparative ecology of respiratory mycotic disease agents. *Bacteriol Rev* 1967; 31:6–24.
17. Goodwin RA, DesPres RM. State of the Art. Histoplasmosis. *Am Rev Resp Dis* 1978; 117:929–956.
18. Hoff GL, Bigler WJ. The role of bats in the propagation and spread of histoplasmosis: a review. *J Wildl Dis* 1981; 17:191–196.
19. Schlech WF, Wheat LJ, Ho JL, et al. Recurrent urban histoplasmosis, Indianapolis, Indiana, 1980–1981. *Am J Epidemiol* 1983; 118:301–312.
20. Graybill JR, Drutz DJ. Ketoconozole: a major innovation for treatment of fungal disease. *Ann Intern Med* 1980; 93:921–923.
21. Bennett JE, Dismukes WE, Duma RJ, et al. A comparison of Amphotericin B alone or combined with flucytosive in the treatment of cryptococcal meningitis. *N Engl J Med* 1979; 301:126–131.

11
Rabies—At Home and Abroad

Daniel B. Fishbein and John W. Krebs

Introduction

Although rabies has been enzootic or epizootic in domestic or wild animals in the United States during most of the twentieth century, the disease has never been a serious problem among people in this country. During the first half of the century, only about 50 cases of human rabies—most caused by dogs—were reported each year (1). Following the control of canine rabies in the 1940s and 1950s, the number of indigenously acquired human rabies cases fell to an average of fewer than two per year during the 1960s and 1970s (2). Between 1980, when potent and safe tissue culture-derived rabies vaccines were introduced in the United States, and 1992, only seven persons are known to have acquired rabies in this country. All but two of these cases were attributed to insectivorous bats (3–7). None of the these cases were definitely attributable to leisure activities, although the exact circumstances of the exposure were sometimes unknown (5,7).

Wild animals are now indirectly responsible for most of both the economic and public health burden of the disease in the United States; since 1960, more wild than domestic animals have been reported rabid in this country. Annual expenditures for rabies prevention and control may exceed $1,000,000 per 100,000 population in some parts of the United States (8). The principal component of these expenditures is the routine vaccination of pets against rabies (8).

In contrast to the situation in the United States, canine rabies remains a serious threat for persons traveling to and living in developing countries. Largely because of the ubiquitous presence of dogs in human society in these countries, rates of human rabies sometimes exceed 1 per 100,000 population per year, and more than 1,000 per 100,000 people receive postexposure treatment each year (9). U.S. residents are at much higher risk of exposure to rabies in these countries than in the United States and have occasionally developed the disease when they failed to receive proper postexposure treatment (10). Four Americans living outside the United States acquired the disease since 1980; one other U.S. resident acquired the disease during a 2-month visit to India (11). In addition, five persons from countries with endemic rabies developed the disease while in the United States; each is believed to have acquired the disease before coming to this country.

Since the animal reservoirs and human risk groups differ so markedly inside and outside the United States, the epidemiology and prevention of rabies in these two areas will be considered separately.

Epidemiology of Rabies in the United States

The marked increase in outdoor activities, suburbanization, and close contact with pets provides countless situations in which humans can come into contact with animals in the United States. For this reason, rabies prevention is usually based on an understanding of the epidemiology of the disease in animals rather than analysis of individual activities that may put persons at risk.

Wild Animals

The number of rabies cases in wild animals has increased markedly since the 1950s. Numbers of rabid wild animals exceeded rabid domestic ones in 1960. By 1991 wild animals accounted for 91% of the 6,974 cases, and cases were reported in one or more wild species in 48 of the 50 states (Table 11.1, Fig. 11.1) (1).* Raccoons (*Procyon lotor*), skunks (*Mephitis mephitis*), and bats (*various species*) were responsible for 83.7% of the cases.

Monoclonal antibody analysis has allowed the rabies virus strains or variants affecting terrestrial wildlife in the United States to be classified into six distinct variants (12). Geographic separation of the outbreaks allows further division into 10 distinct outbreak areas. In each of these areas, other rabid terrestrial animals (including domestic) appear to acquire the disease as a result of spillover from wild animals. Recently, nucleotide sequencing has revealed more diversity of rabies virus strains (13,14).

Raccoons now account for the largest proportion of rabies cases. Although raccoon rabies has been enzootic in the Deep South since the 1950s, the disease was not present in the Mid-Atlantic states until 1978, when raccoons that were presumably incubating the disease were transported from the Deep South to stock hunting clubs (15). In 1990, for the first time, raccoons exceeded skunks as the predominant rabid wild animal. In 1991, the number of rabid raccoons increased 69.1% to 3,079

---

*Rhode Island did not report any cases of the disease; Hawaii reported one imported case of bat rabies but is still considered rabies free.

TABLE 11.1. Rabies in animals and humans, United States, 1991.

Type of animal	Number of states reporting cases	Number of cases	Percent change from 1990
Total	48*	6,975	+42.9
Wild Animals	48	6,354	+11.6
Raccoons	19	3,079	+69.1
Skunks	35	2,073	+31.3
Bats	47	690	+8.3
Foxes	25	318	+61.4
Groundhogs	6	55	+120.0
Mongooses	1	54	+63.6
Coyotes	4	50	+525.0
Deer	5	8	+300.0
Bobcats	4	6	−60.0
Opossums	4	6	+200.0
Beavers	3	3	†
Bears	2	2	†
Otters	2	2	†
Rabbits	1	2	†
Porcupines	1	1	†
Nutrias	1	1	†
Squirrels	1	1	0
Wolves	1	1	−66.0
Badgers	1	1	†
Domestic Animals	36	617	+11.6
Cats	27	189	+7.4
Dogs	28	155	+4.7
Cattle	23	217	+25.4
Horses/mules	18	44	−2.2
Goats/sheep	5	10	+11.1
Llamas	2	2	†
Swine	1	1	−50.0
Humans	3	3	+200.0

* Rhode Island did not report any cases of the disease; Hawaii (which is rabies free) reported one imported case of bat rabies.

cases. Raccoon rabies is now established in or threatens parts of all the Eastern Seaboard states. As this epizootic enters areas previously free of the disease (Philadelphia in 1988, New Jersey in 1989, New York State in 1990, and Connecticut in 1991), the public health community has been forced to allocate limited resources for public education, vaccination programs for domestic animals, and postexposure prophylaxis for humans (8). In spite of the spread of the disease and the marked increase in the number of cases, no raccoon-associated human cases have been reported in the United States.

During the 1980s and 1990s, a new approach to control of rabies in raccoons was developed and is now being field tested in raccoons. Oral

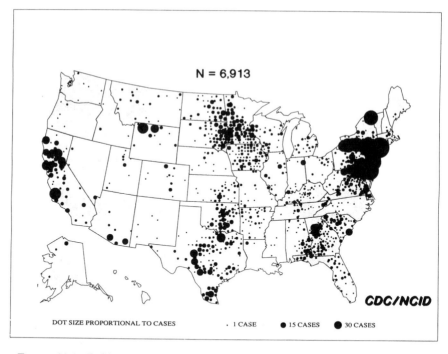

FIGURE 11.1. Rabies in animals in the United States, 1991. Cases by county; dot size proportional to number of cases in county.

vaccines for wildlife have now controlled and apparently nearly eliminated fox rabies in Switzerland and in large parts of Germany and France (16). A recombinant rabies vaccine for raccoons is now being tested in this species in the United States. The vaccine vector is the Copenhagen strain of vaccinia virus; the glycoprotein of rabies virus is inserted in the thymidine kinase region of the virus (17).

Two separate skunk rabies enzootics have been entrenched in the midwestern states since the late 1960s (18). One enzootic stretches from Alberta, Canada, south and east to Tennessee; the other, from Nebraska and Missouri south to (and presumably across) the Mexican border. The rabies virus variant circulating in skunks in northern California is similar to that in the North Central states. Although the number of reported rabid skunks decreased throughout most of the 1980s, there was an increase in the early 1990s (31.3% between 1990 and 1991 alone). This was the result of transmission of the disease from raccoons to skunks in the northeastern United States. The last case of human rabies that appears to have been skunk associated occurred in 1982 (3).

Four human rabies cases that occurred in the 1960s were definitely attributable to exposure during avocational activities. All four occurred in similar circumstances: children sleeping outdoors in an unprotected sleeping bag were bitten by skunks (three cases) or an unknown animal (one case) (19–22). No human cases known to be associated with avocational activities in the United States have been reported since 1970.

Bats are the most ubiquitous rabid animal in the United States. Rabies is present in at least 30 of the 39 species of bats indigenous to the United States and the temperate parts of Canada, and rabid bats are found in all states except Hawaii. Although the vast majority of rabies cases are attributable to the dominant terrestrial species in the area, bats do appear responsible for isolated cases of rabies in other animals (23). Perhaps most importantly, five of the seven human rabies cases known or suspected to be acquired in the United States in the period 1980 to 1992 were attributed to bats on epidemiological grounds, through virologic analysis, or both (4,5,7,24). More remarkably, most of the humans with rabies appear to have been infected by a single bat species, the silver-haired bat (*Lasionycteris noctivagans*). Although none of these cases were attributable to specific avocational pursuits, two spelunkers developed rabies in 1960 (25).

The reason that bats appear to be the animal that poses the most serious threat to humans in the United States since 1980 is unclear (Table 11.2). Although there was a slow increase in the number of bats reported rabid since rabies was recognized in insectivorous bats in the United States in the 1950s, the number of cases of rabies in bats remained fairly constant—between 500 and 1,000 per year—from 1975 through 1991. The number of humans bitten by bats is not particularly large, and rabid *Lasionycteris noctivagans* are not particularly common among bats submitted to state health departments (26). While the reason that bats pose such a serious threat to humans is unknown, it is clear that exposure to these animals must be treated with the utmost caution.

The number of rabies cases in other wild animals is relatively small, although the number of such animals reported rabid has increased markedly in the last few years because of the continuing spread of the raccoon rabies epizootic (Table 11.1). There were 318 rabid foxes reported in 1991; cases were reported from 25 states, reflecting the ability of terrestrial wild animals to infect other species. What appears to be a relatively small focus of fox rabies in northern New York is really the southern border of a large epizootic in Ontario, Canada, that was once connected with the epizootic in Alaska. Antigenically unrelated foci of fox rabies are found in gray foxes (*Urocyon cinereoargenteus*) in western Texas and Arizona (13).

In 1991, woodchucks (*Marmota monax*, one of the largest rodents) accounted for 87.3% of the reported rabies cases in rodents and lagomorphs. Probably because other rodents rarely survive the bite of the larger wild animal that exposes them to rabies, these smaller rodents (such as squirrels, hamsters, guinea pigs, gerbils, chipmunks, rats, and

TABLE 11.2. Human rabies, United States, 1980 to 1992:* location and circumstances of exposure and animal source.[†]

Location and circumstances of exposure	Presumed animal source[†]			
	Bat	Dog	Skunk	Unknown
Exposures in the United States				
In personal residence	2			
In public building	1			
Location/circumstances unknown	2	1	1	
Exposures outside of the United States				
Citizens or residents of the United States				
Traveling outside United States, bitten by stray		1		
Residing outside United States, bitten by stray		1		
Residing outside United States, bitten by pet		3		
Citizens of other countries				
Residing outside United States, bitten by stray		1		
Residing outside United States, circumstances unknown			3[‡]	1

* All laboratory-confirmed cases of rabies in humans who developed the disease in the United States and two U.S. citizens who were exposed to rabies and died of the disease outside the United States.
[†] In some cases where no exposure was known, monoclonal antibodies and/or nucleotide sequencing used to infer probable animal source of infection.
[‡] Three persons who were citizens of other countries when exposed to rabies who developed rabies after moving to the United States.

mice) and lagomorphs (including rabbits and hares) are almost never found to be infected with rabies. Another important rabid wild animal is the mongoose, which is a reservoir of rabies in Puerto Rico as well as other Caribbean islands (27).

Domestic Animals

Only one case of human rabies acquired in the United States since 1980 has been attributable to a domestic animal; the exact circumstances of transmission were never elucidated (6). Although the vast majority of rabies cases occur in wild animals, the vast majority of humans are treated as a result of exposure to domestic animals (28). This explains the tremendous cost of rabies prevention in domestic animals in the United States. While wild animals are more likely to be rabid than domestic ones in the United States, the amount of contact with domestic animals greatly exceeds the amount of human contact between humans and wild animals. Pets are therefore vaccinated to prevent them from acquiring the disease from wild animals and thereby transmitting it to humans. Nonetheless, hundreds of domestic animals acquire rabies from wild animals every year in the United States, and the risk of contact between humans and domestic animals seems to justify the recommendation and cost of vaccinating all dogs and cats. The occurrence of only one indigenously acquired human rabies case possibly attributable to a pet domestic animal in the United States since 1979 attests to the success of current prevention measures (see below).

Rabid domestic animals accounted for only 8.9% of all rabies cases in 1991. As in previous years, approximately equivalent numbers of cases were reported in dogs, cats, and cattle; the majority of these cases were reported from states where the disease is endemic or epidemic in raccoons or skunks. In 1991, 217 rabid cattle were reported, making this animal the most common rabid domestic species. Cattle were also the most common domestic host during most of the 1980s. However, a decrease in rabid cattle has occurred in parallel with a decrease in skunk rabies in the Midwest during this decade. Most cases still occur in areas with enzootic skunk rabies, although an increasingly large proportion are reported from states with raccoon rabies. Although most of the reported 189 rabid cats were from states affected by the raccoon rabies epizootic, 26 states and Puerto Rico reported at least one rabid cat. Dogs were the third most commonly reported rabid domestic animal. The 155 reported cases occurred primarily in states with rabid skunks, but in Texas, the state reporting the largest number of cases (36), most cases occurred in southern counties where an outbreak of dog and coyote rabies began in 1988. This is the only area in the United States where dog to dog transmission of rabies may be occurring. In 1991, cases of rabies were also reported in a few horses and mules, sheep and goats, and swine (Table 11.1). Monoclonal antibody analysis of rabies virus isolates from rabid domestic animals has demonstrated that these animals are almost always infected by the dominant terrestrial wildlife reservoir in the area.

Rabies Outside the United States

In most developing countries of Asia, Africa, and Central and South America, dogs are the major reservoir of rabies. The importance of rabid dogs in these countries, where tens of thousands of people die of the disease each year, cannot be overstated (9). Rates of postexposure prophylaxis in developing countries are about ten times higher than those in the United States, and rates of human rabies, approximately 100 times higher (9). In 1987, according to surveillance conducted by the World Health Organization, dogs were responsible for 91% of all human rabies cases, cats for 2%, other domestic animals for 3%, bats for 2%, foxes for 1%, and all other wild animals for fewer than 1% (29).

Of the 17 cases of human rabies reported in the United States (or in U.S. citizens living overseas) in the period 1980 to 1992, 10 were acquired in other countries (Table 11.2). Five were citizens or residents of the United States who were exposed to rabies abroad. (Each was bitten by a dog in a country where rabies is enzootic.) All of the other victims had come to the United States from countries where rabies is enzootic. One had been exposed to a dog only a few months earlier. The other four had no history of exposure to rabies. However, two had emigrated from Asia years before the onset of illness, and two were citizens of Mexico temporarily working in the United States (30–33). Genetic analysis of the virus strains from three of these five patients showed that the virus strain originated in their native countries and established minimum incubation periods of 1, 5, and 7 years (34).

Although the rate of rabies in persons traveling from the United States to endemic rabies countries is not known, two U.S. Peace Corps volunteers have acquired the disease, a rate in this population of seven per million per year (35). Travelers to countries where canine rabies is endemic are at high risk of exposure to rabies, and have occasionally developed the disease when they failed to receive advice before departure about the risk of exposure, preexposure immunization, or both (35). A second opportunity to prevent rabies is often missed when postexposure treatment is either not administered or administered incorrectly (10).

Apart from dogs and the wild animal species discussed earlier, other important hosts include vampire bats (in much of South America and parts of Central America and Mexico), and mongooses (in Cuba, Puerto Rico, Grenada, and the Dominican Republic) (27,36). In Europe, red foxes (*Vulpes fulva*) are the major host. Black-backed jackals (*Canis mesomelas*) and yellow mongooses (*Cynictis penicillata*) are important hosts in some parts of southern Africa, and wolves (*Canis lupus*) are an important reservoir in Iran and Turkey. In some republics of the former Soviet Union and parts of Poland and Finland, a new wild reservoir, the raccoon dog (*Nyctereutes procyonoides*), has been an increasingly important host.

Prevention of Human Rabies

The marked decrease in the number of human rabies cases in the United States since 1950 was the direct result of the control of canine rabies. Although attributing any of the decrease to the introduction of potent tissue culture-derived vaccines in the 1980s is difficult, the efficacy and extremely low rate of adverse reactions of tissue culture-derived vaccines cannot be disputed.

Prevention and Interpretation of Exposures

Although only seven people are known to have acquired rabies in the United States from 1980 through 1992, tens of thousands of people in the United States are exposed each year to animals capable of carrying the disease. The most effective way to prevent exposure to rabies is to warn the public to avoid contact with all wild animals and unfamiliar domestic animals. In addition, all pet dogs and cats should be vaccinated, and wild animals (many of which are extremely susceptible to rabies) should not be kept as pets. Because of the high incidence of human rabies and postexposure treatments in developing countries—among both residents and visitors—travelers to these countries should be counseled to avoid contact with dogs and other reservoirs of the disease. In addition, persons at risk of unavoidable contact with such animals in enzootic rabies areas (usually those traveling to these areas for more than 30 days) should receive preexposure prophylaxis (37).

Evaluation of humans with possible exposures to rabies

Every year in the Untied States, more than 20,000 persons receive rabies postexposure prophylaxis and approximately 10,000 more receive pre-exposure prophylaxis. Although canine rabies has been controlled, dogs remain responsible for the majority of these antirabies treatments (28). Two unrelated factors explain this anomaly: the close association and frequent contact between dogs and humans, and the unwillingness of the medical and public health community to accept even a minute risk of rabies developing in a person bitten by a domestic animal which cannot be observed or tested for rabies.

Appropriate management of persons who may have been exposed to rabies depends on the rapid interpretation of the risk of infection. Each possible exposure to rabies should be evaluated by a physician; local or state public health officials should be consulted if questions remain. In the United States, the following factors should always be considered: the type of exposure, the local epidemiology of rabies, and the health and vaccination status of the exposing species (37).

Rabies is only transmitted when the virus is introduced into open cuts or wounds in skin or mucous membranes. Thus, if the virus could not have been introduced or the material containing the virus was dry, postexposure treatment is not necessary. Contact such as petting a rabid animal and contact with the blood, urine, or feces (e.g., guano) of a rabid animal, does not by itself constitute an exposure and is not an indication for prophylaxis.

It is useful to divide possible exposure into bite and nonbite types. Any penetration of the skin by teeth constitutes a *bite exposure*. Bites are responsible for almost all rabies cases because a relatively large quantity of virus must be inoculated to cause disease. Although bites carry the highest risk when the face is involved and the lowest risk when the lower extremity is involved, the site of the bite only rarely influences the decision to begin treatment (38).

Scratches, abrasions, open wounds, or mucous membranes contaminated with saliva or other potentially infectious material (such as brain tissue) from a rabid animal constitute *nonbite exposures*. Although occasional reports of transmission by nonbite exposure suggest that such exposures are sufficient reason to begin postexposure prophylaxis, nonbite exposures rarely cause rabies (39). The limited risk of nonbite exposures (such as scratches and licks) to rabid animals is demonstrated by the unusual nature of the two types of exposures most consistently implicated in the nonbite transmission of rabies: corneal transplantation and inhalations. The cases of rabies in recipients of transplanted corneas in Thailand (two cases), India (two cases), the United States (one case), and France (one case) are also the only documented cases of human to human transmission of rabies. Retrospective investigations found that each of the donors had died of an illness compatible with or proven to be rabies. Of the four cases of rabies attributable to aerosol exposures, two occurred in rabies research laboratories and two in bat-infested caves in Texas.

The Exposing Animal

Information about the epidemiology of animal rabies in the geographic area where the exposure occurred is essential to the proper treatment of the patient and prevention of the disease. Exposure to specific domestic and wild animal species are extremely dangerous in some parts of the country and relatively free of risk in other parts.

Carnivorous wild animals (especially skunks, raccoons, and foxes) and bats are the animals most often rabid, and are the cause of most of the indigenously acquired human rabies in the Untied States since 1960 (40). These animals constitute the most important potential source of infection for humans in the United States. All bites by wild carnivores and bats must be considered possible exposure to rabies; in areas where the disease is endemic in these animals, up to 34% of these animals submited for testing are found positive for the disease (41). The signs of rabies in carnivorous wild animals and the period of rabies virus shedding cannot be interpreted reliably; (15) therefore, any such animal that bites or scratches a person should be killed at once (without unnecessary damage to the head) and the brain submitted for rabies testing. If a person is bitten by such an animal, postexposure prophylaxis should be initiated as soon as possible unless the animal has already been tested and found not to be rabid. Treatment can be discontinued if the brain is negative by immunofluorescence.

Many types of exotic pets (such as ferrets) and domestic animals crossbred with wild animals are highly susceptible to rabies and should therefore be considered as wild animals in evaluating the need for treatment. Such animals should not be kept as pets. When the biting animal is a particularly rare or valuable specimen (e.g., exotic pet, zoo animal), public health authorities may choose to recommend postexposure treatment of the bite victim in lieu of killing the animal for rabies testing (42). Since rodents rarely are found rabid, state or local health department officials should be consulted before a decision is made to initiate postexposure antirabies prophylaxis for a person bitten by a rodent.

The likelihood that a domestic animal is infected with rabies varies from region to region; hence, the need for postexposure prophylaxis also varies. In the continental United States, dog rabies is reported commonly along the U.S.–Mexico border, and sporadically from the areas of the United States with enzootic wildlife rabies, especially the Midwest. Rabid cats are now more common than rabid dogs, possibly because of fewer cat vaccination laws, fewer leash laws, and the roaming habits of cats. Most cases of cat rabies have occurred in states affected by the Mid-Atlantic raccoon rabies epizootic.

In areas where canine rabies is not enzootic (including virtually all of the United States and its territories), a healthy domestic dog or cat that bites a person should be confined and observed for 10 days. Any illness in the animal during confinement or before release should be evaluated by a veterinarian and reported immediately to the local health department. If signs suggestive of rabies develop, or the animal is a stray or unwanted dog or cat, the animal should be killed immediately and the head removed and shipped, under refrigeration, for rabies examination by a qualified laboratory (42). If the dog or cat is unavailable for observation, other epidemiological factors should be taken into account. An unprovoked attack by a domestic animal is more likely than a provoked attack to indicate that the animal was rabid. Bites inflicted on a person attempting to feed or handle an apparently healthy animal should generally be regarded as provoked. A fully vaccinated dog or cat is very unlikely to become infected with rabies. In a nationwide study of dog and cat rabies in 1988, only one dog and two cats that were currently vaccinated developed rabies; all three of these animals had received only a single dose of vaccine (43). Rare documented vaccine failures have also occurred in dogs or cats that received two vaccinations (44).

In most developing countries, exposures to dogs carry an extremely high risk (45). In such areas, postexposure rabies treatment should be initiated immediately following exposure. Treatment can be discontinued if the dog or cat remains healthy during the 10-day observation period (37). As stated before, all five of the U.S. residents who acquired rabies while traveling or living outside the country since 1980 had exposures that were not properly managed. In each case, either the victim did not recognize the risk of rabies or obtained incorrect advice regarding treatment (11,46–49). Although dogs are the main reservoir of rabies throughout much of the world, the epizootiology of the disease in other animals differs sufficiently from one region or country to another to warrant the evaluation of all animal bites in these countries.

Postexposure Treatment Regimen

The essential components of postexposure treatment are local treatment of wounds and immunization. Extensive laboratory evidence and field experience in many areas of the world indicates that the combination of local wound treatment, passive immunization, and vaccination is uniformly effective when appropriately administered (50,51). However, rabies has occasionally developed in humans when key elements of postexposure prophylaxis were omitted or incorrectly administered. The two essential components of rabies postexposure prophylaxis are local wound treatment and vaccination, including the administration, in most instances, of both rabies immune globulin (RIG) and vaccine. Treatment should begin within 24 hours after bites by animals strongly suspected of being or proven rabid.

Immediate and thorough washing of all bite wounds and scratches with soap and water is perhaps the most effective measure for preventing rabies; tetanus prophylaxis and measures to control bacterial infection should be given as indicate. In experimental animals, simple local wound cleansing has been shown to markedly reduce the likelihood of rabies (52). The decision to suture large wounds should take into account cosmetic factors, the potential for bacterial infections, and the possibility of inoculating rabies virus deeply into the wound.

The combination of human rabies immune globulin (HRIG) (local and systemic) and vaccine is recommended for both bite and nonbite exposures, regardless of the interval between exposure and initiation of treatment. There have been instances in which the decision to begin treatment was made many months after the exposure because of delay in recognizing that an exposure had occurred and awareness that incubation periods of more than 1 year have been reported.

The first postexposure regimen to include tissue culture vaccines was the one recommended by the World Health Organization in 1977. The regimen, which was based on studies in Germany and Iran, combined passive immunization with a single dose of RIG and active immunization with six doses of HDCV administered over a 90-day period.

When used this way, the vaccine was found to be safe and effective in protecting persons bitten by proven rabid animals and induced an excellent antibody response in all recipients (51). Studies conducted in the United States by the Centers for Disease Control have shown that a regimen of HRIG and five doses of HDCV over a period of 28 days also induced an excellent antibody response in all recipients (50).

Two rabies vaccines are currently available in the United States; either is administered in conjunction with HRIG at the beginning of postexposure therapy. Five 1-mL doses of HDCV or rabies vaccine adsorbed (RVA) should be given intramuscularly. The first dose should be given as soon as possible after exposure; one additional dose should be given on days 3, 7, 14, and 28 after the first vaccination. For adults, the vaccine should always be administered in the deltoid area. For children, the anterolateral aspect of the thigh is also acceptable. The gluteal area should never be used for HDCV injections because administration in this area results in lower neutralizing antibody titers (53).

The recent withdrawal of the only RIG of equine origin from the commercial market in the United States leaves HRIG as the only form of RIG available in this country. HRIG is administered only once, at the beginning of antirabies prophylaxis, to provide immediate antibodies until the patient responds to HDCV or RVA by active production of antibodies. If HRIG was not given when vaccination was begun, it can be given through the seventh day after administration of the first dose of vaccine. From the eighth day on, HRIG is not indicated since an antibody response to cell culture vaccine is presumed to have occurred. The recommended dose of HRIG is 20 IU/kg. This formula is applicable for all age groups, including children. If anatomically feasible, up to one-hlaf the dose of RIG should be thoroughly infiltrated in the area around the wound and the rest should be administered intramuscularly in the gluteal area. RIG should never be administered in the same syringe or into the same anatomical site as vaccine. Because RIG may partially suppress active production of antibody, no more than the recommended dose should be given (54).

For persons who have been previously vaccinated, two intramuscular (IM) doses (1.0 mL each) of vaccine should be administered, one immediately and one 3 days later. "Previously vaccinated" refers to persons who have received one of the recommended preexposure or postexposure regimens of HDCV or RVA, or those who received another regimen and had a documented rabies antibody titer. RIG is unnecessary and should not be given in these cases because an anamnestic antibody response will follow the administration of a booster regardless of the prebooster antibody titer (55).

Postexposure Failures

Although there have been no postexposure vaccine failures in the United States during the 10 years that HDCV has been licensed, seven persons outside the United States have contracted rabies after receiving postexposure treatment with both RIG and HDCV. Six other people have developed the disease after receiving active immunization with other cell culture-derived vaccines and HRIG or antirabies serum of equine origin. However, in each of these cases, there was some deviation from the recommended postexposure treatment protocol (56–59). Specifically, patients who developed rabies after postexposure prophylaxis did not have their wounds cleansed with soap and water or other antiviral agents, received their rabies vaccine injections in the gluteal area instead of the deltoid area, or did not receive passive immunization around the wound site.

Preexposure Vaccination

Preexposure vaccination should be offered to persons in high-risk groups, such as veterinarians, animal handlers, certain laboratory workers, and persons spending time (e.g., 1 month or more) in foreign countries where rabies is enzootic. Persons whose pursuits bring them into frequent contact with rabies virus or potentially rabid dogs, cats, skunks, raccoons, bats, or other species at risk of having rabies should also be considered for preexposure prophylaxis. However, preexposure prophylaxis is not recommended for hunters and other outdoor enthusiasts who may occasionally be exposed to the disease. Such persons should be able to recognize exposures and report them to medical authorities and exposures are rare enough that the cost of administering preexposure prophylaxis to the entire group at risk almost always exceeds that of administering postexposure prophylaxis to those who are exposed (60).

Although administration of rabies preexposure prophylaxis to persons traveling to rabies-enzootic areas may not be strictly cost beneficial, preexposure prophylaxis is recommended for persons traveling to rabies-enzootic countries for more than 30 days. Preexposure vaccination is given for the following reasons: 1) it may provide protection to persons with inapparent exposures to rabies; 2) it may protect persons whose postexposure therapy might be delayed; 3) although preexposure immunization *does not eliminate* the need for additional therapy after a rabies exposure, it simplifies therapy by eliminating the need for RIG and decreasing the number of doses of vaccine needed. This last reason is of particular importance for persons at high risk of being exposed to rabies in areas where immunizing products may not be available or where they may carry a high risk of adverse reactions.

The primary preexposure IM vaccination regimen, consisting of three 1.0 mL injections of HDCV or RVA, should be given in the deltoid area, one each on days 0, 7, and 28. Intradermal (ID) preexposure prophylaxis may be administered with a special syringe developed for that purpose; the 0.1 mL dose is administered in the deltoid area following the same schedule as the IM regimen discussed above (61). Serologic testing is not necessary except for persons suspected of being immunosuppressed. 3-dose 0.1 mL ID dose/route has been recommended by the Immunization Practices Advisory Committee as an alternative to the 1.0 mL IM dose/route for rabies preexposure prophylaxis with HDCV; *RVA should not be given by the ID dose/route* (62).

Chloroquine phosphate (administered for malaria chemoprophylaxis) interferes with the antibody response to HDCV (63). In persons traveling to malaria endemic countries, HDCV should not be administered by the

ID dose/route while the person is receiving chloroquine (64). The IM dose/route of preexposure prophylaxis provides a sufficient margin of safety in this situation (64). For persons who will be receiving both rabies preexposure prophylaxis and chloroquine in preparation for travel to a rabies-enzootic area, the ID dose/route should be initiated at least 1 month before travel to allow completion of the full three-dose vaccine series before antimalarial prophylaxis begins. If this is not possible, the IM dose/route should be used. Although interference with the immune response to rabies vaccine by other antimalarials structurally related to chloroquine (e.g., mefloquine) has not been evaluated, following similar precautions for persons receiving these antimalarials seems prudent.

Because persons who work with live rabies virus in research laboratories or vaccine production facilities are at the highest risk of inapparent exposures, they should submit a serum sample for rabies antibody testing every 6 months. Booster doses (IM or ID) of vaccine should be given, as needed, to maintain a serum titer corresponding to at least complete neutralization at a 1:5 serum dilution by the rapid fluorescent focus inhibition test (RFFIT). Other laboratory workers, such as those doing rabies diagnostic testing, spelunkers, veterinarians and staff, animal control and wildlife officers in areas where animal rabies is epizootic, and international travelers living in or visiting (for more than 30 days) areas where canine rabies is a constant threat should have a serum sample tested for rabies antibody every 2 years. If the titer is less than 1:5 (complete neutralization) by the RFFIT, these persons should have a booster dose of vaccine. Alternatively, a booster can be administered in lieu of a titer determination. Veterinarians, animal control workers, and wildlife officers working in areas of low rabies enzooticity do not require routine preexposure booster doses of HDCV or RVA after completion of primary preexposure immunization.

Summary

Despite widespread epizootics of rabies in terrestrial wildlife, these animals are known to have caused only one human death in this country since 1980. No one avocationally (or vocationally) exposed to rabies is known to have acquired the disease since 1977, when a laboratory worker developed rabies following an accident in a research facility (65). In the 1980s and 1990s, insectivorous bats appear to have been responsible for five of the seven of human rabies cases acquired in the United States, but none of these individuals were in groups known to be at increased risk of exposure. Only three of seven victims appear to have recognized their exposures, and none of these three reported their exposures to medical or public health personnel. Perhaps the most important observation regarding these cases is the difficulty in developing strategies that might have prevented them. All seven indigenously acquired cases appear to be have been almost completely unpreventable. Nonetheless, the thousands of wildlife reported rabid each year serve as reminders that the disease continues to pose a threat to the outdoor enthusiast who may come in contact with these animals. People living in the United States should be advised to avoid contact with wild animals and stray or ill-appearing domestic animals.

Enzootic canine rabies in developing countries is, perhaps, the most serious threat to Americans, although again the casual traveler appears at lower risk than people residing outside the United States. Travelers to such countries can substantially reduce the risk of rabies exposure by avoiding all dogs as well as wild animals; those persons whose risk of exposure cannot be reduced should be educated about rabies and receive preexposure vaccination.

References

1. Held JR, Tierkel ES, Steele JH. Rabies in man and animals in the United States, 1946–65. *Public Health Rep* 1967; 82:1009–1018.
2. Anderson LJ, Nicholson KG, Tauxe RV, Winkler WG. Human rabies in the United States, 1960 to 1979: epidemiology, diagnosis, and prevention. *Ann Intern Med* 1984; 100:728–735.
3. Centers for Disease Control. Human rabies—Oklahoma. *MMWR* 1981; 30:343–349.
4. Centers for Disease Control. Human rabies—Michigan. *MMWR* 1983; 32:159–160.
5. Centers for Disease Control. Human rabies—Pennsylvania. *MMWR* 1984; 33:633–635.
6. Centers for Disease Control. Human rabies—Texas, 1990. *MMWR* 1991; 40:132–133.
7. Centers for Disease Control. Human rabies—Texas, Arkansas, and Georgia, 1991. *MMWR* 1991; 40:765–769.
8. Uhaa IJ, Dato VM, Sorhage FE, et al. Epizootic raccoon rabies: cost of control and economic benefits of an oral vaccine. *J Am Vet Med Assoc* 1992; In press.
9. Bögel K, Motschwiller E. Incidence of rabies and post-exposure treatment in developing countries. *Bull WHO* 1986; 64:883–887.
10. Devriendt J, Staroukine M, Costy F, Vanderhaeghen JJ. Fatal encephalitis apparently due to rabies. Occurrence after treatment with human diploid cell vaccine but not rabies immune globulin. *JAMA* 1982; 248:2304–2306.
11. Centers for Disease Control. Human rabies—California, 1992. *MMWR* 1992; 41:461–463.
12. Reid-Sanden FL, Dobbins JG, Smith JS, Fishbein DB. Rabies surveillance in the United States during 1989. *J Am Vet Med Assoc* 1990; 197:1571–1583.
13. Smith JS. Rabies virus epitopic variation: use in ecologic studies. *Adv Virus Res* 1989; 36:215–253.

14. Smith JS, Orciari LA, Yager PA, Seidel HD, Warner CK. Epidemiological and historical relationships among 87 rabies virus isolates as determined by limited sequence analysis. *J Infect Dis* 1992; 166:296–307.
15. Jenkins SR, Winkler WG. Descriptive epidemiology from an epizootic of raccoon rabies in the Middle Atlantic States, 1982–1983. *Am J Epidemiol* 1987; 126:429–437.
16. Wandeler AI, Capt S, Kappeler A, Hauser R. Oral immunization of wildlife against rabies: concept and first field experiments. *Rev Infect Dis* 1988; 10 (4 Suppl):S649–653.
17. Rupprecht CE, Hamir AN, Johnston DH, Koprowski H. Efficacy of a vaccinia-rabies glycoprotein recombinant virus vaccine in raccoons (Procyon lotor). *Rev Infect Dis* 1988; 10 (4 Suppl):S803–809.
18. Charlton KM, Webster WA, Casey GA, Rupprecht CE. Skunk rabies. *Rev Infect Dis* 1988; 10 (4 Suppl):S626–628.
19. Hattwick MA, Hochberg FH, Landrigan PJ, Gregg MB. Skunk-associated human rabies. *JAMA* 1972; 222:44–47.
20. Gomez MR, Siekert RG, Herrmann EC. A human case of skunk rabies. Case report with comment on virological studies and the prophylactic treatment. *JAMA* 1965; 194:333–335.
21. Bell GR. Death from rabies in ten-year-old boy (one of two cases in United States in 1966). *S D J Med* 1967; 20:28–29.
22. Uhaa IJ, Mandel EJ, Whiteway R, Fishbein DB. Rabies surveillance in the United States during 1990. *J Am Vet Med Assoc* 1992; 200:920–929.
23. Smith JS. Monoclonal antibody studies of rabies in insectivorous bats of the United States. *Rev Infect Dis* 1988; 10(Suppl 4):S637–643.
24. Centers for Disease Control. Human rabies—Texas, 1990. *MMWR* 1991; 40:132–133.
25. Humphrey GL, Kemp GE, Wood EG. A fatal case of rabies in a woman bitten by an insectivorous bat. *Public Health Rep* 1960; 75:317–326.
26. Constantine DG. An updated list of rabies-infected bats in North America. *J Wildl Dis* 1979; 15:347–349.
27. Everard CO, Everard JD. Mongoose rabies. *Rev Infect Dis* 1988; 10 (4 Suppl):S610–614.
28. Helmick CG. The epidemiology of human rabies postexposure prophylaxis, 1980–1981. *JAMA* 1983; 250:1990–1996.
29. Veterinary Public Health Unit. World Survey of Rabies XXII (for years 1984/85). Geneva: World Health Organization, 1987. *Who/Rabies/87.189*.
30. Centers for Disease Control. Human rabies—Texas. *MMWR* 1984; 33:469–470.
31. Centers for Disease Control. Human rabies—California, 1987. *MMWR* 1988; 37:305–308.
32. Centers for Disease Control. Human rabies diagnosed 2 months postmortem—Texas. *MMWR* 1985; 34:700,705–707.
33. Centers for Disease Control. Human rabies—Oregon, 1989. *MMWR* 1989; 38:335–337.
34. Smith JS, Fishbein DB, Rupprecht CE, Clark K. Unexplained rabies in three immigrants in the United States. A virologic investigation. *N Engl J Med* 1991; 324:205–211.

35. Bernard KW, Fishbein DB. Pre-exposure rabies prophylaxis for travellers: are the benefits worth the cost? *Vaccine* 1991; 9:833–836.

36. Lopez A, Miranda P, Tejada E, Fishbein DB. Outbreak of human rabies in the Peruvian jungle. *Lancet* 1992; 339:408–411.

37. Centers for Disease Control. Rabies prevention—United States, 1991. Recommendations of the Immunization Practices Advisory Committee (ACIP). *MMWR* 1991; 40:1–19.

38. Hattwick MAW. Human rabies. *Public Health Rev* 1974; 3:229–274.

39. Afshar A. A review of non-bite transmission of rabies virus infection. *Br Vet J* 1979; 135:142–148.

40. Eng TR, Hamaker TA, Dobbins JG, Tong TC, Bryson JH, Pinsky PF. Rabies surveillance, United States, 1988. *MMWR* 1989; 38(No. SS-1):1–21.

41. Fishbein DB. Rabies. *Infect Dis Clin North Am* 1991; 5:53–71.

42. Centers for Disease Control. Compendium of animal rabies control. *J Am Vet Med Assoc* 1990; 196:36–39.

43. Eng TR, Fishbein DB. Epidemiologic factors, clinical findings, and vaccination status of rabies in cats and dogs in the United States in 1988. *J Am Vet Med Assoc* 1990; 197:201–209.

44. Centers for Disease Control. Imported dog and cat rabies—New Hampshire, California. *MMWR* 1988; 37:559–560.

45. Wilde H, Chutivongse S, Tepsumethanon W, Choomkasien P, Polsuwan C, Lumbertdacha B. Rabies in Thailand: 1990. *Rev Infect Dis* 1991; 13:644–652.

46. Centers for Disease Control. Imported human rabies. *MMWR* 1983; 32:78–80,85–86

47. Centers for Disease Control. Human rabies—Kenya. *MMWR* 1983; 32:494–495.

48. Centers for Disease Control. Human rabies—Rwanda. *MMWR* 1982; 31:135.

49. Centers for Disease Control. Human rabies acquired outside the United States from a dog bite. *MMWR* 1981; 30:537–540.

50. Anderson LJ, Sikes RK, Langkop CW, et al. Postexposure trial of a human diploid cell strain rabies vaccine. *J Infect Dis* 1980; 142:133–138.

51. Bahmanyar M, Fayaz A, Nour-Salehi S, Mohammadi M, Koprowski H. Successful protection of humans exposed to rabies infection. Postexposure treatment with the new human diploid cell rabies vaccine and antirabies serum. *JAMA* 1976; 236:2751–2754.

52. Dean DJ, Baer GM. Studies on the local treatment of rabies infected wounds. *Bull WHO* 1963; 28:477–486.

53. Fishbein DB, Sawyer LA, Reid-Sanden FL, Weir EH. Administration of human diploid-cell rabies vaccine in the gluteal area [letter]. *N Engl J Med* 1988; 318:124–125.

54. Helmick CG, Johnstone D, Sumner J, Winkler WG, Fager S. A clinical study of Merieux human rabies immune globulin. *J Biol Standard* 1982; 10:357–367.

55. Fishbein DB, Bernard KW, Miller KD, et al. The early kinetics of the neutralizing antibody response after booster immunizations with human diploid cell rabies vaccine. *Am J Trop Med Hyg* 1986; 35:663–670.

56. Centers for Disease Control. Human rabies despite treatment with rabies immune globulin and human diploid cell rabies vaccine—Thailand. *MMWR* 1987; 36:759–760,765.

57. Shill M, Baynes RD, Miller SD. Fatal rabies encephalitis despite appropriate post-exposure prophylaxis. A case report. *N Engl J Med* 1987; 316:1257–1258.

58. Wilde H, Choomkasien P, Hemachudha T, Supich C, Chutivongse S. Failure of rabies postexposure treatment in Thailand. *Vaccine* 1989; 7:49–52.

59. Fescharek R, Quast U, Dechert G. Postexposure rabies vaccination during pregnancy: experience from post-marketing surveillance with 16 patients [letter; comment]. *Vaccine* 1990; 8:409.

60. Mann JM. Routine pre-exposure rabies prophylaxis: a reassessment. *Am J Public Health* 1984; 74:720–722.

61. Centers for Disease Control. Rabies prevention: supplementary statement on the preexposure use of human diploid cell rabies vaccine by the intradermal route. *MMWR* 1986; 35:767–768.

62. Center for Disease Control. Rabies vaccine, adsorbed: a new rabies vaccine for use in humans. *MMWR* 1988; 37:217–223.

63. Pappaioanou M, Fishbein DB, Dreesen DW, et al. Antibody response to preexposure human diploid-cell rabies vaccine given concurrently with chloroquine. *N Engl J Med* 1986; 314:280–284.

64. Benard KW, Fishbein DB, Miller KD, et al. Pre-exposure rabies immunization with human diploid cell vaccine: decreased antibody responses in persons immunized in developing countries. *Am J Trop Med Hyg* 1985; 34:633–647.

65. Centers for Disease Control. Rabies in a laboratory worker—New York. *MMWR* 1977; 26:183–184.

12
Eating Yuppie Cuisine

J.K. Griffiths and Gerald T. Keusch

Introduction

Fashions in food have always carried the cachet of class and trendiness; sometimes the cost is illness. As travel has expanded the locales that the traveler may visit, it has also expanded the range of food-related illnesses that may be acquired by the individual on vacation. Moreover, one needn't be traveling to acquire these maladies, as sometimes they travel to you. Tongue-in-cheek, we have named this chapter "Eating Yuppie Cuisine," but of course as fashions in food and travel spread from the trendiest group in society to the society at large, the pool of people at risk increases, including those who do not fill the stereotype of the "yuppie."

Many foods, when eaten in their freshest and tastiest form—such as raw seafood or unpasteurized dairy products—can be a vector for bacteria, viruses, and parasites injurious to the consumer. Some of these pathogens are well-known human pathogens, and some are zoonoses that would not normally infect humans. And while some of the aquatic parasites found in sushi cannot develop into mature forms within humans, but only in marine sea mammals (such as sea lions' unpleasant *Anasakis* parasite), the larvae can cause dreadful symptoms in humans.

With the current trends towards freshness and purity, there has also been a trend towards home production of foods. Some of these, such as yogurt and mayonnaise, are wonderful culture media for specific bacteria (*Staphylococcus aureus, Salmonella* species). For toxin-mediated diseases, cooking or heating the food/culture media may kill a bacterium, but leave the toxin to do its damage. Patterns of food storage also can dispose towards disease; in some parts of the world, such as Africa and Asia, uneaten rice is stored overnight and eaten for breakfast. Unfortunately *Vibrio cholerae*, the etiological agent of Asiatic cholera, has been shown in recent CDC studies (1) to be capable of increasing in number in rice from 10^2/gm to over 10^{10}/gm during storage. The adventurous traveler who partakes of such a breakfast may be greatly surprised, to say the least!

Raw Fish and Seafood: Worms in the Time of Cholera

Perhaps no foodstuff is more stereotypical of yuppie cuisine than sushi, in which the freshest of fish and seafood is matched with rice, pickled vegetables, and other condiments. Originally a Japanese cuisine, it has become universal. Similarly, the Latin American and Caribbean dishes of raw seafood marinated in acidic fruit juices, such as ceviche, have attracted attention in other societies because of their purity of flavor and their novelty. Many cultures have long been attracted to other raw seafoods, such as herring and oysters in Europe, sea urchins in the Mediterranean, etc.

Much attention has been focused of late on anisakiasis, a potentially catastrophic disease caused by the larval stages of the marine nematodes of the family Anisakidae (2), sometimes called "herring worms." These parasites are usually found in the stomachs of large sea mammals: humans are infected as dead-end hosts for the parasite. *Pseudoterranova decipiens*, a common offender, is a pathogen of seals, sea lions, and walruses, while *Anisakis simplex* is a parasite of porpoises and whales. Larvae develop first in small crustaceans, and develop further in fish and squid which serve as transport hosts until the larvae are eaten by the definitive host. Sea creatures that may harbor the parasite include cod, sole, flounder, fluke, salmon, mackeral, herring, octopus, and squid (3). Many of these make delicate sushi and sashimi. Larval forms are ingested when raw fish is eaten, which is the usual manner in which a sea mammal is infected with a larval parasite, although humans may be vulnerable to raw, pickled, salted, or undercooked fish. In surveys, the prevalence of this group of parasites is higher in the Pacific than in the Atlantic Ocean, perhaps reflecting the higher number of sea mammals in the Pacific Ocean.

The hallmark of anisakiasis is acute pain, which may be intermittent or constant, beginning 1 to 12 hours after eating raw fish. Freezing the fish first for 24 hours at $-20°C$ will preclude this, but what self-respecting, bona fide yuppie would eat thawed sushi? Nausea, vomiting, fever, and epigastric pain are common. Not infrequently the worm is regurgitated, which ends the problem (4). Many affected individuals have been operated for presumptive perforation of a viscus, for appendicitis, or tumor. The most severe cases appear to be related to the ingestion of *A simplex*, and milder illness is often caused by *P decipiens*. If endoscopy is performed early on, it is possible to retrieve the slender, long (1 to 4 cm) larval worm. With time, the parasite perishes in the (inappropriate) human host, leaving a granulomatous reaction in the wall of the stomach.

Ikeda and colleagues in Japan, where most cases have been reported, found that in 9 of 19 patients with a syndrome highly suggestive of anisakiasis, one or more stage 3 *Anisakis* larvae could be recovered at endoscopy (5). In all those in whom a larva could be found, pain resolved immediately upon removal of the worm.

Commercial salmon farming is becoming an important economic activity in a number of countries, including Canada, the United States, Scandinavia, and Chile. Concern has been raised about the wisdom of eating pen-reared salmonids given the potential risk of anasikiasis. Deardorff and Kent (6) studied the prevalence of *Anisakis* infection in 50 wild sockeye salmon caught during their spawning migration, and compared this to infection in 237 Atlantic, coho, and chinook salmon raised in commercial pens. All of the wild salmon were infected with *Anisakis simplex* larvae, whereas not one of the commercially raised salmon carried the parasite. Thus, for those who eat raw salmon, farmed fish may be safer than wild caught fish.

Another group of parasites transmitted by sushi are *Gnathostoma* species. Most prominent is *G spinigerum*. Adult worms live attached to the stomach walls of mammals such as felines and dogs; eggs are passed in the feces of the definitive host, and water-living *Cyclops* species are the host for the first and second stage larvae. Fish, frogs, and snakes are the next hosts for third stage larvae. These animals are the usual vectors for transmission to humans, in whom the parasite cannot develop. Instead, larvae unable to complete development migrate through the tissues, sometimes for years.

Gnathostomiasis is a major problem in Thailand and elsewhere in Southeast Asia, where it is considered the most common symptomatic tissue helminth infection. Other reported places of infection include Japan, India, Latin America, and the Middle East (7,8). Worms removed from humans are 2 to 3 mm in length and about 0.5 mm wide; adults in the definitive host are up to 5 cm in length. Clinical manifestations are related to the restless and relentless migration of the parasite through the tissues; most common are cutaneous migrations, evidenced by intensely pruritic swelling and eruptions. Concurrent marked eosinophilia, high IgE levels, and parasite-specific antibody are usually found. Most worrisome are invasions of the central nervous and ocular systems, which may be fatal. Gnathostomiasis can cause an eosinophilic meningitis in association with painful radiculopathy, subarachnoid hemorrhage, and the cutaneous symptoms and signs already mentioned. The latter help to differentiate it from eosinophilic meningitis caused by *Angiostrongylus cantonensis*, the rat lungworm, in which the associated symptoms of *Gnathostoma* infection are not found (9). *Angiostrongylus* eosinophilic meningitis is usually manifested by headache, paresthesias, generalized weakness, and occasionally visual difficulties and extraocular muscle palsies (10). Given the popularity in Thailand of ceviche, sushi, and raw fish and snake, gnathostomiasis may be expected in the adventurous (and traveling) epicure.

Taniguchi et al (11) reported a typical tale of two individuals who ate raw loach fish they had caught in a rice paddy in central Japan. They developed classic symptoms of gnathostomiasis, and a biopsy from one of them revealed typical lesions. Both had reactive sera, and fish from the same rice field had the parasite demonstrated by scanning electron microscopy. This is the usual method of acquisition throughout Asia.

In 1988, Bennish and colleagues (12) presented details of a diplomatic dinner in Dhaka, Bangladesh in which 8 of 12 diplomats who ate a previously frozen, and subsequently marinated (pH 5.0), fish pate developed *Gnathostoma spinigerum* infection. Six of the eight developed intermittent, migratory subcutaneous swellings, and two had systemic symptoms with diarrhea, weight loss, and abdominal and thoracic pain. Serologic studies performed at Mahidol University in Thailand documented antibody titers of $>1:1,600$ in the symptomatic, and $<1:25$ in the asymptomatic, diplomats. Despite multiple courses of thiabendazole and mebendazole, symptoms and migratory swellings persisted beyond 10 months in five of the six. One of the authors of this chapter (JKG) assisted in the care of these patients and can attest to the frustrating lack of effective therapy for this parasite. This outbreak proves the point that the attack rate can be very high when infected fish are consumed. It is clear that freezing of the fish and subsequent marination in a mildly acidic lime juice solution were not sufficient to kill the parasite, although it is not known whether or not a temperature of $-20°$C was reached and sustained.

One may expect that, with time, other parasites will be added to the list of sushi-related diseases. Wittner and colleagues recently reported a case of *Eustrongyloides* infection in a college student (13). This nematode is a parasite of fish-eating birds, and the patient probably was infected by eating raw fish. Larvae are also found in reptiles and amphibians, which may serve as paratenic (transport) hosts (14,15). Presenting with severe right lower quadrant pain and peritoneal signs, thought to be acute appendicitis, the student underwent surgery. A 4.2 cm pink-red worm in the peritoneal cavity was the only abnormality found. Three gentleman who swallowed live minnows in Maryland had a similar disease; in one the disease resolved spontaneously, but the other two underwent laparotomy, and *Eustrongyloides* larvae were found to have perforated their ceca (16). Probably even sushi devotees can be persuaded not to eat live minnows; one wonders if in the era of eating live goldfish these infections were more common.

Diphyllobothrium latum is a tapeworm acquired by eating the raw or undercooked muscle of fish. It is a big problem today, primarily in the sense that it grows to a length of 20 to 30 feet. The adult worm is found in humans, cats, dogs, foxes, bears, wolves, and pigs: animals that eat freshwater and marine fish. Eggs passed in human or animal feces embryonate in water and are ingested by freshwater crustaceans. When the crustacean is eaten by a fish, the parasite penetrates the intestinal wall where it develops into a plerocercoid, which is infectious to carnivores that subsequently eat the infected fish. These plerocercoids are 1 to 5 cm long and visible to the naked eye. Fish species that have been found infected include salmon, whitefish, rainbow trout, pike, perch, turbot, and ruff (17). Areas of endemicity include subArctic and temperate Asia and Europe, the lake regions of the European Alps, the Danube River basin, and many parts of North and South America where human immigration has carried the parasite. About 10% of people in Scandinavia are infected with *Diphyllobothrium*. Salmon spend a portion of their lives in fresh water, and fresh salmon from Alaska were implicated in an outbreak of fish tapeworm disease along the West Coast of the United States in 1979 and 1980 (18). It is presumed that young salmon are infected after hatching in spawning rivers contaminated by infected bears as they are fishing.

Like other physicians trained in New York City, the authors of this chapter were taught to suspect *D latum* infection in any vitamin B_{12}-deficient Jewish immigrant from Eastern Europe who commonly prepares gefilte fish in the traditional way. This ethnic delicacy is made with chopped freshwater fish, and the proper balance of spices can only be made as the (still uncooked) fish dish is being made. Indeed, pernicious megaloblastic anemia is sometimes caused by the special ability of the tapeworm to take up vitamin B_{12} in the proximal small intestine. For reasons that are unclear, this complication of infection is more common in Europe than in the United States, where the worm can be found in Great Lakes fish (19). Other nonspecific symptoms include abdominal pain and weight loss. Diagnosis is made by examination of the stool for proglottids and the oval eggs, which have a characteristic operuculum (20). Several agents, including the time-tested niclosamide and praziquantel, are curative with single-dose treatment.

Other *Diphyllobothrium* species may well be involved in human infection. Curtis and Bylund have discussed the other species thought to infect humans in the circumpolar Arctic region (21), including *D dendriticum, D ursi, D dalliae*, and *D klebanovaskii*. Interestingly, there are no reports of anemia in individuals infected with one of the above mentioned non-*latum* species. It is not possible to speciate different *Diphyllobothrium* infections by stool exam, as the eggs are very similar and the proglottids of the non-*latum* species are easily confused with those of *D latum*. There is some evidence that the fish reservoirs for the different *Diphyllobothrium* species are separable; for example, *D dendriticum* is usually found in salmonid fish such as salmon, trout, whitefish, and Arctic char, and has never been reported in perch and pike. Perch and pike are the usual intermediate hosts for *D latum*, and salmonids rarely harbor *D latum*.

Of note is the intestinal fluke *Nanophyetus salmincola*, which has been reported to cause disease in people who have eaten raw salmon, Pacific steelhead trout, or steelhead roe that was undercooked or smoked (22,23). Unlike many other flatworm infections, the majority of reported cases (13 of 20) had symptoms of abdominal pain, diarrhea, bloating, nausea and vomiting, weight loss, and fatigue. One individual reported fever. Ten of eighteen individuals examined had eosinophilia of $\geqslant 500$ eosinophils per microliter. Diagnosis is made by examining stools for the oval, operculated eggs using concentrated fecal specimens or trichrome-stained stools. Most cases have been reported from the Pacific Northwest region, and praziquantel appears to be an effective therapy. Nanophyetiasis may be the most commonly encountered trematode infection in North America.

Sohn, Chai, and Lee reported a case of *Stellantchasmus falcatus* infection in a 33-year-old man in Seoul who had eaten raw brackish-water fish; after a single dose of praziquantel and a magnesium-salt purge, 17 adult worms were found (24). The affected gentleman had had vague abdominal pain and discomfort. This mild illness pales in comparison to the acute renal failure and hepatitis suffered by 13 Korean people who ate raw carp bile (25). All of the individuals initially reported gut upset after ingestion of the raw carp, followed by oliguria in seven, jaundice in eight, and hematuria in ten. The severity of the symptoms was related to the amount of bile ingested; all recovered with supportive therapy, including dialysis. Biopsy samples of the kidney and liver revealed changes consistent with an acute tubular necrosis produced by nephrotoxins, and those of the liver revealed changes of acute toxic hepatitis. Clearly, lovers of sushi who insist on persisting in the habit should stop short of ingesting raw bile.

Ceviche, as already noted, is the generic name for raw fish dishes prepared in Latin and Central America. Depending upon the locale, the fish may be steeped in lime or lemon juice (and other condiments) for 24 hours before eating, or briefly rinsed in acidic fruit juice on its way to the mouth of the impatient diner. This dish is extremely popular with indigenous populations, and increasingly so with the adventurous tourist or business traveler from abroad. Ceviche, also served in the Pacific Northwest, has been implicated in cases of anisakiasis.

Cholera

Epidemic cholera has recently emerged throughout South and Central America, and is endemic along the U.S. Gulf Coast. It has been epidemiologically associated with the ingestion of raw seafood (26). The Pan-American Health Organization has estimated that since the Western Hemisphere epidemic began in January 1991, 322,562 cases of cholera occurred in Peru in that year alone. Many suspect that this is a conservative estimate. In a well publicized case touching closer to home, 75 cases of acute cholera in 1991 were linked to the ingestion of a cold seafood salad aboard an airliner that flew from Peru to California. Presumably the salad was contaminated with *V cholerae*, either by a handler or from the start, perhaps because preparation was inadequate to kill the bacterium. Similarly, 11 cases of cholera were associated with eating crab smuggled from Colombia into New Jersey. Episodic cases are being reported in U.S. citizens and foreigners returning from South and Central America after eating raw seafood (27). Gulf Coast raw shellfish and crabs have historically been the reservoir for a few cases per year in the U.S.; the risk of cholera from eating raw seafood in the more southern Americas has now become far greater and deserving of a cautionary word to those departing to southern climes. Moreover, given the increasing travel for both business and pleasure to the Caribbean and Latin America, we should also expect cases of imported cholera to appear in locales in the U.S. and elsewhere where little or no indigenous cholera exists. With the transport of raw seafood delicacies across continents to appease the appetites of epicurean yuppies, cholera may appear anywhere.

In an illustrative report, Swaddiwudhipong et al reported on several sporadic outbreaks of El Tor cholera in the northern Chiang Mai region of Thailand (28). Two of the three described outbreaks were associated with infected food handlers [one a butcher, one a food packer]; in the other, six young men ate raw fish from a canal contaminated with *V cholera*. Thus both marine and freshwater fish may carry and transmit cholera.

Cholera is the prototypical dehydrating diarrheal disease. It can lead to death in as little as 6 hours after the onset of diarrhea. The key to treatment (and survival) is rehydration with fluids that contain the salts lost in the diarrheal flux. In the majority of cases, *vigorous* oral rehydration will prevent death and restore euvolemia. Antimicrobials play a secondary role in the treatment of cholera, shortening the duration of illness and stopping further contamination of the environment with viable *Vibrios* (29). It is an error of management and judgement to focus on drug therapy and not on the fluid replacement needs in this disease, which can be prodigious. Disturbingly, there are now reports of antimicrobial resistance in South American isolates associated with the indiscriminate use of tetracyclines, ampicillin, and trimethoprim-sulfamethoxazole.

Raw Beef, Raw Pork, and Dysentery

Raw beef and pork are famous for transmission of the beef and pork tapeworms, *Taenia saginata* and *T solium*, respectively. Those epicures who favor dishes such as steak tartare are protected in some countries by strict public health measures, but in some regions such as Africa and the Middle East, the estimated prevalence of bovine cysticercosis exceeds 10%. In some parts of Europe, eastern and Southeast Asia, and Latin America the rates are 0.1% to 5%. *Taenia saginata* infections are usually asymptomatic, though mild epigastric discomfort, nausea, vomiting, weight loss, and diarrhea may be reported. The most common complaint is the passage per anus of motile, muscular proglottids, which seems rarely to occur at a discrete time or location. Rarely, acute appendicitis, pancreatitis, bowel obstruction, or cholangitis may occur with an obstructing bolus of worm. Tissue invasion with larval forms of *Taenia saginata* is rare, and cysticercosis with this parasite is reportable and publishable.

In contrast, the pork tapeworm *Taenia solium* has a different potential for invasive disease. Though infection in humans with the mature tapeworm form is clinically indistinguishable from *T saginata*, infection with the *larval* form (cysticerci), or cysticercosis, can be extremely unpleasant. This infection has been controlled in many countries by the mandatory freezing of pork before sale is allowed and by rigidly excluding potentially infected foodstuffs from swine feed. The larval stages of the parasite can be hematogenously spread from the gut to the liver, brain, long muscles, subcutaneous tissues, and the eye, amongst other tissues. The cysticerci become surrounded by a connective tissue membrane and can live up to 10 years after the acute infection. When the cysticerci die, antigens may leak into the surroundings and cause inflammation. In Mexico, cerebral cysticerci are found in 10% to 30% of patients undergoing craniotomies, and in about 3% of individuals autopsied. In one series from Mexico City, neurocysticercosis was the main identified cause of adult onset epilepsy (30). Fully half the 100 patients studied had evidence of cysticercal disease as documented by computed tomography, electroencephalography, CSF analysis, serologic testing, and (in some cases) angiography and surgical extirpation. Thirty-six of the 50 individuals had seizures, 41 had parenchymal calcifications, and 15 had two or more lesions.

Seizures, motor deficits, or visual impairment are common in this disease. About 5% of CNS cysticercosis involves the spinal cord. Peripheral eosinophilia is usually absent or low grade, and the CSF may be normal or show nonspecific increases in protein concentration or cell counts, including eosinophils and plasma cells. Computed tomography often shows parenchymal, subarachnoid, or intraventricular cysts, hydrocephalus, and punctate calcifications. Enhancement of the lesions with contrast agents is variable. Serologic studies are positive in only about 80% of individuals. The treatment of choice is praziquantel, although albendazole may be more effective. Steroids may be required to decrease the inflammatory sequelae after killing the parasites with antiparasitic agents, and seizures often warrant the use of anticonvulsants. Shunting procedures may be indicated when ventricular obstruction is present (31–34). Vasquez and Sotelo reviewed the course of seizures after treatment for cerebral cysticercosis (35) and found that treatment was usually associated with a remission or marked improvement in the associated seizure disorder, correlating with a marked decrease in the number of cysts. While a proportion of cysts are destroyed by the host's immune response, scarring at the focus can lead to persistent seizures; in this study, drug therapy was least likely to lead to persistent seizures.

A patient's abstinence from pork should not prevent the clever physician from considering *T solium* infection in the proper clinical setting. Schantz and colleagues investigated an outbreak of neurocysticercosis in an Orthodox Jewish community in New York City (36). Seven of seventeen immediate family members were seropositive for the parasite, and two children had cystic CNS lesions. Of note, the afflicted families had employed housekeepers who were seropositive for the parasite, or in whom stool exams were positive for *Taenia* eggs. The housekeepers were recent immigrants from Latin America, and were the presumed sources of infection for the Orthodox families. If we assume the average yuppie has sufficient disposable income to afford sushi, a BMW car, and a housekeeper, then even the vegetarian yuppie is at risk of neurocysticercosis!

Eating raw pork is well associated with infection by *Trichinella spiralis*, the cause of trichinosis. This disease is found everywhere in the world except for Australia and Puerto Rico. When undercooked meat is eaten, the larvae are released from cysts in the muscle tissue. The larvae move to the intestine, where they mature. Following copulation, the adult female worms burrow into the gut, and the released larvae enter the systemic circulation and are distributed amongst the tissues, primarily skeletal muscle. Female worms are thought to be capable of producing about 1,500 larvae during their lifetime. Larvae enter single cells and encyst within them, remaining viable for months to years. The symptoms of trichinosis relate to both the intestinal stage and the dissemination of the new larvae into the tissues. When only a few larvae infect the host, symptoms may be absent. With heavy infections, diarrhea, cramps, or sometimes constipation result from the original infection of the small bowel. Secondary larval spread causes severe myositis, neurological, pulmonary, and cardiovascular manifestations, including inflammatory myocarditis that can lead to death (37). In addition to the pig, larvae are found in bear, wild boar, walrus, and other carnivorous mammals. Many of these are game and the particular delight of gourmands, be they yuppies or not.

Recent outbreaks associated with eating wild boar meat and pig have been reported from Spain (38). In Italy, wild boar meat has been implicated in 9.4% of the 584 cases diagnosed since 1961, but it is not believed to play a major role in the sylvatic cycle of *Trichinella* in the Piedmont and Liguria; none of 1,508 samples of wild boar muscle were infected during the period 1987 to 1990, whereas 14 of 608 wild foxes were infected (39). Until recently, the U.S. Department of Agriculture had banned the importation of prosciutto and other dried pork products from Europe, to the dismay of their admirers. Satisfyingly, Smith and coworkers in Canada have shown that the appropriate salt curing process of these raw meat delicacies destroys *Trichinella spiralis*, as demonstrated by rat bioassay and pepsin digestion methods, but it probably will not affect confiscation of these delicacies at the airport, or their ultimate human consumption (40).

In some countries, the incidence of trichinellosis remains high, with substantial mortality related to the migration of the parasites through the tissues. These cases represent the tip of the iceberg. For example in Thailand, about 3,000 people are estimated to have been infected with *Trichinella* in the last 25 years, and 85 of them have died. Hill tribe pigs are thought to be the main source of human infections (41). The number of infected humans surely exceeds this figure by several orders of magnitude. To give some historical perspective to this study, epidemics in Germany during the 1800s were associated with mortality rates as high as 30% (42). In contrast, with the implementation of public health measures, the increasing use of frozen pork, and a trend away from home preparation of fresh pork sausage, the incidence has fallen dramatically in some countries. For example, the number of reported cases in the United States has fallen from around 400 per year in the late 1940s, with 10 to 15 deaths yearly, to 57 per year, with 3 deaths, in the 5 years 1982 to 1986 (43). One to two percent of human autopsy examinations of diaphragm muscle are still positive for larvae, however. Pork products are responsible for about two-thirds of U.S. cases, with the rest associated with ground beef and wild animal meat. Cattle are not naturally infected with the parasite, and it is believed that ground beef products are accidentally contaminated with infected pork products. The number of cases attributable to commercial pork sources continues to fall, whereas the number of cases attributed to wild game (bear, wild boar, etc.) has remained relatively constant. There are marked variations in the incidence of infected porcine populations in the U.S.: no infected animals were found in the 3,245 sampled in 1983 to 1985 from the Midwest, whereas 0.73% of 5,315 hogs slaughtered in the New England region were infected.

Special mention should be made of trichinosis in the Arctic regions, where amongst Inuit populations the ingestion of raw walrus and polar bear meat is common. Trichinosis in the Arctic is caused by a nematode that some consider biologically distinct from the temperate and tropical pest, and it has been proposed that the northern variant is a distinct species, *Trichinella nativa* (44). In a variety of surveys, the prevalence of *Trichinella* in polar bears was 45%, in wolves 22.3%, in Arctic foxes 4%, and in walruses 2.6% (45), demonstrating the ubiquitous nature of the parasite in Arctic carnivores. Many cases have been linked to the ingestion of walrus meat which is preferentially eaten raw amongst the Inuit, in contrast to polar bear meat which is most often eaten cooked. A new syndrome has been described in the Arctic, marked by prolonged diarrhea, that is distinct from the classic myopathic form. The group that has described this new entity has presented evidence that it represents a secondary infection in previously sensitized individuals (46).

The classic myopathic disease may begin with abdominal pain and diarrhea thought to reflect the invasion of the gut by the adult nematode females. This intestinal stage usually begins within 7 days of ingestion of the cysts, and symptoms of nausea, vomiting, diarrhea, constipation, malaise, epigastric or right lower abdominal pain, and low-grade fever are common. It is followed by a visceral stage which is manifested by fever, edema, muscle weakness, and myalgias; the latter is the cardinal symptom that has been used in survey work. Chills, cough, diaphoresis, diarrhea or constipation, and pruritis may also be seen. Skin rashes, petechiae, and conjunctivitis may also be noted. Muscle pain and swelling are striking features, with the most commonly affected muscles being the diaphragm, extraocular, masseter, tongue, laryngeal, intercostal, neck, back, and deltoid muscles. Symptoms are related to the specific muscle groups affected; dyspnea with the diaphragmatic and intercostal muscles, dysphagia with the pharyngeal and tongue muscles, etc. CNS involvement results in generalized seizures, focal motor deficits, deafness, and encephalopathy. These neurological symptoms are seen in 10% to 24% of hospitalized patients. Cardiac involvement can lead to myocarditis, arrhythmias, congestive heart failure, and death. Eosinophilia is pro-

TABLE 12.1. Worms in yuppie delights.

Parasite	Therapy (in some infections only scanty data is available)
Anisakidae species	Removal
Diphyllobothrium latam	niclosamide[1] or praziquantel[2]
Eustrongyloides	Removal
Gnathostoma species	None available
Nanophyetus salmincola	praziquantel[3]
Stellantchasmus falcatus	praziquantel[3]
Taenia saginatum	niclosamide or praziquantel
Taenia solium	niclosamide or praziquantel for gut forms
Cysticerosis	praziquantel[4] or albendazole[5] for CNS disease, often with steroids and/or antiseizures medications as indicated. Surgery may be required.
Trichinella spiralis	thiabendazole;[6] steroids if symptoms severe

[1] 2 grams orally once in adults; 11 to 34 kgs, 1 gram orally once; >34 kilos, 1.5 grams once.
[2] 10 to 20 mg/kg orally, once.
[3] unclear what regimen to use.
[4] 50 mg/kg/d in three divided doses for 2 weeks.
[5] 15 mg/kg/d for 1 month; some investigators believe that a 3-day course is sufficient.
[6] 25 mg/kg twice daily (maximum 3 g/d) for 5 days; in some people with AIDS, repeat treatment may be required.

minent, and elevated serum levels of muscle enzymes (CPK, SGOT) are found, sometimes being extraordinarily high in severe cases. Other findings include decreased serum proteins, hypokalemia, leukocytosis, and mild elevations of hepatocellular enzymes. Muscle biopsy is diagnostic, as it shows the larvae within muscle cells. These are observed live and instantaneously by crushing the sample on a slide and viewing under low-power light microscopy. However, given the life cycle, muscle biopsy may not be positive until the third or fourth week of illness. The deltoid and gastrocnemius muscles are preferred tissue sites to sample. Stool examination is usually not helpful, as eggs are not produced by this viviparous worm, and larval or adult worms are rarely seen. Thiabendazole is the treatment of choice, and the administration of steroids may be prudent in severe cases. The convalescent stage is marked by the resolution of fever and myalgias, usually during the third or fourth week of illness. Treatment for this parasite, as well as the others, is summarized in Table 12.1.

In the newly described form of the illness, diarrhea is prominent with ≥10 stools a day at the onset, and persistent diarrhea with 2 to 5 loose motions and prominent abdominal pain are common, accompanied by high level eosinophilia.

An underappreciated consequence of eating poorly cooked beef may be exposure to bacterial pathogens that cause diarrhea and other intestinal complaints. *Escherichia coli* O157:H7 is an enteric pathogen that causes a hemorrhagic colitis and is strongly linked with hemolytic uremic syndrome (HUS) and thrombotic thrombocytopenic purpura (TTP). In a recent study published by the Mayo Clinic in Rochester, Minnesota, it was the fourth most common bacterial pathogen isolated during a 6-month period (47). This organism produces toxins structurally and functionally similar to the prototypical Shiga toxin of *Shigella dysenteriae* type 1 (48); however, it is not enteroinvasive and does not produce the heat-labile or heat-stable enterotoxins associated with enterotoxigenic *E coli*. Wells and colleagues investigated several outbreaks of HUS associated with raw milk consumption in the United States and found that enterohemorrhagic *E coli* (EHEC) such as O157:H7 could be isolated from local dairy cattle (heifers and calves), milk samples, and raw beef samples. Similar results have been obtained in Canada (49) where 10.4% of 225 beef samples were culture-positive, and where 26.4% of the samples harbored bacteria producing the cytotoxin, based upon cytotoxicity assays. Thus, EHEC are present in the food chain (specifically in cattle and dairy products) in areas where HUS occurs.

The direct association between HUS and infection with *E coli* O157:H7 has been illuminated by several recent studies. Chart and colleagues found serologic evidence for infection in 44 of 60 patients with HUS, and in none of 16 controls (50). Tarr and coworkers have published clear-cut evidence that the timing of initial stool cultures in cases of postdysenteric

HUS in the U.S. directly affects the likelihood of isolating *E coli* O157: H7 from the stool, with the highest success rate in the first 6 days of diarrheal illness (51). Thus the pathogen that is linked epidemiologically with HUS is present in dairy cattle and in raw or undercooked meat. The magnitude of the problem is not yet known; however, HUS due to *E coli* O157:H7 is probably the most common cause of acute renal failure in children in the U.S. at this time.

Salmonella, ubiquitously present in animals of commercial food importance such as fowl and cattle, and in some household pets such as turtles, are discussed in Chapters 8 and 9.

Steak Tartare and Toxoplasmosis

While McDonalds, Burger King, and Wendy's are vehicles for EHEC, *Salmonella*, and other organisms, and are the essence of Americana, they are not yuppie cuisine. Hence, we turn to steak tartare, a flavorful concoction of raw chopped beef, raw egg, onion, capers, and a vinaigrette. Unfortunately, other things get into steak tartare, including *Toxoplasma gondii*, the etiological agent of toxoplasmosis. *Toxoplasma gondii* is an obligate intracellular parasite found throughout the world. Infection with the parasite is followed by dissemination into the tissues, most often including the brain, heart, and skeletal muscle. Encysted *Toxoplasma* is usually asymptomatic, and chronic silent infection is the rule. The acute symptomatic infection is less common, accounting for 10% to 20% of infections in adults. Though usually benign and self-limited, and often an infectious mononucleosis-like syndrome, the severe end of the spectrum of clinical manifestations includes myocarditis, pneumonitis, and meningoencephalitis.

Felines are the definitive hosts for *Toxoplasma*, in which both an enteroepithelial and extraintestinal cycle occur; in contrast, only the extraintestinal cycle occurs in other mammalian, avian, and saurian hosts. Tachyzoites are the form found in tissues during *acute* infection, and invade all mammalian cells except red cells. Tissue cysts developing within host muscle cells are the infectious form eaten by epicures ingesting raw meat. The intestinal digestive juices (peptic and tryptic) disrupt the cyst wall, liberating the tachyzoites which invade gut enterocytes. From this focus the parasites disseminate systemically using lymphatic or hematogenous routes, usually setting up new foci in the abovementioned brain, heart, and skeletal muscle, although all tissues can be affected. Once new tissue cysts develop in the newly-infected host, these persistent forms may serve as a source of recrudescent disseminated disease, especially in the immunosuppressed. In felines (of the family *Felidae*), parasites which infect gut cells go through both an asexual cycle (schizogony) and a sexual cycle (gametogony), leading to the development of oocysts which are excreted in feces. The intestinal cycle in cats is primarily in young animals and for a limited time period, with eventual resolution. Oocysts are hardy, environmentally-resistant forms that can survive in warm, moist soil for months to a year. Ingestion of oocysts also causes infection in humans.

Infection is usually acquired by eating food with infectious tissue cysts, by ingesting infectious oocysts, or transplacentally. Rare cases have been reported of infection via contaminated water, transfusion, transplantation, and through laboratory accidents. The prevalence of cysts in raw beef is not well studied; according to Remington and McLeod (52), approximately 10% of lamb and 25% of pork is infected. In the United States and Europe, the highest rates of seropositivity are in young adults, which is thought to be secondary to eating undercooked pork, lamb, or beef. In contrast, in countries such as Burundi, Panama, and Somalia, undercooked meat is rarely eaten (especially pork), and there is widespread environmental contamination with oocysts. Infection is often acquired in early childhood, and children have the highest seropositivity rates (53–55).

Toxoplasmosis has always been of major public health importance because of the congenital disease that can occur (see below). These concerns have increased considerably in the AIDS era. In countries such as Finland and Slovenia where the prevalence of toxoplasma antibody in adults is relatively low, the incidence of infection during pregnancy is around 3 per 1,000 pregnancies (56,57), comparable to the range of 2.5 to 5.5 cases per 1,000 pregnancies in studies conducted in the United Kingdom (58). In contrast, in countries where raw meat is favored—such as France (59), Germany, Pakistan (60), Turkey (61), and Sudan (62)— the toxoplasma antibody seropositive rate is high, as is the seroconversion rate during pregnancy, and it poses more of a public health problem. In screening studies in Paris conducted between October 1981 and September 1983, the standardized prevalence rate in pregnant French women was 71% ± 4%, compared to 51% ± 5% in immigrant women, and the incidence of seroconversion in nonimmune pregnant women was estimated to be 1.6% (59)!

The usual infection in a child or adult results in a mononucleosis-like syndrome, with the most frequent manifestation being lymphadenopathy. Any and all lymph nodes can be involved; with involvement of the abdominal group, abdominal pain and fever can be dominant. The lymph nodes become enlarged and firm, but do not suppurate. Other manifestations include hepatitis and hepatosplenomegaly; myalgias and arthralgias; urticaria and a maculopapular rash that spares the palms and soles; confusion, headache, and meningismus. These symptoms and signs usually resolve without specific therapy—and indeed are rarely recognized as being toxoplasmosis—in the normal host. Unhappily, in some individuals more severe disease may be seen; hepatitis, pneumonitis, meningoencephalitis or encephalitis, pericarditis or myocarditis, and polymyositis.

Special mention should be made of ocular and central nervous system disease. Acute chorioretinitis can produce epiphora, photophobia, scotomas, pain, and blurred vision; if the macula is involved, central vision may be lost. In congenital disease, strabismus, nystagmus, anisometropia, cataracts, small cornea, and microophthalmia may result. In infants, the only site of clinically overt infection may be the eyes, and examination by an ophthalmologist is important; chronic infection and inflammation can cause scarring, vision loss, and optic nerve atrophy. In contrast, in AIDS patients significant inflammatory changes are less common, and necrotic eye disease is caused by the direct effects of the parasite.

CNS disease mainly occurs in two groups: the congenitally infected and those with HIV infection. Women who become infected while pregnant have an increasing risk of transmitting the parasite to the fetus the nearer they are to term; however, the disease is most severe in the first trimester, less so in the second trimester, and rarely problematic in the third trimester. Apparently the parasites cause irremediable CNS and ocular disease in the still developing early fetus, whereas damage to other organs and tissues can often be compensated for. Congenital infection can cause protean manifestations in newborns, affecting all organ systems. In those with signs of active infection at birth, deafness, mental retardation, epilepsy, spasticity, paisies, and blindness may occur. Chorioretinitis will occur in about half of congenitally infected children, including the asymptomatic, and less commonly mental or physical retardation, epilepsy, blindness, and strabismus may result. In a study of 23,000 pregnancies (63), children born to highly seropositive (antibody titer 256 to 512) mothers, had a 60% increase in microcephaly, a 30% increase in low IQ (<70), and a doubling in the rate of deafness. In a subgroup of women with high indirect hemagglutination antibody levels or seroconversions with IgM, there were 15 pregnancies; 2 children had congenital toxoplasmosis, and 3 were stillborn.

In individuals with AIDS, the most common manifestation of toxoplasmosis is recrudescent disease of the brain from old, formerly silent cysts. Acute infection does occur in regions of high prevalence, and can result in a protean disseminated disease. The latter is often fulminant and rapidly fatal, but is less common than the typical CNS presentation. In these patients, symptoms and signs of CNS toxoplasmosis are related to the mass lesions, meningoencephalitis, and encephalopathy that occur; thus seizures, fever, focal neurological deficits, and headache are common. The basal ganglia are most often affected, followed by the frontal, parietal, and occipital lobes; the cerebellum is not often involved. MRI is even more sensitive than contrast-enhanced CT for the detection of lesions. The CSF is usually abnormal, although a lumbar puncture may be contraindicated if cerebral edema exists. CNS toxoplasmosis is the most common CNS opportunistic infection in AIDS (64). It is uniformly fatal if not treated.

There is evidence that treatment of pregnant women with acute toxoplasmosis leads to reduced risk of disease in the fetus. Daffos and colleagues (65) in Paris have reported their experience using pyramethamine and sulfa drugs in 15 women, in a cohort of 746, who developed acute toxoplasmosis in pregnancy and carried their infants to term. Of the 15 infants, 2 had chorioretinitis and the others remained clinically well during follow-up. Members of this same group have published another study in which 52 women with *Toxoplasma* infection acquired during pregnancy were treated with spiramycin and followed to term; 54 live infants were born. Forty three of the 52 women were also treated with pyrimethamine and sulfonamides. Only one infant had severe congenital toxoplasmosis, and this child was the result of one of the nine pregnancies not additionally treated with pyramethamine and sulfa. The researchers recommended that spiramycin be started as soon as the diagnosis of maternal *Toxoplasma* infection during pregnancy was proven or strongly suspected (66). It is less clear that postnatal treatment of the congenitally infected infant is as helpful. Wilson and Remington have recently published suggested treatment regimens for toxoplasmosis in pregnant women and the congenitally infected infant which incorporate their own experience with that of Dr. Jacques Couvreur at the Institut de Puericulture, Paris (67). It is recommended that sulfa drugs be avoided in the first trimester of pregancy and at term, the latter related to the risk of kernicterus.

In individuals with AIDS, a number of treatment regimens have been recognized as efficacious. The standard of treatment is pyrimethamine plus sulfadiazine or trisulfapyrimidines; sulfathiazole, sulfapyridine, sulfadimetine, and sulfisoxazole are less effective. Clindamycin, trimethoprim, trimethotrexate, and 566C80 are also efficacious in human trials or in in vitro and in vivo experiments (68). Sulfa drugs, such as trimethoprim-sulfa, may provide prophylaxis against the development of clinical disease in individuals seropositive for both *Toxoplasma* and HIV (69). Treatment regimens are summarized in Table 12.2.

There is no evidence that treatment is appropriate in the healthy individual with asymptomatic or mildly symptomatic toxoplasmosis.

Unpasteurized Milk Products

Unpasteurized milk products have always enjoyed a reputation for slightly fresher taste and aroma compared to their pasteurized cousins. Previously the provenance of the poor, many of the famous local cheeses of Europe can only be made, in the opinion of the local artisans, with unpasteurized milk, and this belief has been accepted on the far side of

TABLE 12.2. Therapy for toxoplasmosis.

Host	Therapy
Normal Host	None
Pregnant woman[1]	Spiramycin[2] followed by pyramethamine + sulfa + folinic acid; if spiramycin not available: pyramethamine + sulfa + folinic acid.[3]
Congenitally infected infant, overt infection	pyramethamine + sulfa + folinic acid[4] alternating with spiramycin[5] for one year.
Possible congenital infection	pyramethamine + sulfa + folinic acid for one month while testing pursued.
HIV seropositive, healthy	if CD_4 count ≤200, trimethoprim-sulfa as prophylaxis 3 to 7 times weekly; dapsone + pyramethamine may also work in the sulfa-intolerant.
HIV seropositive, clinical disease	pyramethamine + sulfa + folic acid[6]
	alternatives (some experimental and unproven):
	clindamycin + pyramethamine
	spiramycin
	trimethotrexate
	566C80
	azithromycin
	clarithromycin
	Steroids in selected cases with brain edema and mass effect.

[1] Avoid sulfa drugs in first trimester and before birth.
[2] 3 grams per day in divided doses.
[3] Pyramethamine 25 mg po qd or qod; sulfadiazine or trisulfapyrimidines 3 to 4 grams/day divided tid or qid; folinic acid, 5 mg po qd.
[4] pyramethamine 1 mg/kg to maximum of 25 mg qd; sulfadiazine or trisulfapyrimidines 85 mg/kg/d divided bid; folinic acid 5 mg every 3 days IM. If bone marrow toxicity occurs, double dose of folinic acid or hold pyramethamine.
[5] 100 mg/kg/day orally divided bid.
[6] Pyramethamine 25 to 75 mg po qd; sulfadiazine 8 grams/day; 5 mg folinic acid.

the Atlantic. Indeed, the authors of this chapter often enjoy a glass of wine with locally produced, no doubt disease-ridden cheese of artisanal production. Pathogens that can be acquired from eating unpasteurized food products include *Mycobacterium bovis*, *Listeria monocytogenes*, *Salmonella* species, *Campylobacter jejuni*, *Yersinia enterocolitica*, *Brucella abortus*, *Streptococcus zooepidemicus*, and the toxin-mediated diseases of *Escherichia coli* and *Staphylococcus aureus*.

Turista

"Travel expands the mind, and loosens the bowels."—Anonymous

"Turista" is a term that can be used to describe the affliction of the traveler—diarrhea. It is instructive to reflect upon the fact that foreigners who visit "developed" countries such as the United States also suffer from diarrhea; in other words, one needs to accommodate to the indigenous bacterial and viral flora and fauna wherever one might travel.

In some studies, up to 98% of travelers—usually yuppies, of course, who will indulge in ingesting unhealthily raw and delicious foodstuffs—will develop diarrhea during a lengthy trip abroad. In addition to the usual viral offenders, a number of bacteria can wreak havoc with the traveler's bowels: in most studies, enterotoxigenic *Escherichia coli* are high on the list, followed by *Salmonella, Campylobacter*, and *Shigella* species. Avoidance of raw salads, food that is cold or has cooled, and ice cubes when in a hot and tropical clime is indeed difficult, but important nonetheless in avoiding the trots. Cholera has been thankfully rare among healthy, well-nourished travelers. However, as the world pandemic spreads and involves regions frequented by pleasure seekers, we can expect more malignant and profuse turista to occur.

Many of the foodstuffs discussed in this chapter can act as vectors of a diarrheal disease; we only wish to note a few of our personal suggestions. First, we do not recommend prophylactic drug treatment in the absence of diarrhea, but do suggest the avoidance of risky foods, the use of only boiled or bottled beverages—preferably fine wines—and, when appropriate, the use of prophylactic bismuth subsalicylate. When diarrhea is persistent, bloody, or associated with fever, we utilize empiric therapy with a fluoroquinolone such as ciprofloxacin or norfloxacin. We suggest this class of antimicrobial agent because many of the pathogens around the world are resistant to drugs such as trimethoprim-sulfa, ampicillin, or tetracycline, and untreated or mistreated shigellosis is not a mild disease.

The importance of turista should not be underestimated; through the ages nasty tourists have died from turista—the Visigoths at the gates of Rome and the Imperial French army in Haiti after the slave revolt immediately come to mind. Great literature, such as *Love in the Time of Cholera* and *The Horseman on the Roof* (also about a cholera epidemic), may have been conceived by these fertile writers after particulary bad cases of turista.

Summary

You can get an unbelievable number of gross and unpleasant diseases by eating raw or contaminated foods, most of which are delicious and delightful. Enjoy!

Acknowledgments. The authors gratefully acknowledge the expert assistance of Lorianne Fryar in the preparation of this manuscript.

References

1. St Louis ME, Porter JD, Helal A, et al. Epidemic cholera in West Africa: the role of food handling and high-risk foods. *Am J Epidemiol* 1990; 131: 719–727.
2. McKerrow J, et al. Revenge of the sushi parasite. *N Engl J Med* 1988; 319:1228.
3. Kliks MM. Human anisakiasis: An updata. *JAMA* 1986; 255:2605.
4. Lichtenfels JR, Brancato FP. Anisakid larva from the throat of an Alaskan Eskimo. *Am J Trop Med Hyg* 1976; 25:691–693.
5. Ikeda K, Kumashiro R, Kifune T. Nine cases of acute gastric anisakiasis. *Gastro Endoscopy* 1989; 35:304–308.
6. Deardorff TL, Kent ML. Prevalence of larval *Anisakis simplex* in pen-reared and wild-caught salmon (*Salmonidae*) from Puget Sound, Washington. *J Wildlife Dis* 1989; 25:416–419.
7. Daengsvang S. Gnathostomiasis in Southeast Asia. *Southeast Asian J Trop Med Public Health* 1981; 12:319.
8. Ollague W, Ollague J, Guevara de Veliz A, Penaherrera S. Human gnathostomiasis in Ecuador (Nodular migratory eosinophilic panniculitis). *Int J Dermatol* 1984; 23:647.
9. Schmutzhard E, Boongird P, Vejjajiva A. Eosinophilic meningitis and radiculomyelitis in Thailand, caused by CNS invasion of *Gnathostoma spinigerum* and *Angiotrongylus cantonensis*. *J Neurol Neurosurg Psychiatry* 1988; 51:80.
10. Koo J, Pien F, Kliks MM. Angiostrongylus (Parastrongylus) eosinophilic meningitis. *Rev Infect Dis* 1988; 10:1155–1162.
11. Taniguchi Y, Hashimoto K, Ichikawa S, et al. Human gnathostomiasis. *J Cutan Pathol* 1991; 18:112–115.
12. Bennish ML, Sullivan C, Michelson S, et al. A point source outbreak of Gnathostomiasis at a diplomatic dinner. Abstract 1098. In: *Abstracts of the Twenty-Eighth Interscience Conference on Antimicrobial Agents and Chemotherapy, Los Angeles, October 23–26, 1988.* Washington D.C., American Society for Microbiology, 1988.
13. Wittner M, Turner JW, Jacquette G, et al. Eustrongylidiasis—a parasitic infection acquired by eating sushi. *N Engl J Med* 1989; 320:1124–1126.
14. Lichtenfels JR, Lavies B. Mortality in red-sided garter snakes, *Thamnophis sirtalis parietalis*, due to the larval nematode, *Eustrongylides* sp. *Lab Anim Sci* 1976; 26:465–467.
15. Panesar TS, Beaver PC. Morphology of the advanced-stage larva of *Eustongylides wenrichi* Canavan 1929, occurring encapsulated in the tissues of *Amphiuma* in Louisiana. *J Parasitol* 1979; 65:96–104.
16. Centers for Disease Control. Intestinal perforation caused by larval *Eustrongylides*—Maryland. *MMWR* 1982; 31:383–384, 389.
17. von Bonsdorff B, Bylund G. The ecology of *Diphyllobotrium latum*. *Ecol Dis* 1982; 1:21.
18. Centers for Disease Control. Diphyllobothriasis associated with salmon—United States. *MMWR* 1981; 30:331–332, 337–338.
19. Salokannel J. Intrinsic factor in tapeworm anaemia. *Acta Med Scand Suppl* 1970; 517:1–51.
20. Schmidt GD. *Handbook of Tapeworm Identification. Key to the Gerna Taeniidae.* Boca Raton, FL, CRC Press, 1986, pp. 221–227.

21. Curtis M, Bylund G. Diphyllobothriasis: fish tapeworm disease in the circumpolar north. *Arctic Med Res* 1991; 50:18–24.
22. Eastburn RL, Fritsche TR, Terhune CA Jr. Human intestinal infection with *Nanophyetus salmincola* from salmonid fishes. *Am J Trop Med Hyg* 1987; 36:586–591.
23. Fritsche TR, Eastburn RL, Wiggins LH, Terhune CA Jr. Praiquantel for treatment of human *Nanophyetus salmincola (Troglotrema salmincola)* infection. *J Infect Dis* 1989; 160:896–899.
24. Sohn WM, Chai JY, Lee SH. A human case of *Stellantchasmus falcatus* infection. (Kisaengchunghak Chapchi) *Korean J Parasit* 1989; 27:277–279.
25. Park SK, Kim DG, Kang SK, et al. Toxic acute renal failure and hepatitis after ingestion of raw carp bile. *Nephron* 1990; 56:188–193.
26. Loury PW, Pavia AT, McFarland LM, Peltier BH, Parrett TJ, Bradford HB, Quan JM, Lynch J, Mathison JB, Gam RA, Blacke PA. Cholera in Louisiana: Widening spectrum of seafood vehicles. *Arch Int Med* 1989; 149:2079–2084.
27. Ries AA. Cholera epidemic in the Americas—Update #92-13-REVISED. *Memorandum, Centers for Disease Control*, July 22 1992.
28. Swaddiwudhipong W, Akarasewi P, Chayaniyayodhin T, Kunasol P, Foy HM. *J Med Assoc Thailand* 1989; 72:583–588.
29. Keusch GT, Griffiths JK. Cholera. In: Burg FD (ed): *Current Pediatric Therapy*, 14th ed. (in press) Philadelphia, W. B. Saunders, 1993, pp. 634–636.
30. Medina MT, Rosas E, Rubio-Donnadieu F, Sotelo J. Neurocysticercosis as the main cause of late-onset epilepsy in Mexico. *Arch Intern Med* 1990; 150:325–327.
31. Sotel J, Escobedo F, Rodriguez-Carbajal J, et al. Therapy of parenchymal brain cysticercosis with praziquantel. *N Engl J Med* 1984; 310:1001–1007.
32. Earnest MP, Reller LB, Filley CM, Grek AJ. Neurocysticercosis in the United States: 35 cases and a review. *Rev Infect Dis* 1987; 9:961–979.
33. Del Brutto OH, Sotelo J. Neurocysticercosis: an update. *Rev Infect Dis* 1988; 10:1075–1087.
34. Takayanagui OM, Jardim E. Therapy for neurocysticercosis. Comparison between albendazole and praziquantel. *Arch Neurol* 1992; 49:290–294.
35. Vazquez V, Sotelo J. The course of seizures after treatment for cerebral cysticercosis. *N Engl J Med* 1992; 327:696–701.
36. Schantz PM, Moore AC, Munoz JL, et al. Neurocysticercosis in an Orthodox Jewish community in New York City. *N Engl J Med* 1992; 327:692–695.
37. Pawlowski ZS. Clinical aspects in man. In: Campbell WC (ed): *Trichinella and Trichinosis*. New York, Plenum Press, 1983: pp. 367–401.
38. Rodrigues-Osorio M, Gomez-Garcia V, Rodriguez-Perez J, Gomez Morales MA. Seroepidemiological studies of five outbreaks of trichinellosis in southern Spain. *Ann Trop Med Parasitol* 1990; 84:181–184.
39. Rossi L, Dini V. Importance of the wild boar in the epidemiology of wild trichinellosis in Piedmont and Ligura. *Parasitologia* 1990; 32:321–326.
40. Smith HJ, Messier S, Tittinger F. Destruction of *Trichinella spiralis spiralis* during the preparation of the "dry cured" pork products proscuitto, proscuittini and Genoa salami. *Canadian J Vet Res* 1989; 53:80–83.
41. Pozio E, Khamboonruang C. Trichinellosis in Thailand: epidemiology and biochemical identification of the aethiological agent. *Trop Med Parasitol* 1989; 40:73–74.

42. Gould SE. *Trichinosis in Man and Animals.* Springfield, IL, CC Thomas, 1970.
43. Bailey TM, Schantz PM. Trends in the incidence and transmission patterns of trichinosis in humans in the United States: comparisons of the periods 1975–1981 and 1982–1986. (Review article). *Rev Infect Dis* 1990; 12:5–11.
44. Britov VA, Boev SN. Taxonomic rank of various strains of *Trichinella* and their circulation in nature. *Vestn Akad Med Nauk SSSR* 1972; 28:27–32.
45. MacLean JD, Viallet J, Law C, Staudt M. Trichinosis in the Canadian Arctic: Report of five outbreaks and a new clinical syndrome. *J Infect Dis* 1989; 160:513–520.
46. MacLean JD, Poirier L, Gyorkos TW, et al. Epidemiologic and serologic definition of primary and secondary trichinosis in the Arctic. *J Infect Dis* 1992; 165:908–912.
47. Marshall WF, McLimans CA, Yu PKW, et al. Results of a 6-month survey of stool cultures for *Escherichia coli* O157:H7. *Mayo Clin Proc* 1990; 65:787–792.
48. O'Brien AD, LaVeck GD, Thompson MR, Formal SB. Production of *Shigella dysenteriae* type 1-like cytotoxin by *Escherichia coli*. *J Infect Dis* 1982; 146:763–769.
49. Read SC, Gyles CL, Clarke RC, et al. Prevalence of very cytotoxigenic *Escherichia coli* in ground beef, pork, and chicken in southwestern Ontario. *Epidemiol Infect* 1990; 105:11–20.
50. Chart H, Smith HR, Scotland SM, et al. Serological identification of *Escherichia coli* O157:H7 infection in haemolytic uraemic syndrome. *Lancet* 1991; 337:138–140.
51. Tarr PI, Neill MA, Clausen CR, et al. *Escherichia coli* O157:H7 and the hemolytic uremic syndrome: importance of early cultures in establishing the etiology. *J Infect Dis* 1990; 162:553–556.
52. Remington JS, McLeod R. Toxoplasmosis. In: Gorbach SL, Bartlett JG, Blacklow NR (eds): *Infectious Diseases.* Philadelphia, W. B. Saunders, 1992: pp. 1328–1343.
53. Excler JL, Pretat E, Pozzetto B, et al. Sero-epidemiological survey for toxoplasmosis in Burundi. *Trop Med Parasitol* 1988; 39:139–141.
54. Sousa OE, Saenz RE, Frenkel JK. Toxoplasmosis in Panama: a 10-year study. *Am J Trop Med Hyg* 1988; 38:315–322.
55. Ahmed HJ, Mohammed HH, Yusus MW, et al. Human toxoplasmosis in Somalia. Prevalence of *Toxoplasma* antibodies in a village in the lower Scebelli region and in Mogadishu. *Trans Royal Soc Trop Med Hyg* 1988; 82:330–332.
56. Lappalainen M, Koskela P, Hedman K, et al. Incidence of primary toxoplasma infections during pregnancy in southern Finland: a prospective cohort study. *Scand J Infect Dis* 1992; 24:97–104.
57. Logar J, Novak-Antolic Z, Zore A, et al. Incidence of congenital toxoplasmosis in the Republic of Slovenia. *Scand J Infect Dis* 1992; 24:105–108.
58. Ades AE. Methods for estimating the incidence of primary infection in pregnancy: a reappraisal of toxoplasmosis and cytomegalovirus data. *Epidemiol Infect* 1992; 108:367–375.
59. Jeannel D, Niel G, Costagliola D, et al. Epidemiology of toxoplasmosis among pregnant women in the Paris area. *Intern J Epidemiol* 1988; 17:595–602.

60. Bari A, Khan QA. Toxoplasmosis among pregnant women in northern parts of Pakistan. *J Pakistan Med Assoc* 1990; 40:288–289.
61. Cengir SD, Ortac F, Soylemez F. Treatment and results of chronic toxoplasmosis. Analysis of 33 cases. *Gynecol Obstet Invest* 1992; 33:105–108.
62. Abdel-Hameed AA. Sero-epidemiology of toxoplasmosis in Gezira, Sudan. *J Trop Med Hyg* 1991; 94:329–332.
63. Sever JL, Ellenberg JH, Ley AC, et al. Toxoplasmosis: maternal and pediatric findings in 23,000 pregnancies. *Pediatrics* 1988; 82:181–192.
64. McArthur JC. Neurologic complications of human immunodeficiency virus infection. In: Gorbach SL, Bartlett JG, Blacklow NR (eds): *Infectious Diseases*. Philadelphia, W. B. Saunders, 1992: pp. 956–973.
65. Daffos F, Forestier F, Capella-Pavlovsky M, et al. Prenatal management of 746 pregnancies at risk for congenital toxoplasmosis. *N Engl J Med* 1988; 318:271–275.
66. Hohlfeld P, Daffos F, Thulliez P, et al. Fetal toxoplasmosis: outcome of pregnancy and infant follow-up after in utero treatment. *J Pediatrics* 1989; 115:765–769.
67. Wilson CB, Remington JS. Toxoplasmosis. In: Feigin RD, Cherry JD (eds): *Pediatric Infectious Diseases*, 3rd ed. Philadelphia, W. B. Saunders, 1992: pp. 2057–2069.
68. Dannemann B, McCutchan JA, Israelski D, et al. Treatment of toxoplasmic encephalitis in patients with AIDS. A randomized trial comparing pyrimethamine plus clindamycin to pyramethamine plus sulfadiazine. *Ann Int Med* 1992; 116:33–43.
69. Carr A, Tindall B, Brew BJ, et al. Low-dose trimethoprimsulfamethoxazole prophylaxis for toxoplasmic encephalitis in patients with AIDS. *Ann Int Med* 1992; 117:106–111.

13
Traveling Abroad

MARTIN S. WOLFE

Approximately 15 million Americans travel abroad each year and about half of this number go to the developing world. Tourists usually visit these remoter parts of the world for a period of weeks, where they may be exposed to diseases that are not present, or are at best rare, in the United States. Other individuals may be longer-term travelers or residents in the developing world.

In response to the hazards posed to travelers, the medical specialty of Travel Medicine has evolved, and numerous travel clinics are in operation. Travel medicine involves both the prevention of travel-related diseases, and the diagnosis and treatment of exotic, primarily tropical, diseases on the traveler's return (1).

The main areas involved in prevention include pretravel advice; preparation of an individualized medical kit; immunizations; malaria prophylactic measures; and prophylaxis and self-treatment of traveler's diarrhea.

Pretravel Advice

A pretravel physical examination, best performed by a personal physician, is indicated for travelers with serious medical problems and for those planning a long or physically demanding trip. A medical summary, including recent chest x-rays and electrocardiogram, should be carried. A serious medical condition can be summarized on a health card or an engraved bracelet. The names of recognized, preferably English-speaking, physicians or specialists in the countries to be visited should be known by the traveler.

In addition, adequate medical insurance should be obtained to cover conditions acquired abroad, and hospitalization and medical evacuation if required. Those with chronic illness should carry a needed supply of required drugs.

316

Individualized Medical Kit

Items to be included depend on pre-existing and other potential needs. General items could include a thermometer, bandages, gauze, tape, a germicidal soap solution, aspirin, antacids, antimotion sickness medication, and a mild laxative. Particular antibiotic, antifungal, and anti-inflammatory ointments should be included. A sunscreen is indicated for tropical areas. Antibiotics can be carried by travelers to remote areas where medical assistance may not be readily available. Suggested specific items for a medical kit and information on their use can be found in a publication of the American Society of Tropical Medicine, *Health Hints for the Tropics* (2). Specific items are discussed in the various sections which follow.

Immunizations

Vaccine requirements by country are published annually by the Centers for Disease Control (*Health Information for International Travel*) (3) and by the World Health Organization (*International Travel an Health: Vaccination Requirements and Health Advice*) (4). A number of commercial computer programs are also available.

Yellow Fever

Yellow fever is presently the only disease for which vaccine is required for international travel. Yellow fever occurs in tropical Africa and South America and vaccination can be required for entry into countries in these regions, or for travelers entering certain other countries if they have come from a country with regions that are infected (3). Vaccination must be validated in an international Certificate of Vaccination. Yellow fever vaccine requires continuous cold storage and must be used within 60 minutes following reconstitution. Because of this, yellow fever vaccine is given only in approved state licensed official vaccination centers. A single dose is valid for 10 years, and side effects are minimal. The vaccine is contraindicated in those with an altered immune status or known hypersensitivity to eggs, in children below age 9 months, and in pregnant women. These individuals must be advised not to enter any area with active yellow fever infection and should be given a letter of contraindication.

Cholera

At present, no countries officially require a cholera certificate and the vaccine is not recommended, even for travel to areas with epidemic cholera. Currently available vaccines offer only 50% to 70% protection for 6 months and can cause side effects (3). New and improved oral cholera vaccines may be available in the near future.

Smallpox

Smallpox is considered to be eradicated worldwide, and vaccine is no longer required or recommended for any traveler.

Hepatitis B

Vaccination is recommended for travelers who anticipate direct contact with blood, or sexual contact with residents of high-risk areas (3). Three doses are required, and the vaccine is very expensive.

Immune Globulin (Gamma Globulin)

Hepatitis A infection is a very significant risk for travelers to the developing world, where contaminated water and food (particularly shellfish) may be difficult to avoid. Excellent protection can be afforded to travelers of all ages by immune globulin. For travel of 3 months or less, adults receive a 2 mL dose and children receive smaller doses per weight (3). Immune globulin (and hepatitis B vaccine) prepared in the United States is highly purified and totally safe, and has not been implicated in the transmission of HIV or any other infection. A hepatitis A vaccine has been licensed in Europe and is expected to be available in the United States by early 1994 (5).

Influenza and Pneumococcal Vaccines

Travelers at high risk for contracting these infections should receive these vaccines.

Japanese Encephalitis Vaccine

Japanese encephalitis is endemic in much of the Far East, Southeast Asia, and South Asia. Occasional cases have occurred in expatriates, usually in those in long-term residence. A travel clinic should be consulted for indications for this vaccine, which is uncommon for short-term travelers (6).

Meningococcal Meningitis

Epidemic meningococcal meningitis occurs annually in sub-Saharan Africa during the dry winter months (December through June). Recently, outbreaks have occurred in East Africa. Nepal and India are other areas where outbreaks occur. Pilgrims and some visa applicants to Saudi Arabia can be required to have evidence of this vaccination for entry. Vaccine is quadrivalent, consisting of types A, C, Y, and W, and a single dose offers protection for 3 years (3).

Plague

Plague occurs sporadically, usually in remote locations. Vaccine is rarely indicated for the usual vacation traveler, but is particularly indicated for field workers who could have direct contact with potentially plague infected wild rodents in rural plague endemic areas. A recent case of plague imported into the United States by an American rodent collector infected in rural Bolivia emphasizes the importance of vaccine for such workers (7). A primary series requires 3 doses, and periodic boosters are required when exposure risk continues.

Rabies

Rabies is endemic in practically all of the developing world. The usual traveler is at minimal risk, and the expensive 3 dose human diploid cell vaccine preexposure series is rarely indicated in this group. This series can be recommended for such higher-risk groups as young children, joggers, animal handlers, and field workers (3). The preexposure series offers added protection but does not eliminate the need for additional therapy following rabies exposure. All travelers going to rabies endemic areas should not approach or pet stray dogs, cats, primates, and other wild animals.

Tuberculosis-BCG

Although tuberculosis is a potential hazard to visitors to the developing world, the use of BCG vaccine is not usually recommended by American travel medicine specialists because of troublesome side effects and questionable efficacy of available vaccines. Pre- and posttravel tuberculin skin test screening is considered preferable.

Typhoid

Typhoid and paratyphoid fevers are endemic in much of the developing world. There are no available vaccines for paratyphoid, but there are oral and injectable typhoid vaccines. Until recently, only a killed injectable vaccine with considerable troublesome side effects had been available. This vaccine requires a primary series of two doses 4 or more weeks apart and a booster every 3 years thereafter. There is now a live oral typhoid vaccine which is equally effective but has far fewer side effects. This is given as four oral capsules, one every other day (8).

Typhus

No American traveler has contracted epidemic typhus in the last 40 years. Typhus vaccine is no longer recommended and is not available in the United States.

Routine and Childhood Vaccinations

All Americans should be up to date on the routine immunizations regardless of travel plans, and indicated boosters must be given before travel. Boosters of adult tetanus and diphtheria are necessary every 10 years. *Haemophilus influenza* Type B vaccine should be given to all children older than 2 months. Measles/mumps/rubella (MMR) is usually given as a single dose at age 15 months. However, the age of vaccination should be lowered for children traveling to areas where they are at increased risk of endemic or epidemic measles (3). Adult travelers may also be at increased risk of measles infection. Persons born in or after 1957 should be vaccinated with measles vaccine (9); the necessary time intervals between administration of measles vaccine and immune globulin must be considered (10). Polio remains a distinct risk for travelers to the developing world, and unprotected adults are particularly susceptible to paralytic complications. Most travelers have had a basic polio immunization series during childhood, but not all have had a necessary subsequent booster. A single booster dose is recommended for these travelers to areas of increased polio risk. Both an oral live (OPV) vaccine and an enhanced injectable vaccine (eIPV) are now available.

Malaria Prophylaxis

Malaria infection is a very serious risk for travelers to malaria endemic areas. The emergence and continued spread of chloroquine- and other drug-resistant *Plasmodium falciparum* malaria, and the complexities involved with contraindications and toxic effects of available malaria prophlactic drugs, makes it most difficult to offer appropriate advice to travelers. Expert opinion is required to determine the areas of drug resistance and to make decisions on the best drug and antimosquito measures for particular situations.

Chloroquine is the drug of choice for the relatively few malarious areas where *P falciparum* parasites remain sensitive to it (Central America, Haiti, the Middle East, and parts of South Asia). In all other malarious areas, chloroquine-resistant *P falciparum* (CRPF) malaria occurs, and other drugs must be used. Drugs should be started at least 1 week prior to travel to test for tolerance, and should be taken while in and for at least 4 weeks after leaving the malarious area.

Chloroquine tablets are available in the United States and liquid preparations are available abroad. The adult dose is 500 mg salt (300 mg base) once weekly for adults and 5 mg/kg weekly for children. Chloroquine is considered safe for young children and pregnant women (11). Minor side effects are common, but marked intolerance is rare. Retinal toxicity is virtually nonexistent in the recommended malaria prophylaxis dose (12).

Proguanil (Paludrine) may be used by those unable to tolerate chloroquine and can be used in addition to chloroquine in CRPF areas of Africa and India (13). Paludrine is not marketed in the United States but is available abroad. Paludrine has a long record of safety and can be used by pregnant women and young children. The dose is 200 mg daily, with reduced dosages for children.

Mefloquine (Lariam) is the prophylactic drug of choice for all areas of CRPF, and especially for multiple drug-resistant areas such as Southeast Asia, Oceania, and the Amazon region (3). The adult dose is 250 mg weekly. Mefloquine has proved safe for long-term weekly use (13a). There are a number of important contraindications to mefloquine use, including in pregnant women; in young children below 15 kg weight; possibly in those who use beta-blocker drugs and quinidine; and in those with psychiatric problems or a history of epilepsy.

Doxycycline is an alternative for those unable to take mefloquine in areas of multiple drug resistance (3). However, doxycycline cannot be used by pregnant women or children under age 8 years. It may also cause photosensitivity, diarrhea, and yeast infections. The dose is 100 mg daily.

Some other drugs are no longer recommended by American experts because of potentially serious side effects. These include pyrimethamine-sulfadoxine (Fansidar), amodiaquine, and Maloprim.

Primaquine should optimally be taken following completion of the posttravel terminal 4-week course of the drug(s) taken during travel. Practically all malarious areas have *P vivax* or *P ovale* malaria, which have the potential to remain in the liver for up to 3 years following exposure and to enter the blood and cause symptomatic malaria. Primaquine is the only available drug that can eliminate these forms from the liver. Those travelers with longer malaria exposure are more likely than short-term travelers to develop these relapsing forms of malaria, but all travelers have potential risk. The dose for adults is 15 mg base daily for 14 days. Young children receive 0.3 mg/kg for 14 days. Normal glucose-6-phosphate dehydrogenase (G6PD) must be confirmed before giving primaquine, otherwise there is a risk of severe, possibly life-threatening, hemolysis from this drug. Primaquine is contraindicated in pregnant women.

In addition to drug prophylaxis, a number of mosquito avoidance measures should be practiced. Malaria transmission by mosquitoes occurs primarily between dusk and dawn. Measures to prevent mosquito bites during these hours include:

1. Remaining in well-screened areas.
2. Use of mosquito nets. Permethrin can be used to impregnate nets and give added protection (14).
3. Wearing clothes that cover most of the body.
4. Use of DEET containing insect repellents on exposed parts of the

body. An optimal 32% DEET concentration with a stabilizer to lengthen protection is now available (Ultrathon lotion).
5. Application of permethrin (Permanone) repellent to clothing (15).
6. Use of pyrethrum containing flying insect spray.

Traveler's Diarrhea

Approximately 20% to 50% of travelers to the developing world are affected by travelers' diarrhea. This can be caused by bacteria (particularly toxigenic *E coli*), viruses, and, less commonly, by parasites. Infection is usually contracted from contaminated water or food (16).

To prevent travelers' diarrhea, water should be boiled for 5 minutes or treated with chemical such as iodine or chlorine (3). A particularly useful chemical method is the "Water Tech Water Purifier Cup" (Water Technologies Corp.). Foods should be well cooked and hot salads and cold foods should be avoided. Raw or poorly cooked shellfish, unwashed vegetables and fruits, and suspect dairy products should not be eaten.

Prophylactic antibiotics are generally not recommended by experts because of the potential for side effects and widespread bacterial resistance (17). Bismuth subsalicylate (Pepto-Bismol), two tablets four times a day, for up to 3 weeks, has proven to be a safe and effective means of reducing the occurrence of travelers' diarrhea by about 65% (18). Halogenated hydroxyquinolones (such as Mexaform and Enterovioform), recommended as drug prophylaxis for travelers' diarrhea by some physicians abroad, should not be used as they cause subacute myelo-optic neuropathy (19).

Should diarrhea occur during travel, lost fluids should be replaced by drinking water, tea, broth, or carbonated beverages. Oral rehyfration electrolyte mixtures are a more ideal replacement (20). Cramps or moderate diarrhea can be relieved by such antimotility agents as loperamide (Imodium) (21). Pepto-Bismol liquid, one ounce every half-hour for eight doses is useful, particularly for diarrhea due to toxigenic *E coli* (21). If these measures are not adequate, or if fever, chills, or blood or mucus in the stool occur, a physician should be contacted for appropriate diagnosis and treatment. In an emergency, self-treatment, preferably with a quinolone antibiotic, can be taken (22).

Posttravel Management

The most common problems in returning travelers are diarrhea or other gastrointestinal difficulties; fever; unexplained eosinophilia; and skin rashes. Drugs for parasitic infections are summarized in reference 23.

Diarrhea or Other Gastrointestinal Difficulties

Diarrhea and gastrointestinal complaints are the most common problems for travelers, both during the trip and/or following return. The most common cause for acute diarrhea during or just after return is toxigenic *E. coli*, but infection may also be due to a variety of viral, bacterial, fungal and protozoal organisms, or toxic marine organisms (i.e., fish and shellfish poisoning) (24). Symptoms developing sometime following travel are most commonly due to pathogenic intestinal protozoa. Less likely causes are tropical sprue or enteropathy; postinfectious lactose intolerance; or intestinal helminths.

Viral Intestinal Infections

Rotavirus, spread by the fecal-oral route, is a cause of enteric disease worldwide (16). After an incubation period of less than 48 hours, there is the onset of frequent watery diarrhea, nausea, and malaise. Symptoms usually last 5 to 7 days. The viral etiology is usually made from the clinical picture and the absence of other organisms. Specific diagnosis can be made from an ELISA assay in a kit form which detects rotavirus in stool.

Norwalk virus also occurs worldwide, has an incubation period of 18 to 48 hours, and causes a 24- to 48-hour illness (16). There is currently no available diagnostic assay. Treatment of both these viral infections is supportive, with particular emphasis on fluid replacement.

Bacterial Intestinal Infections

Toxigenic *E coli* causes approximately 50% of travelers' diarrhea cases. Other relatively common bacterial etiological agents include *Shigella* and *Salmonella* species, *Campylobacter jejuni*, and *Vibrio parahaemolyticus*. Less common etiologies include other *Vibrio* species (*V cholera* is distinctly uncommon), *Clostridium*, *Staphylococcus aureus*, and *Yersinia enterocolitica* (16).

More severe infections leading to dysentery with fever, chills, and blood and mucus in the stool, are usually caused by large bowel invasive *C jejuni*, *Shigella* species, and certain invasive *Salmonella* species. Other organisms, such as toxigenic *E coli*, are noninvasive and usually cause symptoms by producing an enterotoxin, leading to watery diarrhea and a relatively short self-limited illness. A wet mount of stool stained with methylene blue usually reveals sheets of polymorphonuclear leukocytes and red blood cells with the former more invasive organisms, while these cells are generally absent with noninvasive bacteria colonizing the smaller bowel (16).

Definitive diagnosis is with stool culture, using various media including those for *Salmonella* and *Shigella* and special selective media for *C jejuni* and *Vibrio* species. Noninvasive *Vibrio* and *Salmonella* species are generally self-limited and usually do not require treatment. The other invasive organisms are well treated with a quinolone antibiotic (22).

In a traveler who has recently taken antibiotics, diarrhea may be due to *Clostridium difficile* infection. This is diagnosed by tissue culture assay to detect *C difficile* toxin in the stool. If present, treatment is with metronidazole or vancomycin.

Fungal enteritis

Recent use of broad spectrum antibiotics or metronidazole can eliminate normal intestinal bacteria and allow candidal overgrowth. In some cases, this can lead to diarrhea and other gastrointestinal symptoms. Intestinal candidiasis should be considered as the etiology when budding yeast and mycelial forms are found in large numbers on direct fecal examinations, after antimicrobial treatment. Rapid improvement is seen with oral nystatin (24).

Fish and Shellfish Toxins

Fish and shellfish toxins may initially cause acute diarrhea, which can then be followed by prolonged neurological symptoms. Ciguatera poisoning from ingestion of large marine reef fish (including grouper, snapper, and barracuda) containing ciguatoxin, is the most common form of fish poisoning (25).

Intestinal Parasites

Pathogenic intestinal protozoa commonly affecting travelers include *Giardia lamblia* (most freqnently recognized), *Entamoeba histolytica*, and *Dientamoeba fragilis*. Less common are *Cryptosporidium* and *Isospora belli* (16). As the incubation period of these organisms is generally considerably greater than that for viruses and bacteria, initial symptoms frequently do not develop until late in a trip or following return. Symptoms can also be more prolonged or recurrent.

Giardia lamblia is a worldwide threat to travelers (26). Infection is usually from contaminated water, and the incubation period is approximately 12 to 15 days. Typical symptoms include recurrent or persistent soft, foul smelling stools and flatus, intestinal bloating and gurgling, belching, indigestion, weight loss, and fatigue. Diagnosis is usually from a series of stool specimens, best collected in a preservative. However, up to 30% of those infected can be "low excretors" of the parasite, and can be difficult to diagnose by stool examination. A new ELISA test to detect *Giardia* antigen in stool is now available (27), but it remains to be proven that this test is consistently positive in stool-negative low excretors. Other methods which can be used to confirm infection include examination of upper intestinal fluid obtained with a nasogastric tube or with the "Enterotest" duodenal string test, examination of a biopsy impression smear, or histological examination of a small bowel biopsy specimen. In some cases with typical travel and exposure history and typical *Giardia*-like symptoms, it is not possible to confirm infection. In this situation, empiric treatment is advocated. Available drugs in the United States include metronidazole, quinacrine (Atabrine), and furazolidone (Furoxone). The former two drugs are about 90% effective. Tinidazole (Fasigyn), which can be administered in a single dose, is available outside of North America. Lactase deficiency is common with giardiasis and may persist after successful treatment, giving symptoms mimicking persistent giardiasis (26).

Entamoeba histolytica is also contracted worldwide by travelers. Many of those infected are asymptomatic cyst passers, who may have nonpathogenic strains of the parasite, but the technology to differentiate pathogenic versus nonpathogenic strains is not yet readily available (28). At the other extreme, amoebic dysentery is uncommon. Intermediate nondysenteric symptoms include alternating constipation and diarrhea, lower abdominal cramps, bloating and flatus (not foul smelling), and fatigue. Diagnosis is by finding typical cysts or trophozoites in the stool. In cases of dysentery, proctoscopic examination reveals typical ulcers; scrapings or biopsy of these ulcers can reveal *E histolytica* trophozoites. Amoebic serology is usually positive with invasive amoebic bowel disease. In mild cases, a nonabsorbed luminal drug such as paromomycin (Humatin) or iodoquinol is usually curative. Moderate to severe (dysenteric) symptoms require initial metronidazole, followed by a luminal drug (29).

Dientamoeba fragilis is an amoeba-like noninvasive flagellate of the large bowel found worldwide. This protozoa has no cyst form and occurs only in the very labile trophozoite form. To confirm this parasite, stools must be collected in preservative and permanently stained slides must be examined. Not all those infected have symptoms, but diarrhea, abdominal bloating, flatulence, and fatigue may occur (30). Treatment is with paramomycin, with iodoquinol as an alternative (29).

Cryptosporidium is usually associated with AIDS patients, but infection can occur in travelers with normal immune systems (31). The incubation period can be as little as 4 days, and symptoms can mimic those of giardiasis. Diagnosis may require special stool concentration texts and staining. There is no available treatment, and infection in nonimmunosuppressed persons is usually self-limited within 7 to 30 days.

Isospora belli is a rarely diagnosed parasite which can give symptoms similar to those of giardiasis (32). *Blastocystic hominis* is a ubiquitous parasite whose pathogenicity is debated. It is frequently present in asymptomatic travelers. In one careful study of individuals with only *B hominis* parasites, most patients were later found to have another difficult to recognize pathogenic protozoa (33). A number of nonpathogenic intestinal protozoa must be differentiated from pathogenic parasites. This requires fecal smears permanently stained with iron hematoxylin or trichrome. Intestinal helminths seldom cause chronic diarrhea; a major exception is *Strongyloides stercoralis*.

Travelers with chronic diarrhea who have had relatively pro-longed residence in South Asia and Southeast Asia and parts of the Caribbean may have tropical sprue (34). This malabsorption syndrome is rare in short-term travelers. It should be considered in those with a history of geographic exposure who have persistent diarrhea, in-digestion, flatulence, and weight loss, when no pathogenic organism can be found.

Fever in the Returned Traveler

Many febrile illnesses in the traveler have a cosmopolitan rather than an exotic etiology, and are frequently self-limited. The major exotic tropical fevers occurring in travelers include malaria, enteric fever, hepatitis, amoebic liver abscess, and rickettsial and arboviral infections (35).

Malaria

A febrile traveler returning from an area endemic for malaria must first and foremost be considered to have possible malaria. Most malaria infec-tions occur in those travelers who have had no, irregular, or inappro-priate chemoprophylaxis. However, all febrile travelers from a malarious area must be examined for malaria, since no chemoprophylactic regimen can be considered fully protective. Potentially lethal falciparum malaria usually occurs within 4 weeks after leaving a malarious area. *Plasmodium vivax* and *P ovale* malaria may occur up to 3 years after exposure, if primaquine has not been taken to eliminate persistent latent parasites in the liver. *Plasmodium malariae* does not have a latent liver phase and is the least common species seen in travelers. Typical malaria symptoms are high fever, shaking chills, sweats, headache, and myalgias. Symptoms may be modified or masked depending on the malaria immune status (as in an immune native of an endemic area) or by the use of prophylactic antimalarial drugs. Severe *P falciparum* infections can rapidly lead to such lethal complications as cerebral malaria, renal failure, severe hem-olysis, and adult respiratory distress syndrome (36).

Diagnosis is by appropriately prepared and carefully examined Giemsa-stained thin and thick malaria smears. A single negative set of smears cannot rule out malaria, and smears should be repeated at 6 hour in-tervals for at least a 24-hour period.

Falciparum malaria contracted in one of the relatively few areas with chloroquine sensitive malaria can be treated with chloroquine alone. Initially, one gram of chloroquine phosphate salt (600 mg base) is given orally. Six hours later 500 mg salt (300 mg base) is taken, and this dose is repeated 24 and 48 hours later. For falciparum malaria contracted in chloroquine resistant areas, with a low parasitemia (less than 1%) and no complications, oral treatment can be given. Mefloquine (Lariam) in a single adult 1,250 mg dose can be used for those without a contraindication to this drug. Vomiting and neruopsychiatric side effects can occur in a small percentage of those so treated. Alternatively, oral quinine, 650 mg salt t.i.d. for 3 days can be used, to be followed by oral tetracycline 250 mg q.i.d. for 7 days (37). Patients with severe or complicated falciparum malaria must be hospitalized and managed with intensive care, immediate intravenous antimalarial drug treatment, and necessary supportive management (36). In the United States, intravenous quinine is not available, and treatment must be with intravenous quinidine (38). A continuous infusion of quinidine gluconate is recommended. A loading dose of 10 mg of quinidine gluconate salt (equal to 6.2 mg quinidine base) per kg body weight is given over 1 to 2 hours, followed by constant infusion of 0.02 mg quinidine gluconate salt per kg per minute. This regimen is highly effective and well tolerated in monitored patients. Quinidine is given for 3 days and is then followed by tetracycline, as above. In patients with malaria parasitemia greater than 10%, or with marked clinical deterioration, exchange transfusion along with constant quinidine infusion can be life saving (39).

Plasmodium malariae, P vivax, and *P ovale* can be treated with chloroquine alone, as per chloroquine sensitive *P falciparum.* With *P vivax* or *P ovale,* this should be followed by primaquine 15 mg base daily for 14 days, after normal G6PD status is established.

Enteric Fever

Typhoid and paratyphoid fevers can be contracted from contaminated food or water in the developing world, where the prevalence of these bacteria is high. Currently available typhoid vaccines offer protection to no more than 70% of recipients. Enteric fever should be suspected in travelers returning from an endemic area with fever, headache, abdominal pain, diarrhea, or cough. Symptoms may not develop until several weeks after return. Diagnosis is confirmed by positive blood, stool, or urine cultures. Febrile agglutin (Widal) tests may be useful. *Salmonella typhi* organisms worldwide have developed multiple antibiotic resistance, and a quinolone may now be the drug of choice (40). Paratyphoid organisms are generally sensitive to amoxicillin or trimethoprim/sulfamethoxazole.

Hepatitis

Travelers to the developing world who have not received immune globulin or the new hepatitis A vaccine, run a significant risk of contracting hepatitis A from contaminated water or food. Rare cases of hepatitis E have been contracted in South Asia and elsewhere, and this type of hepatitis is not be protected against by immune globulin (41). Hepatitis B is usually contracted from sexual contact and is uncommon in travelers. In the preicteric phase of acute hepatitis, fever, chills, myalgias, and fatigue may occur, and this syndrome can mimic malaria and other acute tropical fevers. Hepatitis serologic testing can confirm infection, but when these tests are negative in a patient with apparent hepatitis, cytomegalovirus or mononucleosis infection should be considered.

Amoebic Liver Abscess

A period of acute diarrhea frequently precedes development of an amoebic liver abscess. A returned traveler with fever and right upper quadrant pain should be suspected of this disorder. Sonography or CAT scan of the liver will show a filling defect, and an amoebic serology test will confirm infection. Needle aspiration is seldom required for diagnosis or treatment. There is usually very rapid clinical response to oral or intravenous metronidazole. Follow-up treatment should be given with paromomycin or iodoquinol (as per intestinal amoebiasis) to eliminate any bowel cysts and prevent relapse. Abscess cavities may take some months to fill in.

Rickettsial Infections

Tick typhus can be contracted in West, East, and South Africa, and in the Mediterranean littoral. Infection typically begins with a skin eschar at the tick bite site, fever, chills, headache, and, in a few days, a diffuse papular rash develops. Epidemic, scrub, and murine typhus are much less commonly contracted by travelers. The Weil-Felix agglutination battery can be used for initial screening, and confirmation can be obtained from indirect fluorescent antibody tests for specific rickettsial organisms. Tetracycline is a highly effective and rapid treatment (42).

Viral Fevers

Dengue fever is endemic in most parts of the tropical world and is the most commonly imported arbovirus infection (43). Symptoms include fever, headache, body aches, and eye pain. Typically, a diffuse rash appears on the third to fifth day as other symptoms abate. Japanese B encephalitis is a rare infection of travelers to rural areas of the Far East (6). A number of other rarer acute viral illnesses have been imported from endemic areas, including lethal Lassa and Marburg fever viruses from West and Central Africa (44). Diagnosis is usually confirmed serologically and treatment is generally supportive.

Less Common Febrile Illnesses

African trypanosomiasis was contracted by 15 American travelers from 1967 through 1987 (45). Although the actual risk is low, even short-term travelers to game parks of East and Central Africa should take precautions against tsetse fly bites. Travelers should inform their physicians of exposure history if symptoms such as trypanosomal chancre at a bite site, fever, evanescent rash, headache, and lethargy develop up to 4 weeks following return.

Tuberculosis remains a threat worldwide. Although infection in travelers is uncommon, any returnee with fever, cough, and suggested chest radiographic evidence of pulmonary disease, should be evacuated for tuberculosis. Pre-and posttravel tuberculin skin testing is an optimal recommendation.

Brucellosis is contracted from contaminated raw goats' or cows' milk or soft cheese. Presentation can be with fever, chills, sweats, body aches, headache, monarticular arthritis, weight loss, fatigue, or depression. Generalized lymphadenopathy and splenomegaly are common. Diagnosis is by blood culture and specific agglutination tests (46).

Leptospirosis is common in the tropics, but is rarely contracted by travelers. Infection is acquired through direct or indirect contact with infected animals. Most infections are aniceteric and mild. Initial symptoms can include high remittent fever, chills, headache, myalgias, nausea, and vomiting. No more than 10% of cases develop jaundice. Diagnosis is usually made with serologic techniques. Early therapy with penicillin or tetracycline is usually beneficial.

Anthrax is very rarely contracted from contact with contaminated animal byproducts such as hides and wool. Most infections occur on the face or arms after a minor abrasion, presenting as an initial painless papule which vesiculates and becomes hemorrhagic, necrotic, and covered with an eschar. Treatment is with penicillin or tetracycline.

Melioidosis is an uncommon infection in travelers to Southeast Asia. Presentation resembles acute pulmonary tuberculosis. Less commonly, chronic infection may develop.

Histoplasmosis is a cosmpopolitan disease, and has rarely infected travelers to Latin America. Visitors to caves contaminated with bat droppings are at particular risk. Consideration should be given to possible histoplasmosis in a returned traveler with pulmonary or, less likely, disseminated disease.

Visceral leishmaniasis (kala-azar) is extremely rare in American tourists, though European travelers have been infected around the Mediterranean littoral. Symptoms include fever, hepatosplenomegaly, and wasting. Diagnosis is confirmed by demonstrating leishmanial organisms in a biopsy specimen of liver, spleen, or bone marrow.

American trypanosomiasis (Chagas' disease) is very common in Latin America, and travelers engaged there in hiking, camping, and archaeological projects can be exposed. However, naturally-acquired, documented infection is extremely rare in travelers.

Lyme disease occurs in Europe and may also be present in other parts of the world. Hikers in particular should take precaution against tick bites in any recognized endemic area.

HIV infection is a particular hazard from sexual contact, blood transfusion, or contaminated needle or syringe contact in highly endemic areas of the tropical world. A number of disposable syringes and needles can be carried by travelers who might possibly need injections while traveling in areas where only nondisposable products are used. HIV serology screening should be done on any traveler with the above exposure.

Eosinophilia in the Returned Traveler

A returned traveler with eosinophilia greater than 5% who has been in the developing world should be considered to have possible helminthic infection. With some exceptions, protozoal infections do not cause eosinophilia. Allergic problems usually cause an eosinophilia of less than 15%, but some drug reactions can cause a much higher eosinophilia (47).

Helminth Infections

High eosinophilia, up to 80%, can occur during the acute stage of certain helminth infections, particularly those with a tissue larval migration.

Adult intestinal helminths can cause mild to moderate (6% to 30%) eosinophilia. Patients are usually asymptomatic with *Ascaris lumbricoides*, hookworms, *Trichuris trichiura*, *Enterobius vermicularis* (pinworms), and various tapeworms. Diagnosis is by finding typical eggs or tapeworm segments in the stool. Pinworm eggs are best diagnosed by applying sticky paddles or scotch tape to the perianal area. Treatment is with mebendazole (Vermox). *Ascaris* and hookworms have an early larval migration through the lungs which can give pulmonary symptoms and infiltrates and quite high eosinophilia.

Strongyloides stercoralis and the much less commonly acquired *Trichostrongylus* species infect through the skin. *S stercoralis* can complete its life cycle without leaving the host, and infections persisting for over 40 years have been recognized. Eosinophilia is particularly high during the early years of infection, but in long-established infections eosinophil counts can be normal. Many infections are asymptomatic, but some individuals may have epigastric pain, diarrhea, cough, and urticarial rashes occurring on the buttocks and thighs (related to larval migration from the anus). Unsuspected asymptomatic infections can become generally disseminated throughout the body in the presence of immune suppression, steroid treatment, or with cancer therapy. Definitive diagnosis is by finding larvae in the stool, but larvae will not be present in all cases. Special stool concentration tests or examination of duodenal fluid may be required to find larvae. An ELISA serologic test (available at the Centers for Disease Control) is very useful in making a presumptive diagnosis (48). Treatment is with thiabendazole (Mintezol).

Schistosomiasis is acquired through contact with freshwater snails which are intermediate hosts. *Schistosomiasis mansoni* occurs in northeastern South America, certain Caribbean islands, Africa, and the Middle East. *Schistosomiasis hematobium* occurs in Africa and the Middle East. *Schistosomiasis japonicum and S mekongi* are present in the Far East. *S intercalatum* is an uncommon intestinal infection in West and Central Africa. Acute schistosomiasis (Katayama syndrome) is usually associated with *S mansoni* and *S japonicum* infections, and symptoms occur 4 to 8 weeks after exposure when adult worms begin producing eggs. Symptoms include hypereosinophilia, fever, chills, pulmonary complaints, headache, abdominal pain, and urticaria. The majority of established schistosome infections are asymptomatic and eosinophilia seldom exceeds 3,000 eosinophils/mm^3. Intestinal infection with *S mansoni*, *S japonicum*, *S mekongi*, and *S intercalatum*, can cause abdominal pain, diarrhea, and fatigue. *S hematobium* can give hematuria and other urinary tract symptoms. Diagnosis is by finding eggs in the stool or urine, depending on the geographic area of exposure, symptoms, and species. Infection in travelers is often light and eggs can be missed on routine stool and urine examinations. Special concentration tests of stool or urine and rectal or bladder biopsy may be required to confirm infection. Serologic tests may be used to screen travelers with an exposure history. Treatment is with praziquantel (Biltricide) (49).

Liver flukes in their early acute phase can cause hypereosinophilia, painful liver, and fever. *Fasciola hepatica* occurs almost worldwide and is contracted from eating watercress containing infective stage metacercariae. *Clonorchis sinensis* and *Opisthorchis viverrini* occur in Southeast and East Asia and are contracted from eating raw fish containing metacercariae. In early infections, eggs may not occur in the stool and diagnosis is by suggested filling defects in the liver; diagnosis for *F hepatica* is a positive serologic test. In chronic infections, which are frequently asymptomatic, eggs may be found in the stool, and mild eosinophilia may be present (50). *F hepatica* is best treated with bithionol, and *Clonorchis* and *Opisthorchis* with praziquantel.

Trichinosis and echinococcus are extremely rare in travelers.

A number of filariae infect man and can cause quite high eosinophilia (51). *Wuchereria bancrofti* and *Brugia malayi* are rare in travelers; long-term residence in a highly endemic area seems necessary for infection. *Mansonella perstans* is a common parasite in tropical Africa and is the most commonly diagnosed filarial infection in the United Kingdom. Loa

loa and *Onchocerca volvulus* are the two most commonly diagnosed filaria infections in the United States, usually in longer-term residents from tropical Africa. The incubation period can be from 6 months to 1 year, and symptoms may develop some time after return from an endemic area. Classic presentation of Loa loa is the migration of the adult worm across the eye and/or subcutaneous evanescent swellings (Calabar swellings) on the arms or legs associated with hypereosinophilia. Orchoceriasis usually presents with a very pruritic maculopapular eruption on the hips, back, buttocks, and thighs, in the presence of hypereosinophilia. Filariasis should be suspected in travelers from endemic areas with hypereosinophilia and suggested signs and symptoms. Microfilariae should be searched for in the blood, or in the case of onchocerciasis, in skin snips or biopsies. Filariasis serology is not readily available at present. If infection is confirmed or strongly suspected, diethylcarbamazine is the treatment of choice for all species except onchocerciasis. Onchocerciasis is treated with an investigational drug in the United States, ivermectin.

Intestinal Protozoa

Eosinophilia is distinctly uncommon in pure infections with *Entamoeba histolytica* and *Giardia lamblia*. Eosinophilia has been associated with other pathogenic intestinal protozoa, *Dientamoeba fragilis* and *Isospora belli*.

Skin Disorders in the Returned Traveler

The most common skin disorders acquired by travelers are cutaneous mycoses. *Tinea versicolor* is frequently contracted in the tropics, and depigmentation of the lesions may persist for some months after effective treatment. *Tinea pedis* ("athletes' foot") is particularly common in moist climates, as is *Tinea cruris* ("jock itch"). The former can be prevented by regular use of foot powder and dry socks, while the latter can be prevented by use of a drying powder and frequent change of clothing. Superficial mycoses are diagnosed from skin scrapings in potassium hydroxide or by culture. Treatment is with a broad spectrum antimycotic preparation.

Cutaneous myiasis is contracted by travelers to Latin America (*Dermatobia hominis*) and by travelers to Africa (*Cordyloba anthropophaga*—the "tumbu fly"). The latter infection occurs from eggs being deposited on clothes which are air dried and unironed. Larvae hatch in a few days and penetrate the skin, causing persistent, pruritic, and sometimes painful furuncular lesions with central necrosis. These lesions can often be confused with bacterial infections. A larva, which can be extracted, is seen in the center of the lesion and healing is generally rapid.

The sand flea, *Tunga penetrans*, invades the skin (often around the toes) when walking barefoot. These are easily removed with fine forceps.

Scabies or lice are cosmopolitan infections and are contracted when hygiene is poor. There is usually severe pruritus. Infection is confirmed by observing moving lice, or in the case of scabies by examination of scrapings of scabetic burrows or papules. Scabies are treated with topical 5% permethrin or lindane (Kwell). Lice can be similarly treated.

Dog and cat hookworms deposited in sandy soil can penetrate exposed skin and lead to cutaneous larva migrans (creeping eruption). This leaves migrating pruritic serpiginous tunnels in the epidermis. *Strongyloides stercoralis* can cause a particular form of hive-like cutaneous lesions, usually on the buttocks or thighs. These lesions can be treated with locally applied thiabendazole, or this drug can be taken orally.

A number of cutaneous ulcers are contracted in the tropics. Most common is cutaneous leishmaniasis transmitted by sandflies in the Middle East, the Mediterranean littoral, and in parts of Asia, Africa, and Latin America (52). The incubation period can be 1 to 3 months, rarely longer. Typically, a papule develops which gradually enlarges and ulcerates into a painless sore with rolled edges. The causal Leishman-Donovan parasites can be identified in Giemsa-stained preparations, in cultures of aspirate, or biopsy specimens from the edge of the ulcer. Treatment is with pentavalent antimonial compounds. Similar, but rare, ulcers may occur in hot, dry tropical areas, caused by *Corynebacterium diphtheriae*.

A generalized macupapular eruption can be seen with various typhus infections. Most common is tick typhus contracted in Africa, which often presents with an eschar at a tick bite site associated with rash, fever, chills, and headache. This is very responsive to tetracycline.

Routine Posttravel Screening

Posttravel evaluation is usually not necessary for the short-term traveler who remains well while traveling and after return. However, ill travelers and their physicians must be aware of the long latent period of some infections. Prior travel must then be considered in the presence of symptoms beginning some months or even a few years after travel or residence in the developing world. Longer-term travelers or residents from the tropics should have certain routine screening tests following return. These can include: complete blood count, urinalysis, liver function tests, hepatitis B and HIV testing, tuberculin skin test, stool examinations for ova and parasites, and serologic testing for schistosomiasis if possible exposure has occurred (53).

References

1. Wolfe MS. Travel medicine and travel clinics. *Inf Dis Clin N Am* 1991; 5:377–391.

2. Wolfe MS. (ed): *Health Hints for the Tropics*, 10th ed. Bethesda, Maryland, American Society of Tropical Medicine and Hygiene, 1989. (revised 11th edition in 1993)

3. Centers for Disease Control. *Health Informational for International Travel*, 1993. HHS Publication No. (CDC) 93–8280, Washington D.C., Government Printing Office.

4. World Health Organization. *International Travel and Health Vaccination Requirements and Health Advice*. Geneva, World Health Organization, 1993.

5. Midthun K, Ellerbeck E, Gershman K, et al. Safety and immunology of live attenuated hepatitis A virus vaccine in seronegative volunteers. *J Infect Dis* 1991; 163:735–739.

6. Centers for Disease Control. Inactivated Japanese encephalitis virus vaccine. Recommendations of the ACIP. *MMWR* 42/No. RR-1/January 8, 1993.

7. Wolfe MS, Tuazon C, Schultz R. Imported bubonic plague—District of Columbia. *MMWR* 1990; 49:895–901.

8. Typhoid vaccination: Weighing the options. *Lancet* 1992; 340:341–342.

9. Hill DR, Pearson RD. Measles prophylaxis for international travel. *Ann Int Med* 1989; 111:699–701.

10. Wolfe MS. Measles and immune globulin prophylaxis for travelers and hepatitis A. *Ann Int Med* 1990; 112:235.

11. Wolfe MS, Cordero JF. Safety of chloroquine in chemosuppression of malaria. *Br Med J* 1985; 290:1466–1467.

12. Appleton B, Wolfe MS, Mishtowt GI. Chloroquine as a malarial suppressive: Absence of visual effects. *Milit Med* 1973; 138:225–226.

13. Fogh S, Schapera A, Bygbjerg IC, et al. Malaria chemoprophylaxis in travelers to East Africa: A comparative prospective study of chloroquine plus proguanil with chloroquine plus sulfadoxine-pyrimethamine. *Br Med J* 1988; 296:820–822.

13a. Lobel HO, Miani, M, Eng T, et al. Long-term malaria prophylaxis with weekly mefloquine. *Lancet* 1993; 341:848–851.

14. Drawing the curtain on malaria. *Lancet* 1991; 337:1515–1516.

15. Insect repellents. *Med Lett Drugs Ther* 1989; 31:45–47.

16. Wolfe MS. Acute diarrhea associated with travel. *Am J Med* 1990; 88(Suppl 6A):345–375.

17. Gorbach SL, Edelman R (eds): Travelers' Diarrhea: National Institutes of Health Consensus Development Conference. *Rev Infect Dis* 1986; 8:S109–S227.

18. DuPont HL, Ericsson CD, Johnson PC, et al. Prevention of travelers' diarrhea by the tablet formulation of bismuth subsalicylate. *JAMA* 1987; 257:-1347–1350.

19. Wolfe MS, Mishtowt GI. Enterovioform in travelers' diarrhea. *JAMA* 1973; 220:275–276.

20. Oral fluids for dehydration. *Med Lett Drugs Ther* 1987; 29:63–64.

21. Johnson PC, Ericsson CD, DuPont HL, et al. Comparison of loperamide with bismuth subsalicylate for treatment of acute travelers' diarrhea. *JAMA* 1986; 255:757–760.

22. Taylor DN, Sanchez JL, Candler W, et al. Treatment of travelers' diarrhea: Ciprofloxacin plus loperamide compared with ciprofloxacin alone. *Ann Int Med* 1991; 114:731–734.

23. Drugs for parasitic infections. *Med Lett Drugs Ther* 1992; 34:17–26.
24. Danna PL, Urban C, Bellin E, et al. Role of candida in pathogenesis of antibiotic associated diarrhea in elderly inpatients. *Lancet* 1991; 377:511–514.
25. Dembert ML. Common diseases of fish and shellfish ingestion: Hazards of overseas travel and an underseas appetite. *Travel Med Int* 1988; 6:1–9.
26. Wolfe MS. Giardiasis. *Clin Microbiol Rev* 1992; 5:93–100.
27. Addis DG, Matthews HM, Stewart JM, et al. Evaluation of commercially available enzyme-linked immunosorbent assay for *Giardia lamblia* antigen in stool. *J Clin. Microbiol* 1991; 29:1137–1142.
28. Weinke T, Friedrich-Jänicke B, Hopp P, et al. Prevalence and clinical importance of *Entamoeba histolytica* in two high risk groups: Travelers returning from the tropics and male homosexuals. *J Infect Dis* 1990; 161:1029–1031.
29. Wolfe MS. The treatment of intestinal protozoa. *Med Clin N Am* 1982; 66:707–720.
30. Turner JA. Giardiasis and infections with *Dientamoeba fragilis*. *Ped Clin N Am* 1985; 32:865–880.
31. Garcia LS, Current WL. Cryptosporidiosis: Clinical features and diagnosis. *Crit Rev Clin Lab Sci* 1989; 27:439–460.
32. Shaffer N, Moore L. Chronic travelers' diarrhea in a normal host due to *Isospora belli*. *J Infect Dis* 1989; 159:596–597.
33. Markell LK, Udkow MP. *Blastocystis hominis*: pathogen or fellow traveler? *Am J Trop Med Hyg* 1986; 35:1023–1026.
34. Klipstein FA. Tropical sprue in travelers and expatriates living abroad. *Gastroenterol* 1981; 80:590–600.
35. Wolfe MS. Diseases of Travelers. *CIBA Clinical Symposia* 1984; 36(2):1–32.
36. World Health Organization. Severe and complicated malaria. *Trans Roy Soc Trop Med Hyg* 1990; 84(Suppl 2):1–65.
37. Hoffman SL. Diagnosis, treatment, and prevention of malaria. *Med Clin N Am* 1992; 76:1327–1355.
38. Centers for Disease Control. Treatment with quinidine gluconate of persons with severe *Plasmodium falciparum* infection: Discontinuation of parental quinine from CDC Drug Service. *MMWR* 1991; 40:No. RR-4,21–23.
39. Miller KD, Greenberg AE, Campbell CC. Treatment of severe malaria in the United States with a continuous infusion of quinidine gluconate and exchange transfusion. *N Engl J Med* 1989; 321:65–70.
40. Rowe B, Ward LR, Threlfall EJ. Treatment of multiresistant typhoid fever. *Lancet* 1991; 377:1422.
41. Centers for Disease Control. Hepatitis E among U.S travelers, 1989–1992. *MMWR* 1993; 42:1–4.
42. McDonald JC, MacLean JD, McDade JE. Imported rickettsial disease: Clinical and epidemiologic features. *Am J Med* 1988; 85:799–805.
43. Centers for Disease Control. Imported dengue—United States, 1991. *MMWR* 1992; 41:725–732.
44. Centers for Disease Control. Viral hemorrhagic fever; Initial management of suspected and confirmed cases. *MMWR* 1983; 32:275–395.
45. Bryan RT, Waskin HA, Richards FO, et al. African trypanosomiasis in American travelers: A 20-year review. In: Steffan R, Lobel HO, Haworth J, et al (eds): *Travel Medicine* Berlin, Springer-Verlag, 1988: p. 384–388.
46. Young EJ. Human brucellosis. *Rev Infect Dis* 1983; 5:821–842.

47. Wolfe MS. Eosinphilia in the returning traveler. *Infect Dis Clin N Am* 1992; 6:489–502.
48. Pelletier LL, Baker CB, Gam AA, et al. Diagnosis and evaluation of treatment of chronic strongyloidiasis in ex-prisoners of war. *J Infect Dis* 1988; 157:573–576.
49. Mahmoud AAF (ed): Schistosomiasis. *Clin Trop Med and Comm Dis*. Vol. 2, No. 2. London, Bailliere Tindall, 1987.
50. Barrett-Connor E. Human fluke infections. *South Med J* 1972; 65:86–90.
51. Wolfe MS. Filariasis. *Med N Am* 1981; 9:1014–1022.
52. Maguire JH, Gantz NM, Moschella S, et al. Case Report. Leishmanial infections: A consideration in travellers returning from abroad. *Am J Med Sci* 1983; 285:32–40.
53. Wolfe MS. Medical evaluation of the returning traveler. In: Jong EC, Keystone JS (eds): *Travel Medicine Advisor*. Atlanta, American Health Consultants, 1991: p. 26.1–26.15.

Index